Does losing weight—and keeping it off—
get harder with each passing year?

When you eat a full breakfast, do you get hungry
before it's time for lunch?

One you begin to eat starches, snack foods,
or sweets, is it hard to stop?

Do you get unexplainably tired in the middle
of the afternoon?

Do you become sluggish after a large meal?

Do you take insulin, female replacement
hormones, or medication for high blood pressure
or cholesterol problems?

**If you answered yes to two or more
of these questions and you are over 40,
this program was made for you!**

For more than a decade, RICHARD F. HELLER, M.S., Ph.D., and RACHAEL F, HELLER, M.A., M.Ph., Ph.D., each held two professional appointments and conducted research at Mount Sinai School of Medicine in New York City and in the Department of Biomedical Sciences at the Graduate School of the City University of New York. Richard holds a third appointment as Professor Emeritus at the City University of New York. They are coauthors of the bestselling *Healthy for Life* and *The Carbohydrate Addict's Diet* as well as *The Carbohydrate Addict's Program for Success*, *The Carbohydrate Addict's Gram Counter*, and *Carbohydrate-Addicted Kids*.

Visit the Drs. Heller at their official website: http://www.carbohydrateaddicts.com.

Richard F. Heller, M.S., Ph.D.

Professor, Mount Sinai School of Medicine, New York, retired;
Professor, Graduate Center of the City University of New York,
Department of Biomedical Sciences, retired;
Professor Emeritus, City University of New York

and

Rachael F. Heller, M.A., M.Ph., Ph.D.

Assistant Clinical Professor, Mount Sinai School of Medicine, New York, retired;
Assistant Professor, Graduate Center of the City University of New York,
Department of Biomedical Sciences, retired

The Carbohydrate Addict's
LifeSpan
Program:

A Personalized Plan for Becoming Slim, Fit, & Healthy in Your 40s, 50s, 60s & Beyond

A PLUME BOOK

PLUME
Published by the Penguin Group
Penguin Putnam Inc., 375 Hudson Street, New York, New York 10014, U.S.A.
Penguin Books Ltd, 27 Wrights Lane, London W8 5TZ, England
Penguin Books Australia Ltd, Ringwood, Victoria, Australia
Penguin Books Canada Ltd, 10 Alcorn Avenue, Toronto, Ontario, Canada M4V 3B2
Penguin Books (N.Z.) Ltd, 182–190 Wairau Road, Auckland 10, New Zealand

Penguin Books Ltd, Registered Offices:
Harmondsworth, Middlesex, England

Published by Plume, an imprint of Dutton Signet,
a member of Penguin Putnam Inc.
Previously published in a Dutton edition.

First Plume Printing, January, 1998
20 19

Ⓟ REGISTERED TRADEMARK—MARCA REGISTRADA

The Library of Congress has catalogued the Dutton editon as follows:

Heller, Richard F. (Richard Ferdinand).

The carbohydrate addict's lifespan program : a personalized plan for becoming slim, fit, &
healthy in your 40s, 50s, 60s & beyond / Richard F. Heller and Rachael F. Heller.

p.   cm.

ISBN 0-525-94174-6 (hc.)
ISBN 0-452-27838-4 (pbk.)

1. Low-carbohydrate diet. 2. Health. 3. Physical Fitness. 4. Middle aged persons—Health and
hygiene.   I. Heller, Rachael F. II. Title.
RM237.73.H453   1997

613.2 8—dc20   96-23305
                                                                                     CIP

Printed in the United States of America

BOOKS ARE AVAILABLE AT QUANTITY DISCOUNTS WHEN USED TO PROMOTE PRODUCTS OR SERVICES. FOR
INFORMATION PLEASE WRITE TO PREMIUM MARKETING MEMBER, PENGUIN PUTNAM INC., 375 HUDSON
STREET, NEW YORK, NEW YORK 10014.

This book is dedicated to the untold numbers of carbohydrate addicts who, for far too long, have been wrongly judged and unfairly blamed, and who ask only for their well-deserved freedom.

CONTENTS

PART IV   RECIPES AND MEAL PLANS: EATING YOUR WAY TO FREEDOM

APPENDIX

Beyond the Fen-Phen Dilemma

"It was my last chance, or so I thought, and when it didn't work out, I was devastated. There was nothing left for me to try. Everything else had failed and I knew that, once again, there was nothing for me to do but to sit by, helplessly watching myself gain pound after pound, unable to control myself and desperate to stop it from happening. I was tired of struggling but terrified of going back to the way things were."

We have heard this story literally thousands of times and we have lived it ourselves. For Rachael, like so many others, one more failed promise brought her to the brink of suicide. And the headlines and news reports reflect the latest failure in the parade of "miracle cures":

DISPIRITING DILEMMA FOR DIETERS IN U.S.
New York Times, September 17, 1997

THE DARK SIDE OF DIET PILLS   *Time,* September 22, 1997

WHAT THE DIET-DRUG RECALL MEANS TO PATIENTS
Wall Street Journal, September 16, 1997

RECALL OF DRUGS LEAVES MANY DIETERS HOPELESS
New York Times, September 17, 1997

What these headlines do not reveal, however, is the depth to which we can plunge when, once again, we are left hopeless and helpless and unfairly blamed—a deadly combination.

We know. We have been there. And as sure as you are reading this page, we have found the way out.

If you are addicted to carbohydrates, if your body drives you to crave starches, snack foods, junk food, or sweets—even when you don't want to be eating them—if you find that the more you eat the more you want, you are, most likely suffering from a physical imbalance called carbohydrate addiction. And chances are, you suspected it all along.

The good news is we know what causes an addiction to carbohydrates and we know how to correct it, without weighing or measuring or counting ever again, and without pills or injections or silly packaged meals that no one can live on. It is simply a balanced way of eating that, like Fen-Phen, stops the cravings and takes your body out of its fat-making mode—without the drugs. It is easy and, most of all, it works. So maybe it is a miracle after all.

ACKNOWLEDGMENTS

We wish to express our deep appreciation to the following people:

Deb Brody, our editor, whose insightful suggestions and sage advice have always proven invaluable, and to Jennifer Moore, her most diligent and conscientious assistant.

Lisa Johnson, our director of publicity, whose intelligence, excellent judgment, and very hard work combine to bring our message to those who can best use it.

Tracey Guest, our publicity manager, whose creativity and diligence have helped us spread the good news.

Elaine Koster and Arnold Dolin, our publishers, for their continued integrity and commitment to bring their readers the very best in publishing.

Mel Berger of the William Morris Agency, the best agent and advisor in the world. His years of experience, thoughtful and incisive advice, common sense, creativity, and hard work have helped to make our lives both successful and happy.

Claudia Cross, Mel Berger's unfailingly committed, intelligent, and thoroughly capable assistant.

Norman Katz (whose office we share), Supervising Technologist of Electron Microscopy, Department of Pathology, Mount Sinai Medical Center, and his wife, Madeline, whose suggestions, challenging comments, and encouragement prove most valuable.

Professor Alan L. Schiller, M.D., chairman, Department of Pathology, Mount Sinai School of Medicine, for his insights, enthusiasm, and support.

Professor Paul Gilbert, M.D., associate professor, Mount Sinai Medical Center, one of the finest minds and best hearts in medicine, for his insightful advice and recommendations, and for providing us with the best health care possible.

Irwin Neus, D.D.S., and his staff, whose interest, support, comments, and contributions to our research are always valued.

Ana Luisa Vazquez, Sharon Althea Smith, and Audrey Stedford—the finest of research assistants—whose industriousness, intelligence, commitment, and unending hours in the library made our research possible and our lives most enjoyable.

Deborah Heller DeLisa, the love of our life and her talented husband, Chris, for their careful thought, encouragement, caring, intelligent insights, wonderful advice, and unfailing support.

The Apple Computer company and their repair staff, for development and care of the powerful, user-friendly Powerbook 170 and 180 computers, which can be taken on planes, trains, buses, and out under the apple tree in our backyard, and for their repair team who make sure our Powerbooks stay in good working order. Our Powerbooks have been invaluable tools in the preparation of all our written and graphic materials as well as in the compilation and organization of research data. Without Apple's hard work, our work would never have been the same.

A STAR IS BORN

For more than a decade, in addition to our continuing research program, we have been called to work with some of the biggest names in Hollywood, in the entertainment industry, in journalism, broadcasting, and the arts.

Some of the people with whom we have worked are considered to be the most "beautiful people in the industry"; some are the highest paid, most respected, or most powerful. Some are all of these.

They may be stars to their audiences, but to us they are real people with real problems. Many of them struggle with exhausting time and schedule constraints, family concerns and conflicts, crucial career decisions, as well as the unique stresses of crazy directors, impossible producers, and ever-present press photographers. Still, the one most consistent problem with which these stars must cope is the impact that getting older has on their weight, their looks, and their health.

Their reputations may call for them to act as if their perfect bodies and glowing good health come naturally, effortlessly; we, and they, know better. Many of them have worked hard and, in the past, they have struggled with their eating and their weight as well as with their addiction to carbohydrates and, fortunately, most have found freedom and success with this program.

These "stars" are more like all of us than you would imagine; their challenges, like their rewards, are bigger than life, but fundamentally we are all the same.

Perhaps instead of, or in addition to, a critical sister-in-law who stands guard watching for any sign of added pounds, they have millions watching them as they arrive at the Academy Awards. Instead of worrying about wearing that two-piece bathing suit to the beach, they have to contend with baring it all in the love scene of their next movie. Long days mean no time with the kids or spouse, or certainly for themselves, and on the set of a film, as in the TV studio's dressing rooms and green rooms, food is always, always, present. For us, as for them, time stands ready to take its toll in many ways but most crucially in a metabolism that seems bent on making all of us fat.

We originally developed The Carbohydrate Addict's LifeSpan Program™ for these stars' special needs. It had to be:

Simple and easy to follow,

Targeted to eliminate their cravings and weight concerns that grow with each decade; designed to keep them looking good, feeling good, young, and healthy,

Adaptable to their constantly changing schedules, their personal preferences as well as their professional challenges, and

Rewarding, so as to compensate for the impossible demands with which they live on a regular basis.

We have visited our stars on the set, in their homes, in the studio, and as they performed. We have encouraged them and counseled them and, in the end, together we have learned a great deal.

We now bring the fruits of our labor to you; for all who live with constantly changing schedules, silent concerns, and seemingly impossible demands that seem to grow more challenging as we all grow older:

A personalized weight-loss program that is simple, targeted to *your* lifestyle and your decade of life, adaptable to *your* needs, and rewarding—every day;

A program that offers freedom from fear and deprivation, a program that corrects the cause of your cravings and weight gain, and, best of all, offers you a lifetime of well-deserved success.

IN SEARCH OF A STAR

RACHAEL'S AND RICHARD'S STORIES

The Greatest Freedom of All: Rachael's Story

Though I was almost forty years old, the doctor's words made me feel like a five-year-old once again.

"So, why do *you* think you're so fat?" he asked bluntly. He continued to write up the results of my physical examination, never looking up from his notes as he asked his question. Yet the impact of his words resounded through my entire body. I had been waiting a lifetime for someone to ask me the cause of my overweight condition. I had asked myself a million times. I hesitated as he continued to look down at his writings; his eyes never rose to mine. *Just as well,* I thought. *He's seen enough of me.*

> **The physician's examination had exposed the huge expanse of abdominal fat that formed my belly.**

The physician's examination had exposed the expanse of pale flesh that formed my belly—like a great white whale, I reminded myself—and the roll of fat that rose from the sides of my waist and pushed out from the confines of the back of my bra. While he had witnessed the breadth of my huge white thighs, he had seen my legs only as I lay on the examining table. I was silently grateful that he had not been witness to gravity's effect on the great expanse of fat that made up my thighs.

I recounted each unpleasant image as I desperately sought to find the words that would answer his question. I had lived with the thought for so long, it had become almost invisible to me. But now I must grasp it and bring it out to him. Now someone would listen. I forced the embarrassment down and reached inside.

**"It's not my fault," I wanted to explain.
"When I start to eat, something takes hold of me.
At times, no matter how hard I try, I just lose control."**

"It's not my fault," I wanted to explain. "There really is something different about me. When I start to eat, something takes hold of me and, no matter how hard I try and how much I want to control myself, sooner or later . . ."

I imagined how I would sound to this confident and knowledgeable man. How could I explain that it was *not* just a matter of self-control? How could I convince him that it really wasn't my fault. It was as if I were almost . . . almost addicted to food. Once I started eating, I couldn't stop. Not all the time, but more times than I cared to remember. I had often wished there was a detoxification center, like those for alcoholics and drug addicts, where I could go to get off food.

**I had often wished there was a detox center,
like those for alcoholics and drug addicts,
where I could go to get off food.**

Throughout the decades I had tried every diet known—low-fat, low-carbohydrate, the Grapefruit Diet, the Rice Diet, Overeaters' Anonymous, hypnosis, behavioral therapy, all of the commercial programs, over and over. I had tried everything. I had given up carbohydrates for a year and a half and, literally, almost died. In one fit of desperation, I had fasted on nothing but water and diet soda for forty-two days. Everything worked—at first. Then the hunger and cravings would return and slowly but surely I would watch myself undo all the hard work and sacrifice I had endured.

> **"Jeez, you're gaining it all back again.**
> **And you were doing so well. What a shame."**

As the pounds returned, friends and family would stop praising my efforts and a few would voice what I did not need to hear. "Jeez, you're gaining it all back again. And you were doing so well. What a shame."

But the shame was already in me because no matter how hard I tried something simply drove me to the food. The more I ate, the more I wanted and each new diet ended in failure and an even deeper self-loathing.

So here I sat, weighing over 300 pounds, as the doctor waited for me to explain my sad state of affairs. I had to come up with something . . . come up with some "acceptable excuse" that would sum up the reason for my visible shame. I did not dare try to ask him to understand that my hunger was greater than others, a recurring demand for food that grew if I fed it but would not let me rest if I did not. He would only ask me where the hunger was coming from and that I did not know.

> **Suddenly, I was filled with a deep, almost bottomless sadness.**
> **This doctor saw only a 300-pound glutton who was,**
> **he assumed, totally to blame for her condition.**

Suddenly, I was filled with a deep, almost bottomless sadness. This man saw only a fat woman who was a glutton, who was, he assumed, totally to blame for her unpleasant and, for him, inconvenient condition. I could never succeed in making him see that I was no more to blame for my problem than one who had unknowingly contracted a contagious disease or who had the misfortune of having been struck by a hit-and-run car. I could barely convince myself of my innocence; how could he find me guiltless?

The doctor looked up and sighed a small but audible breath of impatience. I had sometimes pictured my day of judgment; imagining St. Peter demanding that I explain why I had wasted my precious gift of life. I fantasized turning the tables and calling St. Peter himself to task—insisting that he explain why I had been given a life of torture, a body that called for food in a world that did not understand. Why, I would ask, are some women who are naturally thin but mean and selfish given love and understanding while my only crime was that of being fat?

Now my judgment day had come, far earlier than anticipated, but there was no one to answer my demands—only me left to explain. I summoned all the "acceptable" reasons that I had heard the experts espouse on the many talk shows. The reasons cascaded through my mind: I was abused—well, that was true, but some abused kids never became fat. I could explain that my parents never let me have the food I wanted. That wouldn't work. I somehow always managed to get the food I needed and, had they given me all I wanted or not, I knew that the hunger was not a reaction to their restrictions. I didn't eat for attention, nor to get even, nor to control. I ate because I was hungry. It was as simple as that. And it never occurred to me to demand that the doctor explain *to me* the cause of my recurring hunger and cravings.

"Well, my parents owned a grocery store, you see . . . ," I began.

"So what does that have to do with it?" he cut in. "They don't own one now."

I sat mute.

"You are fat for one reason and one reason only," he said. "You eat like a pig. You look like a pig because you eat like a pig."

"You are fat for one reason and one reason only," he continued. "You eat like a pig. You look like a pig because you eat like a pig and you will continue to look like a pig until you stop eating like a pig. Your blood pressure is at stroke level. Your triglycerides are twice normal. Your knees are collapsing from the burden of carrying all of that weight around. If you look like this at forty, can you imagine what you'll look like in twenty years?

"Don't bother," he continued, without waiting for a response. "You'll never make it that far."

He pursed his mouth in disgust and handed—no, threw—to me a sheet of paper detailing the food exchanges allowed on his one-size-fits-all weight-loss regimen.

"Follow that and you'll lose weight," he concluded as he handed me the printed diet. "Don't and you'll keep gaining weight—till you blow up or drop dead," he added coldly. And without another word, he rose and left.

There was no one to blame for this mess but me, right? Wrong. Absolutely, positively wrong!

My face hot with shame, I dressed, slipped from the examining room, paid the receptionist, and never, ever thought of complaining. After all, he was right, I assumed. He was the doctor. I must be the cause of all my problems. There was no one to blame for this mess but me, right? Wrong. Absolutely, positively wrong!

This physician failed at every level—as a healer and as a person. Had I come to him with asthma or a pain in my leg or a rash, he would have sought a physical cause to my problem. He would never have told me not to wheeze or blamed me for the pain or rash. He would have helped me to isolate the reason for my condition or discomfort and together we would have eliminated the cause as well as the problems that stemmed from the cause. But prejudice against overweight is so strong that it obscures this very basic tenet of treatment.

> **If you told your doctor that you lost a great deal of weight and you didn't know why, your doctor would look for a physical cause. Why is it that when we gain weight, they don't do the same?**

If you were to go to your physician and complain of having no appetite and losing weight, the doctor would most certainly seek the cause. Why is it that when we admit to having recurring and intense food cravings and to gaining weight, the same approach is abandoned and, instead, they blame *us*?

The diets that we are given are all the same—in the past they have been low-carbohydrate or low-calorie. Today they are low-fat. Like clothes, diets come in and out of fashion and, unfortunately, without much more reason behind them.

We are given instructions on which foods to avoid or to decrease so as to reduce our weight. But the *cause* of our being overweight is never addressed. In other countries it is recognized that as we get older, keeping slim and trim is far more difficult than it was when we were younger. Thirty years ago, we all understood that a "slowing metabolism" made it "normal" to put on some weight as we grew older. But now, it is assumed that an increased appetite is the result of some personal character or moral flaw, that the fact that many of us seem to grow more efficient at storing fat with each passing decade is little more than an excuse, and that the many disorders or diseases that we may encounter as a result of being overweight are clearly our own doing.

Yet nothing could be further from the truth!

> **In this book, you will learn about a hormonal imbalance that may literally be turning your body into a fat-making machine.**

In the pages that follow, you will learn what scientists now know about a prevalent hormonal imbalance that leads to carbohydrate cravings and weight gain—literally turning your body into a fat-making machine. You will discover why, in many of us, this imbalance tends to get worse with each passing decade and how to correct this imbalance easily so that you, too, can become slim and healthy—for life, and without sacrifice.

My addiction to food robbed me of almost four decades of life. I did not marry until I was past forty. I lived through two terribly abusive relationships that I would never have endured had it not been for being so overweight. My addiction robbed of my dignity and my self-respect. I learned to hold back my feelings for fear of what others might think or, even worse, say. In relationships, I lived in terror of being left for a thinner lover. To this day, I am nicer, more apologetic, and far more concerned for the feelings of others than is often called for. I am more unsure of myself than I need to be—in all areas other than this!!

Your hunger, cravings, and weight problems are not your fault. As the pounds fade, so will your guilt and self-blame.

If you are carbohydrate addicted, this book will give you the information you need to literally eliminate your cravings for starches, snack foods, or sweets and get control over your eating and your life—at any age, through all the decades to come—and without sacrifice. You will be able to lose weight and greatly decrease your risk for virtually all of this country's top killer diseases. You will get the guidance you need to make the lifestyle change you have been waiting for so long. And, in addition, you will gain the courage and conviction that your hunger, cravings, and weight problems are not your fault, and as the pounds fade, so will your guilt and self-blame.

I had always dreamed of being thin. The idea of being normal-weight had filled virtually every waking moment of my childhood. When I reached seventeen years of age and my weight topped 300 pounds, I tried to convince myself that the freedom I sought was impossible. But something inside me would not give up.

My dreams were filled with images of flying free—free of the body that held me prisoner all during my waking moments. Each new diet gave me hope of attaining that freedom but, in the end, each new diet—like all the others—would fail me. As time went on,

I sought a cause for the hunger and cravings that ruled my life. I scoured the women's magazines and newspapers for scientific breakthroughs. I searched medical journals and textbooks. If I could not be thin, at least I hoped for some reprieve from my recurring and intense carbohydrate cravings.

It was this quest that changed my life for, without knowing it, when I found the key to my cravings, I uncovered the *cause* of my problem as well. For the carbohydrate addict, excess weight is but a symptom of an important underlying hormonal imbalance. Weight gain is often the first symptom to be seen but, almost without fail, it is followed over time by a whole host of other medical problems.

> **Cravings for starches, snack foods, or sweets as well as the tendency to gain weight easily are often symptoms of a *physical* imbalance.**

A recurring or intense craving for starches, snack foods, or sweets is but another symptom and, though I did not know it at the time, my only chance at freedom lay in uncovering the underlying hormonal imbalance that was causing both the cravings and the weight gain.

In the end, by keeping meticulous records along with the help of some pure dumb luck, I was able to isolate which foods triggered my hunger and to discover how I could still enjoy these foods without triggering either cravings or weight gain. Later, I was to discover that these same basic guidelines would help over half a million others in their quest for ideal weight and health.

> **I have maintained my 165-pound weight loss, without struggle, for more than a decade!**
> **Today, I am completely free of the cravings that once ruled my life.**

Today I am a svelte size six; half the size I ever dreamed of being. I have been this size for over twelve years. Even more important, I maintain my 165-pound weight loss without struggle. I have the freedom of a normal life, free of imprisonment—physical or mental. I am free of the cravings that once ruled my life. I eat the foods I love without measuring or worrying. My blood pressure and blood-fat levels place me in the lowest coronary risk category. I am healthy and happy. Most of all, I live without the fear of gaining the weight back as the years go by. Because I have corrected the cause of the problem, I no longer live in fear of the cravings, or the pounds, returning. They are gone for life.

> **No weight-loss success holds any joy unless you feel confident that you will never gain it back. This is by far the greatest freedom of them all.**

No weight-loss success holds any joy unless you feel confident, all the way through, that you will never gain it back. Of all the freedoms this program provides, this is by far the greatest of them all.

In Search of a STAR: Richard's Story

I am sixty years old and slim, fit, and healthy. My weight, my blood pressure, and my blood-fat levels would make a man half my age jealous. I take no medications, follow no involved exercise regimens, and eat virtually all the foods I love every day.

"Good genes," you may assume. You couldn't be more wrong. Twenty years ago, I was fat, flabby, and well on my way to a heart attack.

It was the summer of my fortieth birthday and I was in for an unexpected and most sobering experience. As I walked from a beach house clad only in my bathing trunks, I passed a newly installed full-length mirror. I glanced at the middle-aged man's reflection with interest. He looked familiar. . . . Then I realized that this heavy-set man, who vaguely resembled my father, was me! My excess weight had added another decade and a half to my appearance, mostly around my middle, and it was not a pretty sight.

In a brave show of commitment, I endured a day without my usual two or three visits to the refreshment stand. By evening, I was famished. My resolve buckled under a dinner replete with two desserts and an evening of nonstop snacking. The image in the mirror followed me into bed and when I declined my then-wife's advances (a rare but usually more-than-welcomed treat), she insisted on an explanation.

In an unusually honest exchange, I shared my fear that my eating and my weight had gotten out of hand. She admitted that the added pounds had become more noticeable and, though she only voiced concerns about my health, I knew that she was purposely avoiding mentioning the decline of my appearance. I resolved to lose the weight "once and for all," though my past failures should have told me something.

As a child, I had been a stocky kid, and though I was always the last one picked for any team sport, I chose to pretend it didn't much bother me at all.

As a teenager, I became painfully aware of my protruding tummy and love handles and I shrank from wearing a bathing suit and never went without a shirt unless it was absolutely necessary. Still I had many male friends, and by concealing my excess weight under overly large sweaters and open jackets, I was able to enjoy my share of girlfriends as well. I was tall and the excess pounds, though they were concentrated around my middle, did not, at the time, greatly interfere with my happiness.

My appetite was (and is) renowned.

My appetite was (and is) renowned. I was always hungry, it seemed, but, again, because I was a "growing boy" it was never cause for alarm at my house. My mother kind of shrugged and even seemed somewhat pleased at cooking almost as much for me as she did for herself, my father, and my brother put together. Though my brother won more than one bet on how much his kid brother could eat, the true impact of earning the title of "the human garbage can" did not make itself felt until I was in my late thirties.

My kids and my then-wife took to scraping all of the excess food from their dinner plates onto mine.

By then my ten or fifteen excess pounds had turned to twenty-some and the love handles had become a spare tire. My chin was softening as it made room for a second one and I was getting far too comfortable with the paunch that stuck out in front. My kids and then-wife took to scraping all of the excess food from their dinner plates onto mine; no need to ask if I wanted it—there was always room for a little more.

As the marriage went from bad to dreadful, it seemed that each transfer of extra food carried with it a message of judgment and disgust.

"How can you eat like that?" both my wife and the kids seemed to be saying, and the state of the food as well as the way in which it was piled onto my plate took on a far less friendly feel.

> **I tried to convince myself it was nothing to worry about but I could not deny the fact that my excess weight added more than a decade to my appearance.**

So there I was, forty years old, and though I wanted to deny it, I knew that my eating and my weight were indeed out of control. I told myself that it was natural—my father had a belly—never extreme, and it was nothing to worry about.

Still, I didn't like what I saw in the mirror. I thought back to my attempts at weight loss as a teenager and young man; from commercial programs and traditional diets to quick-fix home remedies. They all had several things in common: they all worked—for a time; then I gained all the weight back (and some extra as well). No diet seemed to help me keep my weight off and, after a while, they all became virtually impossible to stick to.

Still, I ignored what my forty years of experience had shown me. This time, I told myself, my commitment would win out over everything. So, once again, I joined a commercial program and started anew with yet another food-exchange plan. It lasted a week and I felt great—until our first party. I remember standing in front of an hors d'oeuvres tray and trying to figure out how many fat exchanges and bread exchanges and . . . I just gave up and started stuffing it in. My then-wife's angry glare gave me just the excuse I needed to feed my rebellion and I ate and drank the evening away in splendid defiance.

The next day, I refused to get on the scale and continued my debauchery with a brunch that would have fed a small third world country. My fourth decade consisted of this scene repeated more times than I now care to remember. Diet after diet, failure after failure. And each time, my weight would end up a few pounds higher than before.

**Her angry glare gave me just the excuse I needed
to feed my rebellion
and I ate and drank the evening away in splendid defiance.**

When all else failed, I turned to exercise. "At least I'll be able to eat more if I burn it up," I reasoned, in an attempt to compensate for my slowing metabolism. I threw myself into my regimen with a vengeance. Each day started off with a six- or seven-mile run. Every day, rain or shine.

My legs got muscular, my breathing somewhat easier, but my weight never gave a pound. I pushed on, through walls of pain and demotivation, but by the end of the second year I had to admit that it just was not making any difference. I was, perhaps, holding my weight in check a bit, but only barely, for although the weight gain had slowed down, I was already forty pounds overweight and I clearly was not losing. Also, I wondered, how long could I keep up this insane schedule of activity, and, beyond that, what would happen when I had to stop?

By the third year of running, the strain of the daily pounding on my knees put an end to my running career and I was once again back on the diet merry-go-round.

After additional diet failures, I tried to convince myself that it was "natural" to put on a "few pounds" as I got older and that people could either "take it or leave it."

After a few more failures, I tried to convince myself that it was "natural" to put on a "few pounds" as I got older. I told myself that I worked hard and long and that I needed food to keep up my energy, and, furthermore, I just didn't have time for this foolishness. It didn't matter what anyone said, I was what I was, and that was all there was to it, so—I said silently—the whole world can take it or leave it.

I forced myself to ignore my wife's well-placed comments about other men's bodies. I felt alone and misunderstood and certainly unappreciated, and I was caught on a roller-coaster of diet and rebound that I could not escape except for short periods of denial.

As I approached fifty my body put an end to the madness. Undeniable chest pains forced me to my doctor. He told me what I already knew. My blood pressure was dangerously high and my cholesterol was "through the ceiling." My weight was climbing and I was well on my way to a heart attack by age fifty. I had to take the weight off just as nature seemed intent on putting it on.

As I approached fifty, my body put an end to the madness.

I tried to make my physician understand the difficulties that I had encountered with most diets: "They're so complicated," I explained. "You have to measure this and count that. I just want to be able to eat real food that I can enjoy and feel satisfied. Besides," I went on, "those diets are so rigid. They don't make room for parties or vacations or 'time off.' I eat differently on weekends than during the week and I want to be able to enjoy myself sometimes. You know?" I asked rhetorically.

He looked unconvinced. I continued with my denunciation. "I start off okay but after a while it just becomes impossible. You can't possibly stay on those diets *forever*," I explained, "and when you go off, you gain back all the weight—and more."

He said nothing so I tried a different approach. "Let me ask you something," I queried. "Why is it that some people can eat all they want and still be thin?"

"Metabolism," he offered, succinctly.

"Well, what does that actually mean?" I asked. "Shouldn't a diet raise your metabolism rather than take as a given the fact that our metabolisms slow down with time?"

He remained unimpressed. "This is what we have," he responded, glancing at the pile of food-exchange sheets on his desk. "You're a scientist. What would you recommend?" he asked tersely, then without waiting for an answer, added, "If you don't like it, you come up with something better."

A part of me felt stupid and childish at venting my frustration at him about something that was, most certainly, not his doing, but at the same time something in me stirred at his challenge.

I was a scientist, a trained researcher—a far cry from the kid who, in total desperation, had fasted on lemon water. I could use my own body as a laboratory and I. . . . No, I told myself. That was stupid. If there was a better way, someone else would have found it.

"The oldest excuse in the world," I reminded myself. Maybe it was audacious to think I could come up with a better diet for everybody, but I could, at least, see if something better would work for me.

Though I barely believed my own intent, I still gave it the best I could. As a trained scientist, I began to observe my own body—my hunger, my cravings, my weight, my reactions to food, to tiredness, to stress. I kept notes as if I were studying any other natural phenomenon. Within a few days, I began forming some ideas and I was ready to test them.

I found that bread, pasta, chips, and Chinese food triggered my cravings.

I found that certain foods, like bread, pasta, chips, and Chinese food seemed to trigger more hunger. I would be fine for a short time after eating them, but a little while later my cravings would return with a vengeance. I realized that some "healthy" or "diet" foods like fruit and juice and even diet soda would call me to eat or drink more of the same, and that when I ate junk food like burgers with fries I would eat amazingly large amounts. Sweets, particularly ice cream, would start me on a roll—and I would nibble myself into a snacking frenzy, stopping only when I fell into a sleepy stupor.

**Sweets, particularly ice cream, would start me on
a "carbohydrate roll";
I would nibble myself into a snacking frenzy
and then fall into a sleepy stupor.**

All these foods had one thing in common: they were rich in car-bohydrates and they made my body release insulin—the "hunger hormone," I reminded myself. Things were beginning to come clear as to what might be the cause of my problem, but the solution seemed nowhere in sight. While my knowledge of physiology proved helpful, returning to my own experience gave me the key I needed.

Though we were barely talking by then, my wife and I still managed to be civil about the children. We shared in their care and she reminded me to be certain that our youngest daughter ate her breakfast. "She gets hungry and weak if she doesn't eat a full meal," my wife cautioned. There was something about her words that lay unresolved in my mind all day.

**If I had a full breakfast—with bread and
juice or cereal—I was hungrier
before lunch than if I had nothing to eat at all.**

As I reached for the peanut butter crackers that constituted one of my several daily snacks, I suddenly realized why my wife's words had struck such an odd note in me. My daughter became hungry and weak if she did *not* eat breakfast—most people did—but the opposite was true for me! If *I had* a full breakfast, I was *hungrier* before it was time for lunch than if I had skipped breakfast alto-gether or, perhaps, had only a cup of coffee. Given this fact, I asked myself, why was I routinely eating a full breakfast each morning only to fight my hunger for the rest of the day?

I had been taught that a good breakfast was essential to good nutrition, but I had a hard time believing that I would simply fade away if I didn't have it every morning. Besides, truisms such as that simply didn't seem to work for my body. Perhaps it was time—more than time—to listen to my own body instead.

The next morning I embarked on what seemed like a daring adventure. Rather than my typical breakfast, I ate only foods that were low in carbohydrates—protein-rich and high-fiber foods. By eleven o'clock in the morning the difference was obvious. My energy was high and for the first time I wasn't counting the minutes until lunch. It was too soon to tell but there did seem to be a difference. I extended my experiment to lunch. More protein, more salad. The difference was startling. No midafternoon slump or cravings and no desire to snack while making dinner. I felt terrific. This was no battle—my cravings, as well as the fight to control them, were gone.

At first, deciding which foods to include in my dinner seemed to present a problem. I knew that it was unhealthy to eat only low-carbohydrate foods, even if they would reduce my cravings and increase my energy, and—to tell the truth—the pasta and garlic bread I was making looked far more appealing than a meal of meatballs and salad. I decided to indulge and for this one meal have carbohydrates along with the protein and vegetables. I even allowed myself a small piece of cheesecake for dessert. In fact, I was surprised to find that I wanted no more than a reasonably sized slice and that evening, for the first time in years, I didn't have my usual pint of Häagen-Dazs ice cream before bed. "I'm not in the mood," I told myself. "Not in the mood?" I could have asked. "Who said that?"

**"I'm not in the mood for ice cream," I told myself.
"Not in the mood?" I asked myself, shocked. "Who said that?"**

The next morning the scale revealed what would have been my fondest hope. My weight had dropped. "This can't go on," I told myself. "This is crazy. Look at the dinner I had last night." But hoping against hope, I repeated my approach the next day; high-protein and fiber-rich foods for breakfast and lunch and a well-balanced feast for supper.

> **Within days, my cravings literally disappeared,
> my energy increased,
> and my weight continued to drop, at a *steady* rate.
> That was well over ten years ago.**

Within days, my cravings literally disappeared, my energy increased, and my weight continued to drop, at a *steady* rate. That was well over ten years ago.

Today I weigh 168 pounds and I maintain that weight without struggle or deprivation, using the same program. I take no medications and my blood pressure and blood-fat levels are that of a twenty-year-old, if he's lucky. Rachael and I share in the joy of everything from gourmet meals to occasional junk-food splurges, at home or out, any day we want. No foods are restricted. No counting or measuring or exchanges are ever involved. I have found a program that is Simple, Targeted to my needs and my decade of life, Adaptable to my lifestyle, and one that Rewards me with the food I love; what I call my STAR Program, a personalized weight-loss program for the carbohydrate addict that provides me with the weight loss and the health I always wanted—for life and without deprivation.

> **If you are carbohydrate addicted,
> The Carbohydrate Addict's LifeSpan
> Program was designed
> so that you, too, can live healthfully *and* happily.**

If you are carbohydrate addicted, The Carbohydrate Addict's LifeSpan Program is your STAR program too; literally designed to help you lose weight and to keep it off for life—to eliminate the *cause* of your cravings and your tendency to gain weight and to give to you—as it has given to Rachael and myself—the rewards and freedom of a program with which you can truly live, healthfully *and* happily.

PART I
CARBOHYDRATE ADDICTION: THE SILENT VILLAIN

CHAPTER 1

CARBOHYDRATE ADDICTION BY THE DECADE

Addict: from the Latin *addicere,* to surrender or to be captured into slavery.

—*Webster's Dictionary,* 2nd ed.

Carbohydrate Addiction: A compelling, recurring or, at times, escalating craving for starches such as bread, pasta, rice, or potatoes, or for snack foods such as chips, popcorn, or pretzels, or for sweets such as cookies, cakes, pies, donuts, muffins, or chocolate.

A tendency to gain weight easily or, over time, to regain weight that has been lost by dieting.

*C*arbohydrate addiction often leads to a loss of eating control (regularly or on occasion) and, along with a tendency to gain weight easily, often leads to repeated failure at attaining a permanent weight loss.

If you are carbohydrate addicted or "sensitive" to carbohydrate-rich foods, you may find that your carbohydrate cravings as well as your body's tendency to gain weight increase with each passing decade. As you grow older, you may find that you prefer smaller meals composed of sandwiches and snack foods rather than large, sit-down meals. Though you may not actually eat more food than those who are "naturally slim," as you grow older weight gain may become easier and easier and weight loss, more difficult.

Carbohydrate addicts often vacillate between blaming themselves or their "metabolism," never realizing that their addiction or "sensitivity" to carbohydrates has taken over their eating, their weight, and, for many, their lives.

Your body's tendency to gain weight easily will tend to increase "naturally" with each passing year, as changing hormonal levels make your body more efficient at storing food energy in the form of fat.

Overweight carbohydrate addicts *do not* necessarily consume more food than do naturally slim people; sometimes the carbohydrate addict eats far less.

Stress, emotional upheavals, or loss, menopause, some medications, and smoking cessation can also increase your cravings for carbohydrates, your body's ability to store food energy as fat, or both.

It is important to understand that, at any age, many carbohydrate addicts who are overweight do not necessarily consume more food than do naturally slim people; carbohydrate addicts often eat far less. The carbohydrate addict's body, however, may be much more efficient at turning food energy into fat. For many, weight gain may not be the direct result of having repeatedly consumed excess amounts of food but, rather, a body that readily turns much of the food that is eaten (in particular, carbohydrates) into fat.

The idea of food addiction is not new. As early as the 1940s, scientists began reporting that some people could become "addicted" to certain kinds of foods and in 1963 Dr. J. Kemp was the first scientist to use the term "carbohydrate addiction," observing that many overweight individuals showed intense and recurring cravings for high-carbohydrate foods (starches, snack foods, or sweets).

Many researchers followed on Kemp's heels and about ten years ago, along with the discovery of brain chemicals such as serotonin, there was a virtual explosion of research into the processes that underlie carbohydrate addiction.

Finally, so many people who might have suspected all along that they were indeed addicted to carbohydrates were free to identify themselves as victims of this physically based problem. But in the 1980s much was still to be learned about the cause and, most certainly, the correction of this disorder, for although it was one thing to identify a problem it was another, altogether, to understand and to be able to correct it.

The Seven Most Common Signs of Carbohydrate Addiction

1. A difficulty in stopping, once you start to eat starches, snack foods, or sweets.
2. A tendency to gain weight easily or to regain weight that has been lost through dieting.
3. A desire to snack or eat again about two hours after eating.
4. Extreme sluggishness or tiredness after a large meal.
5. Signs of low blood sugar (hypoglycemia), including one or more of the following, about two hours after eating, :

hunger	dizziness
weakness	disorientation
headache	lack of concentration
irritability	lack of motivation
sweating	

6. Hunger and/or tiredness in the midafternoon, on a regular basis.
7. Hunger or cravings in response to stress, tiredness, or boredom.

What Causes Carbohydrate Addiction?

We now understand that an addiction to carbohydrates is often a simple result of an excess of the hormone insulin. Dr. Judith Rodin of Yale University nicknamed insulin the "hunger hormone" because of its power ability to stimulate appetite. In the past, insulin was most often associated with diabetes, which is how it was first identified, but more current research shows that insulin may indeed be the key hormone in regulating a great deal of what we refer to as "the metabolism."

An addiction to carbohydrates may be a simple result of an excess of the "hunger hormone" insulin.

Among its other jobs, insulin works hard at helping your body to conserve food energy and it does this in three main ways.*

1. Insulin "calls" your body to eat. It signals you to seek out starches, snack foods, or sweets. If you follow these cravings, insulin rewards you by causing you to experience these foods as exceptionally satisfying.
2. Insulin ushers the food energy (which has been turned into blood sugar) to wherever it is needed in the body and signals the liver to turn any extra energy into blood fat (triglycerides), so that it can be stored in the fat cells.
3. Insulin signals the body to keep the food energy locked into the fat cells, storing it for use at a time when no food is available.

This insulin regulation works well as long as you have just the right amount of insulin present in your body, which explains why some people eat when they are hungry and at other times have no desire for food. Their bodies self-regulate, and problem eating and excess weight never seem to become an issue for them.

But for those of us who are carbohydrate addicted, this insulin balance becomes an imbalance. Some carbohydrate addicts simply produce too much insulin. When they see, eat, smell, or even think about starches, snack foods, or sweets, their bodies overrelease insulin into their bloodstreams.

Some carbohydrate addicts have bodies that are insulin resistant. Their bodies do not allow insulin into the cells as readily as it should; their cells resist the insulin and the excess insulin that cannot get into the cells remains in the bloodstream.

Some carbohydrate addicts have bodies that do both—their bodies overproduce the insulin and the cells in their bodies resist taking it in.

In all three cases, the result is the same—too much insulin in the bloodstream—a condition that scientists call *hyperinsulinemia*. If you have too much insulin in your bloodstream, insulin does all three of its jobs too well.

---

*The complex workings of this system has been simplified for ease of understanding.

First, instead of calling you to eat an appropriate amount of starches, snack foods, or sweets, if you are hyperinsulinemic, you will be driven to eat these foods over and over again—and the more you eat, the more you will want. The result: intense and/or recurring cravings for starches, snack foods, or sweets.

Second, instead of bringing the blood sugar where it is needed throughout your body and depositing the leftover food energy into your fat cells, an excess of insulin or a body that is insulin resistant will result in too much blood sugar being swept out of your bloodstream and being turned into blood fat and channeled into your fat cells. The result: raised blood-fat levels, a tendency to gain weight easily, and/or symptoms of low blood sugar (hypoglycemia) about two hours after eating. These symptoms may include headaches, tiredness, weakness, disorientation, lack of motivation, sweating, irritability, cravings, and/or hunger.

Third, an excess of insulin often results in the body's inability to use the energy it has stored in the fat cells. Instead of being able to call on its stores, the body senses that it is starving and drives you to get more food. The result: difficulty in losing weight and/or maintaining weight loss as well as repeated cravings for carbohydrate-rich foods.

Many people are carbohydrate addicted in their youth, but while they are still young their bodies are able to "burn up" excess calories. They may tend to ignore or shrug off their carbohydrate cravings. "I eat all the junk I want," they may say, half bragging, "and I never gain an ounce." Nevertheless, many are sitting on time bombs and, as the years pass, they may find the pounds mount more quickly than the years.

As all of us grow older, changes typical of the aging process "naturally" increase our tendency to store food energy in the form of fat. With each passing decade, the body's need to build and grow decreases and with it growth hormone levels drop. Although insulin levels may not actually increase, the body monitors the growth-hormone-as-compared-to-insulin relationship and, as growth hormone levels drop, the body often falsely perceives that insulin levels have increased. Wrongly concluding that there is an abundance of insulin present, the body remains in a "fat-making mode."

In addition, years of exposure to insulin make our muscles and organs more insulin resistant, a process that could be compared to our tendency to grow used to someone's loud chatter. After a while, it takes an even higher level of communication to get our attention. In the same way, as the years go by, our bodies appear to require higher levels of insulin in order to use food energy appropriately.

The body's need for nutrients also changes as we grow older, and with each passing decade our bodies are less likely to get enough chromium, an essential element in helping insulin do its job. When the body gets less chromium than it needs, in hopes of compensating it releases extra insulin to make up for the missing chromium.

In the carbohydrate addict, all three of these processes appear to be exaggerated, greatly increasing the body's tendency to release excessive amounts of insulin, which, in turn, fuel our carbohydrate cravings as well as our tendency to gain weight, making it easier and easier to gain weight and harder and harder to maintain an ideal weight with each passing year.

Insulin causes you to crave carbohydrate-rich foods, ushers the food energy into your fat cells for storage, then locks it into your fat cells.

Recent scientific experiments have revealed that excess insulin seems to have far more serious consequences, playing an important role in the development of high blood pressure, stroke, undesirable blood-fat levels, heart disease, adult-onset diabetes, gout, certain forms of cancer, polycystic ovary disease, and more.*

But whether we are talking about health risks, cravings, or weight gain, one thing remains clear: an addiction to carbohydrates—and the excess insulin that causes it—is *not* a matter of willpower, it is a matter of biology, pure and simple.

Carbohydrate addiction is *not* a matter of willpower— it's a matter of biology, pure and simple.

---

*(See Chapter 4, Your Health-Promoting Bonus, for more information on the health risks associated with hyperinsulinemia and the risk-reducing, health-promoting benefits of this program).

If you are carbohydrate addicted, you are no more to blame for your condition than you are for the color of your eyes, or your skin, or your hair. That is not to say that there are not many things you can do to correct the problem of carbohydrate addiction—there most certainly are and we'll tell you how—but the fact that you have these cravings, this tendency to put weight on easily and an increased risk for certain health problems is *not your fault.* That's right, it's not your fault. Chances are you suspected as much all along, but now, with this book in hand, you will have the scientific research to prove what you probably already knew: Your cravings and your weight are a result of your biology—not some character or moral flaw.

There is a clear and simple reason why some people can eat all they want and never gain weight or why some people just don't crave these foods at all. What used to be called "a slow metabolism" has a new and usable name and its name is "hyperinsulinemia"—an excess of the metabolism regulator hormone insulin.

**There is a reason why some people eat all they want and never gain weight
or why some people just don't crave these foods at all.**

If you are carbohydrate addicted, you have too much insulin running the metabolic show in your body and, chances are, the problem remains unidentified and undiagnosed. The bad news is that you have probably had the problem for a while and, most likely, you have been fighting a long and hopeless battle all alone. The good news is that we now know what causes it and, best of all, we know how to correct it—easily, and without sacrifice or deprivation.

Why Is It Called an "Addiction"?

There are some people who may challenge the word "addiction," saying that use of the term releases an individual from responsibility for his/her own actions. We believe that underlying prejudices play a large part in this society's reticence to recognize that some eating problems have a physical basis, but, as scientists, it is important for us to demonstrate that our use of the term "addiction" is absolutely appropriate.

> **There are many people who may challenge the word "addiction."**

In our 1984 research article, published in the journal *Medical Hypotheses*, we demonstrated that carbohydrate addiction met all five of the criteria set down by the American Psychiatric Association in their Diagnostic and Statistical Manual of Mental Disorders (DSM). These criteria included: (1) the increased use of a substance (in this case, carbohydrate-rich foods) in greater amounts or over a longer period of time than the person intended, (2) the continued use of the substance in spite of a persistent desire to cut down or control its use, as well as (3) the continued use of the substance in spite of the knowledge that it causes or makes worse an individual's social, psychological, or physical problems.

Almost all carbohydrate addicts recognize their own experience in these first three criteria as well as in a description of "withdrawal symptoms" that may include recurring or escalating carbohydrate cravings or an intense "drive" to eat. The magnitude behind these cravings for carbohydrates is often described as being quite different than simple feelings of hunger.

"When I'm hungry," many carbohydrate addicts will explain, "I'll eat almost anything. It's a clear, pure feeling. But when I crave carbohydrates, on the other hand, I want only those foods. I may not be hungry but I feel like I *have* to have them. It's much more of a compelling feeling than hunger and I can't find peace until I get my 'fix.' "

In addition to carbohydrate cravings, withdrawal symptoms may also take the form of disorientation or confusion, feelings of anxiety, physical weakness, headaches, or a lack of control or motivation. Many have reported an irrational sense of doom.

> **In other forms of addiction, the person recognizes that there is a underlying *physical* problem that keeps them "hooked," but carbohydrate addicts are told that it's just a matter of willpower.**

While in other forms of addiction, the person is aware that he or she is "hooked" on a substance, carbohydrate addicts are rarely aware of the fact that, for them, carbohydrate-rich foods—eaten in the wrong ways—can act as an addictive substance. As reported in Harvard's 1991 Conference on Obesity, food addicts may find themselves "caught up in a cycle of dieting, withdrawal (excessive hunger), overeating, weight regain, and a return to dieting."

To break this fruitless cycle, then, it is essential to educate carbohydrate addicts so that they can understand that the feeling of relaxation that they feel when they satisfy their cravings is a relaxation of withdrawal symptoms. Because these foods are available 24 hours a day, and because low-fat diet recommendations generally tout carbohydrates as "healthy" foods for everyone, carbohydrate addicts must empower themselves with an understanding that it is not what is in the food that is important but, rather, what the food does to them that can make a world of difference.

> **You must empower yourself with the understanding that it is *not* what is in the food that is important but, rather, what the food does to *you*.**

Let's look at some other ways of defining addiction. An addiction has been described as a drive for a substance which affects one or more of the following:

1. Health
2. Family life
3. Social life
4. Work life
5. Physical appearance
6. Feelings of self-worth or value

and from which the individual feels or demonstrates that he/she is unable to break free. It usually involves an underlying physical imbalance (as we describe in this chapter and in the chapters to come) which grows worse with repeated exposure to the substance.

These ideas may seem interesting at a distance, but in order to truly take back control of your eating, your weight, and your health, you will need to embrace them at a very personal level—with a strength of commitment that will keep you going when others tell you, "It's just a matter of willpower."

Those who challenge the idea that you can be "addicted" to carbohydrates are, most likely, not addicted themselves.

Those who will challenge the idea that you can be "addicted" to carbohydrates are, most likely, not addicted themselves.* For these fortunate individuals, eating starches, snack foods, or sweets is simply a matter of indulgence. When they have not had a "goodie" for a while, they indulge with a normal-size portion (or maybe two of the foods they most desire), they enjoy the food, feel good about eating it (or, at most, just a bit guilty); then, finishing the food, they go on with the rest of their lives.

What these indulgers fail to realize, however, is that not all of us are blessed with the same comfortable response to these foods. Once carbohydrate addicts start eating starches, snack foods, or sweets, they have a far more difficult time stopping than if they had never started. Rather than being stimulated to eat these foods by not having them, carbohydrate addicts find that the less they have, the less they need, and, vice versa, the more they have, the more they need (the basis of any addiction).

In addition, while indulgers enjoy their "goodies," carbohydrate addicts experience more of a "sense of relief" when consuming carbohydrate-rich foods, which is, in fact, a relaxing of the withdrawal symptoms. Many carbohydrate addicts explain that they may not even enjoy the food but simply feel that they "have to eat it." Try explaining that to a person who says carbohydrate addicts overeat because they are gluttons!

---

*Some doubters may be carbohydrate addicts themselves, but remain intent on pretending that they—and you—can retain control.

INDULGENCE VERSUS CARBOHYDRATE ADDICTION:
THEY ARE *NOT* THE SAME!

Carbohydrate Indulgence	Carbohydrate Addiction
A desire for starches, snack foods, or sweets is stimulated by a *lack of exposure* to these foods. (You want some if you haven't had any.)	A powerful desire for starches, snack foods, or sweets is stimulated by *exposure* to these foods. (The more you have, the more you want.)
Carbohydrate consumption is an enjoyable experience.	Carbohydrate consumption may be experienced as enjoyable or as a feeling of relief at warding off a drive for food. Repeated carbohydrate consumption may be experienced as *unpleasant*, but regularly, or on occasion, the individual is unable to stop.
Free choice remains.	The *illusion* of free choice may keep the individual from admitting that his/her eating is out of control. When loss of control is acknowledged, panic may be replaced by self-condemnation.
There is little or no blame from others and self although current social sanctions may make any food indulgence a cause for some sense of shame.	Blame from self and others is high.

> **Millions of people in this country have a physical imbalance that drives their cravings, their eating, and their weight gain.**

Literally thousands of scientific experiments have resulted in an overwhelming amassing of evidence that report that millions of people in this country have a physical imbalance that makes their bodies respond abnormally to carbohydrate-rich foods and to use food energy far more efficiently than others. Still there remains in this country such an incredible prejudice against the overweight that it influences the media, the medical profession, and even the scientific community itself. In the end, many of the scientific discoveries related to the processes that underlie carbohydrate addiction, remain unread and, certainly, unused.

Though the scientific evidence continues to mount, leading the former Surgeon General of the United States, C. Everett Koop, in his report to the nation on Health and Nutrition, to acknowledge that some individuals are carbohydrate-sensitive individuals—the prejudice against those who are victims of a carbohydrate addiction remains.

> **If you are carbohydrate addicted, you must refuse to accept the idea that it is your fault.**

If you are carbohydrate addicted, you must become strong!—not in your commitment to "control" your eating or your addiction (we will provide you with a program that has been designed to correct the cause of your cravings, your weight gain, and the addiction itself so that within a matter of days, your cravings will be virtually eliminated) but, rather, in your commitment to your own experience and an understanding that while there is much you can do, your addiction—and it *is* an addiction—is *not* your fault.

> **We offer you this challenge . . .**

If you are one of the few who still remain unconvinced that you are truly addicted to carbohydrate-rich foods, we offer you this challenge. Take the test that follows in the next chapter. If your test results do, indeed, indicate that you are carbohydrate addicted, begin the Basic Plan as described on page 107. After *one week* on the Program, we believe that the incredible freedom from cravings that you experience will make you a believer.

Who Does It Affect?

Our research indicates that up to 75 percent of the overweight and as many as 40 percent of the normal-weight are carbohydrate addicted. Other researchers have reported similar numbers or varying numbers depending on the age, gender, and ethnic differences of the people they have studied.

One thing remains clear: millions of people are carbohydrate addicted and their problem often goes unrecognized, undiagnosed, and, of course, untreated.

Far more relevant than the fact that so many people share this "silent epidemic," however, is whether or not *you* are carbohydrate addicted, for if no one, or everyone else agreed or denied its very existence, your cravings, your experience, and your battles are what count. They must be taken seriously, and the cause, rather than blame, must be fixed and addressed.

It matters little how many others share your problem; what matters is that you have a right to help rather than to condemnation.

In a world full of people with 20/20 vision, the person who cannot see without the aid of glasses is an easy victim. It is important for you to know that it matters little how many others share your problem, or who agrees that such a problem even exists; what matters is that you have a right to attain the help you need rather than to condemnation.

Why Can't I Eat The Way I Did When I Was Young Without Gaining Weight?

If you think that you gain weight on the same amount of food that kept you slimmer when you were younger, it is *not* your imagination. The change in "metabolism" to which this phenomenon is attributed is yet another example of the impact of insulin.

If you think that you gain weight on the same amount of food that kept you slimmer when you were younger, it is *not* your imagination.

While you may not be eating any more than you did when you were younger, your body has gone through a normal change as part of the maturation process. Growth hormone levels, needed for channeling the food energy to muscles and organs in the young, naturally decrease as we grow older. At the same time as you grow older, your muscles and organs become more "resistant" to insulin so that the insulin in your blood, along with the food energy it brings along with it, has little place to go other than into your fat cells. The end result is a body that has a tendency to put weight on more easily as it gets older.

Add to this natural metabolic shift the impact of insulin-releasing triggers* such as relationship or work-related stress, financial or personal concerns, medications and over-the-counter remedies, menopause, female hormone replacement therapy, the emotional challenges of job change or retirement, personal loss, dental problems, cessation of smoking, and family restructuring, and it is no surprise that eating and weight issues may suddenly spring to life with a vengeance.

Suddenly the pounds seem to accumulate on their own. But remember, while this tendency to gain weight is natural, it is *not* inevitable.

---

*For more information on insulin-releasing triggers see Chapter 3, "Loaded Guns, Ready Triggers, and Time Bombs."

Suddenly the pounds may seem to accumulate on their own and to stay put—in the least desirable places. But take heart, while this tendency to gain weight is natural, it is not inevitable. Both of us are slimmer in our fifties than we ever were in our twenties or thirties—so are thousands and thousands of others on this Program—all while enjoying the foods we love the most. So can you.

While you must be realistic in your weight goal (pre-pregnancy adolescent weights may not be ideal for the sixty-five-year-old woman), a slim, healthy body is easily attainable—at any age.

How Do I Know If I'm Carbohydrate Addicted, and If I Am, What Do I Do About It?

Read on! In the chapters to come, a simple quiz will help you determine if you are, indeed, carbohydrate addicted, and The Carbohydrate Addict's LifeSpan Program's Basic Plan and Options will guide you in finding freedom from carbohydrate cravings and weight problems—for life.

Other chapters that follow will help you to individualize the Program to meet your personal preferences and, with the help of simple shortcuts, you will be able to make lifestyle changes virtually without effort. A wide variety of meal plans and recipes will help you select from the literally limitless food choices that are available to you, and special suggestions have been included for those on low-fat, low-salt, or vegetarian diets.

So relax and enjoy! The Program that follows is one that will make your life happier, healthier, and more enjoyable. The hardest part was getting here—from now on, we'll be with you every step of the way.

So relax and enjoy! We'll be with you every step of the way.

CHAPTER 2

ARE YOU CARBOHYDRATE ADDICTED?

If you make the right diagnosis, the treatment is easy.
—J. Burns Amberson, 1890

*T*he Carbohydrate Addict's LifeSpan Quiz has been designed to help you determine if you are, indeed, carbohydrate addicted, and will help you take advantage of the ease and success offered by The Carbohydrate Addict's LifeSpan Program. The quiz that follows has been designed to detect a long-standing addiction to carbohydrates as well as an addiction that may have grown slowly over the years or come about in response to stress, smoking cessation, menopause, or lifestyle change.

**This program is *not* for everyone;
it is *not* a one-size-fits-all diet.**

The LifeSpan Program has been designed to correct the *cause* of your cravings and your weight gain.

The Program that follows is not for everyone—it is *not* a one-size-fits-all diet. One-size-fits-all diets usually assume that losing weight is just a matter of willpower and, because they do not correct the cause of the carbohydrate addict's cravings and weight gain, they offer the same tried and untrue recommendations that have failed over and over and over again.

Like any remedy that is meant to correct the cause of a physical disorder or imbalance, we must first determine if you do indeed have the problem that the remedy, our program, was designed to correct.

The Carbohydrate Addict's LifeSpan Quiz, which is designed to test for that underlying imbalance, comes from a larger evaluation that has been revised and verified several times over the past ten years. To the original quiz, we have added personal and familial risk factor indicators adapted from The Surgeon General's Report on Nutrition and Health, along with the finest medical research available.

When compared with the most exhaustive and expensive blood testing procedures, the LifeSpan Quiz has been shown to reliably indicate the presence of *postprandial reactive hyperinsulinemia*, which is the scientific term for carbohydrate addiction.

Each week, we receive many inquiries as to where one can go to get a blood test that will determine whether or not they are addicted to carbohydrates. Our response is simple and always the same: You can either get an extensive, expensive, and invasive five-hour Glucose Tolerance Test, which uses a standard carbohydrate-rich mixed meal and which samples insulin and glucose levels at alternating half-hour periods, then get a knowledgeable researcher to compare your test results to a norm of nonaddicted persons of similar weight, gender, and age, or, if you prefer, you can take the simple quiz that follows. Most people prefer to just take our quiz.

We have done the work for you. Your quiz score will indicate whether or not you are carbohydrate addicted as accurately as the most difficult and expensive blood tests mentioned above.

A single blood test that measures your *fasting* insulin level *cannot* tell you whether or not you are carbohydrate addicted.

Most important: Don't be fooled by one-time blood tests. A single blood sample that measures your *fasting* insulin level cannot tell you whether or not you are carbohydrate addicted. When you are carbohydrate addicted, your body releases too much insulin or is unable to use the insulin in your bloodstream. This insulin imbalance occurs *after* you have eaten carbohydrate-rich foods. Since you do not eat for many hours before taking a single fasting insulin blood test, its results may *not* show the abnormal insulin rises that mark the carbohydrate addict. Our research, presented in 1994 and 1995 at the Annual Meetings of the American Institute of Nutrition, illustrated that fasting levels of insulin did not predict whether or not subjects would show abnormal insulin responses after eating. Fasting insulin levels, then, should not be used to determine whether or not someone is carbohydrate addicted.

We have found the quiz that follows offers a far more reasonable—and reliable—alternative to the invasive, expensive, and exhaustive blood testing.

Before You Begin

The Carbohydrate Addict's LifeSpan Quiz will take only a few minutes to complete. Like The LifeSpan Program itself, you will find that the test that follows is Simple (to take), Targeted (to the decade-by-decade changes of the adult carbohydrate addict), Adaptable (to your lifestyle), and Rewarding (giving you immediate, clear, and definitive results). And, although the LifeSpan Quiz consists of just fifteen questions, it will take into account the contribution of your family genetics, your personal medical history, your environmental influences, and your physical responses to food. Our job may have been complicated but yours is very simple.

The Carbohydrate Addict's LifeSpan Quiz will take only a few minutes.
Just answer yes or no to each of the fifteen questions that follow.

Just answer yes or no to each question that follows.
Be as honest as you can and, please, don't judge yourself.

Remember: You are *not* responsible for the way your body responds to food—so stop feeling guilty and let's get you some real help!

INSTRUCTIONS

1. Please take the Carbohydrate Addict's LifeSpan Quiz alone, in a quiet place, where you can be sure of not being disturbed.
2. For each of the questions answer yes, if it *usually* applies to you, and no, if it *usually does not.*
3. Answer every question. If you aren't sure whether or not to answer yes because the question is sometimes true and sometimes not, answer yes if it is often true.
4. Answer each question as if it stands by itself. Don't worry if one answer seems to contradict another. You are not a simple yes-no person and the quiz is designed to accommodate the reality of a complex human being's responses.
5. Answer as if you were *not* on a diet nor worrying about what you eat or what you weigh. We are looking for your *natural* response, not how well you can control yourself.

It is important to take the Carbohydrate Addict's LifeSpan Quiz without worrying about defending your responses. This is your test and you don't have to explain your answers to anyone. The LifeSpan Quiz is based on statistical research in the area of response patterns to food. It is designed to compensate for your guesses, so you don't have to be overly concerned about giving the "right" answer. The accuracy of the LifeSpan Quiz will not be influenced by a guess, or two, or even three. Just be as honest as you can and trust your responses.

The Carbohydrate Addict's LifeSpan Quiz
Answer yes or no to every question.

1. _____ After eating a full breakfast, I get hungrier before it's time for lunch than I would have if I had nothing for breakfast at all or just a cup of coffee.

2. _____ I get tired and/or hungry in the midafternoon.

3. _____ I get very sluggish or tired after a large meal.

4. _____ I sometimes put off plans for evening tasks or activities because I lose motivation after dinner.

5. _____ I have more difficulty stopping once I start to eat starches, snack foods, or sweets, than I have in not eating any at all.

6. _____ About two hours after eating I sometimes get tired, hungry, irritable, shaky, disoriented, unmotivated, _or_ find that I have a headache. Sometimes a snack may make me feel better.

7. _____ Stress makes me want to eat, either immediately or after the stress is somewhat diminished.

8. _____ Foods that include table sugar, fruit sugar (fructose), or artificial sweeteners are included in most of my meals.

9. _____ As I get older, I seem to gain weight more easily.

10. _____ At least one of my blood relatives is overweight.

11. _____ I do not lead an active lifestyle.

12. _____ I am under some stress at home or at work on a pretty regular basis.

13. _____ I have been told that I have one or more of the following: high blood pressure, undesirable blood-fat levels (high total cholesterol or triglycerides, low HDL or high LDL levels), or adult-onset diabetes.

14. _____ One or both of my parents had any of the following: high blood pressure, undesirable blood-fat levels (high total cholesterol or triglycerides, low HDL or high LDL levels), adult-onset diabetes, heart disease, atherosclerosis, vascular disease, or a stroke.

15. _____ I receive female hormone replacement therapy, take stool softeners on a regular basis, or take medication (or over-the-counter remedies) for one or more of the following: high blood pressure, undesirable blood-fat levels (high total cholesterol or triglycerides, low HDL or high LDL levels), adult-onset diabetes, water retention, heartburn, or indigestion.

Scoring the Carbohydrate Addict's LifeSpan Quiz

To determine your score, add the values for each question to which you answered yes.

Different questions have been assigned different values depending on how strongly they indicate an addiction to carbohydrates; the higher the value for a question, the stronger its indicator value.

Question	Value
1	6
2	2
3	1
4	4
5	5
6	3
7	3
8	1
9	3
10	3
11	3
12	3
13	5
14	4
15	4

Total Possible Score: 50

Sample Scoring

If you answered yes to questions 1, 2, 3, 5, and 9, for instance, circle the numbers for those questions on the chart above. Now read across the line to find the value for each question (question 1 is worth 6 points; question 2 is worth 2 points; question 3 is worth 1 point; question 5 is worth 5 points; and question 9 is worth 3 points). Add the values (6, 2, 1, 5, and 3 produce a total score of 17).

What Your Score Reveals

Your score indicates whether you fall into the doubtful addiction, mild carbohydrate addiction, moderate carbohydrate addiction, or strong carbohydrate addiction range. (More detailed descriptions follow.)

In general, the higher your score, the greater your addiction to carbohydrates and the greater the underlying insulin imbalance that is causing that addiction. While in general a high score indicates that weight struggles have become a central issue in your life, there are always exceptions: even a mildly carbohydrate-addicted person can be pulled into the battle of the bulge as the years, stress, and pressures mount and, likewise, even a strongly addicted person can sometimes succeed at maintaining near-normal weight against all odds and at great cost.

In all cases of carbohydrate addiction, whether you are mildly, moderately, or strongly addicted, unless a weight-loss program addresses the excess insulin levels that are causing your cravings and weight gain and the impact that the years, medications, stress, and lifestyle demands can have, it is almost certain to end in failure—and leave you to unjustly blame yourself for your lack of success. On the other hand, a program that corrects your insulin imbalance, and thus reduces or eliminates your cravings and your tendency to gain weight, will be one that you can easily follow and on which you can succeed—for life.

Doubtful Addiction	(13 or less)
Mild Carbohydrate Addiction	(14 to 22)
Moderate Carbohydrate Addiction	(23 to 35)
Strong Carbohydrate Addiction	(36 to 50)

Doubtful Addiction

A score of 13 or less is usually a sign that eating and weight issues are not a significant source of concern or, if they do present difficulties, they do not appear to be related to an underlying insulin imbalance. If you scored 13 or less and you are unhappy with your eating patterns or weight level, it would seem appropriate that you consult with your physician to determine the cause of your problem.

A score in the doubtful addiction range does not mean that you cannot follow The Carbohydrate Addict's LifeSpan Program; many people who have a doubtful addiction find that the Program is easy to follow and gives them the weight reduction they seek. And while those with a doubtful addiction may enjoy and benefit from The LifeSpan Program, we simply want you to understand that this program was designed, specifically, to reduce the cravings and weight problems of those in the mild, moderate, or strong addiction range.

Mild Carbohydrate Addiction

A score in the 14 to 22 range indicates that your cravings and the weight problems you may be encountering appear to be related to a mild but significant underlying physical imbalance. The levels of excess insulin you may be experiencing, as well as your body's inability to use the insulin appropriately, may at times overpower your attempts at self-control.

You may experience episodes of eating greater amounts of starches, snack foods, or sweets than you had intended or find that you are at times unable to refrain from eating these foods altogether. Foods that are high in both fat and carbohydrates, such as ice cream, chocolate, pizza, or Chinese food may prove to be extraordinarily tempting.

Fatigue and stress may contribute to your overeating, although you probably eat "out of habit" or when bored as well. You may find that you reward yourself with food, especially when you are unable to take time off for other pleasures or, more important, for rest.

The sight or smell of food may stimulate you to eat when you would otherwise be able to "control" yourself.

You may sometimes be uncertain as to whether or not you are indeed a carbohydrate addict as opposed to "someone who just really likes food." Your test score, however, indicates you do exhibit signs of a hormonal imbalance. Under extreme stress, upon giving up smoking, at menopause or pregnancy, upon taking certain medications and over-the-counter remedies, or simply as you grow older, this underlying imbalance may have worsened considerably—leaving you far more vulnerable to strong and persistent carbohydrate cravings as well as to weight gain than you had been in the past.

Although it is doubtful that your weight is a central and major issue of concern, you may want to take off some weight for health and appearance reasons. If this is the case, chances are you have found diets that involve calorie or fat gram counting, food exchanges, or food or portion restrictions, are simply not worth the effort. You might have told yourself that if you were to use a little more willpower, you would be able to accomplish your weight-loss goals. When you summoned the energy and motivation to attempt that approach, however, the long-term results were in most likelihood disappointing. Rather than realizing that a hidden hormonal imbalance was sabotaging your efforts, you might have wrongly concluded that you did not try hard enough, or that it was the wrong time to attempt such an endeavor, or that your excess weight was not such a problem as to be worth the trouble of the diet.

The Carbohydrate Addict's LifeSpan Program can help on all levels. By correcting the underlying physical cause of your cravings and your tendency to gain weight, The LifeSpan Program makes counting, measuring, and exchanges unnecessary. Weight problems resolve easily and naturally as the desire to eat frequently or to eat large amounts literally disappears. Your body's natural ability to burn food energy—rather than storing in the fat cells—is restored.

By helping to control and correct the excess levels of insulin in your body, The LifeSpan Program can help you avoid the increased cravings, weight gain, and health risks that so often come with stress, medications, menopause, or the simple act of aging.

Best of all, because The Carbohydrate Addict's LifeSpan Program is Simple to follow, Targeted to your needs, Adaptable to your lifestyle, and Rewarding in both pleasure and weight loss (a STAR plan, personalized for you), no longer will you be forced to choose between a happy life and a healthy one.

Moderate Carbohydrate Addiction

A score of 23 to 35 indicates that you experience recurring hunger and carbohydrate cravings that can at times escalate in intensity. Chances are, they have made dieting difficult in the past, although it is likely that when you have been unable to continue on traditional diets and commercial programs, you have blamed yourself rather than the diet or program.

You have probably vacillated in your approach, sometimes "holding out"—trying to completely refrain from eating the foods you craved. At other times, although you have tried to maintain control of the size of your portions or the foods you chose, the effects of stress or cessation of smoking, premenstrual or menopausal changes, fatigue, or the simple act of growing older, may have seemed to rob you of your ability to effectively manage your eating and your weight.

Foods that are high in both fat and carbohydrates, such as ice cream, chocolate, pizza, or Chinese food, may at times prove to be irresistible. Even when you manage to summon super-human self-disciple, you may find yourself rewarded with minimal weight loss, or none at all.

It is essential you understand that, without knowing it, you have been fighting a virtually insurmountable *physical* problem. Medications and over-the-counter remedies, menstrual changes, personal loss and change, illness, and the very act of aging can intensify the insulin imbalance and the cravings and weight gain that stem from it. Ironically, the foods that you have been eating, the way you have been eating them, and the stress from the negative judgments you have made about your loss of control and yourself have in all likelihood been making the physical problem even worse.

The goods news is that if you are moderately carbohydrate addicted, The Carbohydrate Addict's LifeSpan Program can bring to you a freedom from cravings and weight concerns that you never thought possible. Your sometimes insurmountable or escalating desire for starches, snack foods, or sweets will often disappear within a matter of days. As your insulin levels normalize, the need to "cheat" will, in all likelihood, literally disappear. As an added bonus, as your blood sugar levels stabilize, your energy levels will increase proportionately, as will your motivation and your ability to think clearly. In its own way, it can help turn back your "metabolic clock." Though it is not magic, it is, we hope, as one reader put it, "just good science, long overdue."

Most important, as you watch your body normalize, simply by eating all the foods you love in ways that will reduce your excess insulin levels, your sense of self-blame and shame will be eliminated. You will no longer feel embarrassed about something which has never been your fault but which you now find you are able to correct.

You will be able to lose weight and keep it off, for, rather than taking away your freedom or enjoyment, this is a program that adds to the quality, joy, and pleasure of your life.

Strong Carbohydrate Addiction

A score of 36 to 50 indicates that your eating and/or your weight is being powerfully influenced by a hormonal imbalance of which you may have been unaware. If you are strongly carbohydrate addicted, chances are that your recurring cravings for starches, snack foods, or sweets and your concern about your weight has been impacting on your health, your happiness, and your very life. Foods that are high in both fat and carbohydrates, such as ice cream, chocolate, pizza, or Chinese dishes may at times prove to be especially addictive and/or cause you to gain weight more easily.

You may have been drawn to carbohydrate-rich foods in your youth but now find that, with the added years, eating the same foods can lead to added pounds.

For you, traditional diets and commercial programs are literally made to fail. While they may have succeeded in the past for a limited time (a testament to your willpower and motivation), in the end they often worsen the physical imbalance that is causing your cravings and weight problems in the first place. In all likelihood, you will not be able to stick to traditional diets and commercial programs for life and sooner or later, as your old eating patterns return, so will the pounds and with it the self-blame.

As your blood sugar levels sharply rise then fall, you may experience mood swings, irritability, nervousness or anxiety, tiredness, listlessness, and lack of motivation. You may sometimes feel like you are "living in a fog," unable to break free or to think clearly and to get your life in order. You may at times feel trapped, hopeless, and—certainly—out of control. You may try to deny that there is any help and attempt to resign yourself to the feeling that this is your lot in life—but your desire to live and succeed will often not let you give up.

Strongly addicted persons may hide their feelings or, at the very least, refuse to talk about their despair and pain. They may seem to resent friends' and family members' attempts to help, but in fact they are simply tired of trying and failing over and over again.

The strongly addicted are often blamed by others, particularly many in the medical profession who unfairly describe them as "killing themselves." Nothing could be farther from the truth. If you are strongly addicted to carbohydrates, only you know how hard you have tried and how difficult is the battle.

For you, the strongly addicted carbohydrate addict, The Carbohydrate Addict's LifeSpan Program should be easier to follow than any weight-loss program you have ever encountered. This program has been designed to correct the *cause* of your cravings and weight gain—it is *not* a diet of deprivation or sacrifice, but, rather, a correction for the hormonal imbalance that caused your eating and weight problems in the first place. Most people happily report that they succeed simply because they have no *desire* to cheat, and that, we believe, is how it should be.

Medications, over-the-counter remedies, stress, stopping smoking, menstrual changes, and the simple act of aging often increase the hormonal imbalance that leads to an addiction to carbohydrates. Though you are strongly addicted now, you may have been mildly or moderately addicted in the past but found that any of these "triggers" have made it harder for you to maintain control over your eating or your weight (or both). The Carbohydrate Addict's LifeSpan Program will help remove the influence of these triggers, now and in the future, and help you live your life more like one of those amazing creatures who have been blessed with a metabolism that keeps them "naturally slim."

Beyond Words: Beth's Story

"I've never been accused of not being able to express myself," Beth G. began. "When I was a kid, my mother used to call me motor mouth." We cringed at her self-condemnation, but before we could object, she went on. "I've often said that I should be a writer so that I can get paid by the word but . . ." She hesitated, and as she struggled to continue, tears overflowed onto her flushed cheeks. Though she was forty-five and the mother of two teenage girls, she looked like a vulnerable adolescent herself.

Beth continued. "I have to tell you what it has meant for me to realize that it wasn't my fault," she faltered, and the tears continued to form in her eyes. "I always knew, deep inside, that I was really doing my best; it really wasn't my fault."

We didn't need to ask Beth for clarification; we knew only too well what "wasn't her fault." We had heard it thousands of times before, at book signings, in letters, even at chance meetings on the street. Our readers told us of the years that had been wasted on self-blame and recrimination; souls that had been searched and pronounced guilty of some unknown crime; then, after learning of the physical cause of their cravings and weight gain, a transformation of confirmation and vindication that had taken place.

Even before the Program had begun to reverse the physical imbalance that lay silently within, the simple knowledge that the recurring and powerful cravings and excess weight were not a sign of some moral or psychological weakness but the result of a simple hormonal imbalance brought a freedom from self-blame that for many was overwhelming.

"I have been saying it for years and no one ever believed me," Beth continued. "My husband, my doctor, even my mother—and she has the same problem! They would just say I should try harder, but no matter what I did, I always gained it back. But this is about more than just the weight, you know," she said, looking up, "it's about it not being my fault. I mean you're really saying that, aren't you?" She barely paused for confirmation.

We assured Beth that this was exactly what we were saying, and added that even though her weight problem was not her "fault" there was a great deal she could do about it.

"I'm just so glad you understand" she added in a choked voice. And we waited while the tears of relief ran down her cheeks. For Beth, as for so many carbohydrate addicts, the pain, as well as the wish for freedom, is beyond words.

Fuzzy Lines

Though it is helpful to understand the level and severity of your addiction to carbohydrates, remember than these categories are not carved in stone. A sudden stress may turn a mild carbohydrate addict into a moderately or strongly addicted person. Likewise, a particularly relaxing vacation may help, for a time, to reduce an addiction. Medications, over-the-counter remedies, stopping smoking, and getting older will most certainly make your addiction levels rise, causing you to crave foods more often or more intensely or, even when you do not eat any more food, to gain weight more easily.

The lines between addiction levels are fuzzy and, though we move back and forth across them many times in a lifetime, two things must remain clear: First, you are not to blame for your addiction to carbohydrates, and, second, you cannot cure the problem until you correct the cause.

We share with you the struggles of the past. It has been a long-fought battle; our addictions have been mighty adversaries. They have taken their toll in emotional and sometimes physical pain. Perhaps they have made us a bit more sensitive and caring for others. Perhaps they have made us more humble. We have learned our lessons very, very well. Now is the time for freedom. Heaven knows, we have all earned it.

CHAPTER 3

LOADED GUNS, READY TRIGGERS, AND TIME BOMBS

CARBOHYDRATES, AGE, STRESS, MEDICATIONS, AND MORE

For every disease there is a cause; for every cause, a cure.
—Dr. Henry E. Sigerist, *A History of Medicine*, 1934

*Y*ou most certainly have heard someone say "he is of two minds" to describe a person who has two different thoughts, feelings, or purposes, both at the same time. What you probably did not know is that you, every moment of every day, are of two bodies. At all times, two different systems within your body are at work in two different ways to achieve two different, and often opposite, physical purposes.*

Every moment of every day, you are of two bodies.

---

*The complex workings of these systems have been simplified for ease of understanding.

One part of you is intent on using all of your energy to build, repair, and fuel the organs and systems of your body; to keep you going, and to keep you at your best. This is your "spending system." Its sole purpose is to spend the food energy you take in, to keep you alive and in top condition.

The other part of you is intent on storing for the future as much of your energy as possible, putting it away for "a rainy day" when food may not be so available. This is your "saving system." Its main purpose is to tuck as much food energy away as is possible, for future needs, in the form of body fat.

Under ideal conditions these systems work in harmony. In Chapter 1, you learned that insulin, the "saving hormone," is released when you eat carbohydrate-rich foods such as starches, snack foods, or sweets. Insulin urges you to eat more of these foods by making them taste good to you, and after you eat your body turns much of the food you have just eaten into blood sugar (also called blood glucose). Then insulin ushers the blood sugar where it is needed throughout the body and signals the liver to turn any excess blood sugar into blood fat (triglycerides), which is then stored in your fat cells. With most of its work done, insulin tells the body to keep the fat stored away for a while until the food energy is needed later.

**Insulin can "bully" other hormones
and help block fat from leaving your fat cells.**

After doing all of this work, much of the insulin in your blood is "used up," and after a while, when no more food is taken in, your insulin levels drop even further.

Now a second hormone, glucagon, comes into action. This is the "spending hormone." Its job is to bring out the food energy that has been stored away as fat in your fat cells and to move it to the muscles and organs that will burn it for fuel and rebuilding.

When both of these important hormones are in balance, everything works smoothly. Insulin helps the body to get the energy it needs and to store the excess energy away. When food is not available, glucagon helps bring the stored food energy out of the fat cells to be used.

But here's the problem. Insulin and glucagon are not equal partners. Many researchers and medical educators, including Drs. Jay and Helen Tepperman in their textbook *Metabolic and Endocrine Physiology*, report that when insulin is present in sufficient quantity (helping the body to save), glucagon is not released to do its job (to help the body spend).

An excess of insulin may be responsible for virtually all of the carbohydrate addict's eating and weight problems.

An excess of insulin, then, along with its ability to limit the release of glucagon, may be responsible for virtually all of the carbohydrate addict's eating and weight problems.

In the carbohydrate addict, the normal workings of insulin go "overboard" and much of insulin's power overwhelms the body. First, remember that insulin makes carbohydrate-rich foods taste better, but when too much insulin is released you may find that starches, snack foods, or sweets taste so exceptionally good to you that it's hard to keep from going back for more and more.

Second, when your insulin levels are too high, your organs and muscles will often defend themselves against the excess insulin by "shutting down" to it. Your organs and muscles no longer allow enough of the insulin (and the blood sugar that it brings with it), into their cells. In scientific terms, this is called *insulin resistance*. Since insulin cannot get enough of the blood sugar into organs and muscles that need it, insulin acts as if the blood sugar remaining in the bloodstream is excess and signals the liver to turn the blood sugar into fat and to store it in your fat cells.

If you are carbohydrate addicted, this resistance of your muscles and organs to insulin explains why you may get tired easily (not enough blood sugar where your body needs it) and why even if you do not eat very much you may tend to gain weight more easily than others (easy storage in the fat cells). Insulin resistance increases as we grow older, one of the insulin-related reasons why we put weight on more easily with each passing year.

> **Insulin can sweep too much blood sugar
> out of your bloodstream,
> leading to symptoms of low blood sugar (hypoglycemia).**

In addition, many fine medical textbooks, such as *Modern Nutrition in Health and Disease* by Dr. J. T. Devlin and Dr. E. S. Horton, now teach young physicians that insulin can sweep too much blood sugar out of the bloodstream too quickly. If you are carbohydrate addicted, this means you that are more likely to experience some of the symptoms of low blood sugar (hypoglycemia) after eating. You may notice that you feel weak, tired, shaky, confused, lose motivation, get headaches, or become irritable about two hours after eating. These signs are not "in your mind"; they are clear signals that you may be not getting the food energy you need to function well and they often go along with a tendency to gain weight easily (because the food energy is being channeled into your fat cells).

> **If it is difficult for you to lose weight at a steady rate
> or to keep it off once it is lost,
> you may be seeing the effect of insulin's tyranny.**

If you find that it is very difficult for you to lose weight at a steady rate or to keep it off once it is lost, you may be seeing the effect of insulin's tyranny over glucagon once again. Too much insulin in your bloodstream is keeping glucagon from being released, and without glucagon, you cannot spend—burn up—the energy that has been stored in your fat cells.

We want you to understand insulin's enormous impact so that you can appreciate that many of the personal eating preferences, experiences, and problems with weight you may have assumed were your own are, in fact, the simple consequence of this hormone's powerful influence.

Later in this chapter you will discover a whole host of environmental and physical changes that can greatly increase insulin's control over your body. These changes include the ways in which you eat carbohydrate-rich foods as well as some of the medications and over-the-counter remedies you take, the physical changes that your body goes through as it gets older as well as changes in stress levels.

> **We will show you how to stop insulin's tyranny—
> here and now.**

The good news, however, is that we will also show you in the chapters that follow how The Carbohydrate Addict's LifeSpan Program can help you to stop insulin's tyranny—here and now. In addition, in other chapters to come, we will reveal insulin's far more insidious contribution to high blood pressure, undesirable blood fats, heart disease, adult-onset diabetes, stroke, vascular disease, some forms of cancer, and more. And we will show you how the same program that can help you become slim and fit can help you reduce your risk for all these killers.

But first, it is essential for you to understand why *your* body produces more insulin than it should (while other people's bodies may not).

Your Thrifty Gene

Although we talk about an insulin "imbalance" in your body, it is important to understand that there is nothing wrong with your body; it is in perfect working order—for about a million years ago.

> **You have the perfect body—for about a million years ago!**

Your body was built for a time of feast and famine, and in prehistoric times your body probably would have kept you alive and well when almost everyone else would have faded away. Carbohydrate-rich foods were rare then, and when there was an unusual find of fruit or berries or wild grain, your rising insulin levels would have signaled you to eat great amounts of these scarce and essential foods. You would have efficiently stored away the food energy, and when times of famine followed, a drop in insulin levels would have allowed you to fall back on the energy in your fat cells to keep you alive.

**If you release too much insulin,
a "thrifty gene" may be responsible.**

Scientists are beginning to discover that if you release too much insulin, a "thrifty gene" seems to be responsible. Many scientists, from Dr. J. V. Neel in 1962 to current researchers such as Dr. E. Ravussin and Dr. C. Bogardus of the National Institutes of Health, believe that this gene may be a leftover from prehistoric times, when its very presence would have made the difference between life and death. In a world of continual feast—or what your body perceives of as continual feast—your thrifty gene may no longer be working to keep you alive but may actually be increasing your risk for obesity and ill-health.

**Your ability to stay slim, fit, and healthy depends on
learning how to change the messages your body is getting.**

Rather than thinking that there is something "wrong" with you, it is important to understand that your ability to stay slim, fit, and healthy depends on learning how to change the messages that your body gets from the food you eat (and the way you eat it), the medications and over-the-counter remedies you take, as well as the physical changes and stress that you experience throughout your lifetime.

Come with us now as we look at the Loaded Guns, Ready Triggers, and Time Bombs that are taking your excellent body and throwing it out of kilter, then learn how to bring it back into balance and keep it there—for life.

Loaded Guns

There are some things you can change and others you simply cannot. One of the greatest mistakes people make in trying to lose weight is that they repeatedly attempt to change those things they cannot change and fail to change those things they can.

Most people try to use will power to override their cravings and their bodies' increased ability to store fat.

These people are almost certainly bound to fail. Sooner or later nature will win out.

Most people try to use willpower to override their cravings for food and their bodies' increased ability to store the food they eat in the form of fat. But intense and recurring carbohydrate cravings, as well as the body's heightened ability to store fat, come from a *physical* cause, an excess of insulin. Willpower does not change your body's *physical* workings, and while you may override your body for a time, sooner or later nature will win out.

Ironically, when people fail to lose weight and to maintain their weight loss through attempts involving willpower and self-control, rather than reevaluating what they did wrong, they blame themselves—or accept blame from others—and then give up for a while. After some time, they begin the hopeless diet cycle all over again. It is no wonder that up to 98 percent of people who engage in this futile battle will fail.

So let's begin by looking at what you can and what you cannot change about your body and the way in which your body handles food.

Ready Triggers

If you are carbohydrate addicted, you cannot change your body's *predisposition* to release too much insulin—that is a loaded gun that comes, literally, from the genes you inherited from your parents. But this genetic message is only a predisposition—a primed weapon that is *waiting* to go off. It will not go off unless you pull the trigger—and pulling the trigger is something that *you*, most certainly, *can control.* So, while your body may be set up to release too much insulin—which in turn will make you crave carbohydrates and gain weight easily—you can keep the cravings and weight gain from occurring, in the first place, if you know how to avoid triggering the release of the excess insulin.

Your body is a loaded gun—ruled by your genetics— but it cannot go off if you don't pull the trigger.

If you are carbohydrate addicted, there are several important triggers that you must learn to identify, and there are easy ways to avoid setting off the loaded genetic gun that has caused you to gain weight in the past.

Essentially, each of the Guidelines that you find in The Carbohydrate Addict's Basic Plan, as well as in its Options, will help you avoid setting off the triggers that can stimulate your body to release too much insulin. When you do not pull the trigger, the loaded genetic gun cannot go off and your cravings and your weight struggle can, literally, become a thing of the past. Best of all, as you learn how to avoid triggering your addiction to carbohydrates, you may finally be able to enjoy living as a naturally slim person.

Constant Carbos

The most common and the strongest carbohydrate addiction trigger by far is the frequent intake of carbohydrate-rich foods. In our research, we have found that carbohydrate addiction is a two-step process.

First, if you are born with a thrifty gene, the more often you eat carbohydrate-rich foods such as starches, snack foods, or sweets (including fruit and fruit juice), the greater will be your insulin response. This high level of insulin will cause you to crave more and more of these same foods.

Second, as you continue eating these carbohydrate-rich foods on a frequent basis, your muscles and organs will start to become insulin resistant, and both the insulin, and the blood sugar it escorts, will be "channeled" *away* from the muscles and organs that need it and preferentially stored in your fat cells. In the first stages of insulin resistance, you may have a much greater tendency to gain weight but, over time, even the fat cells become insulin resistant and the insulin and blood sugar stay trapped in the bloodstream, which may eventually lead to adult-onset diabetes. If you continue to eat carbohydrate-rich foods frequently, the cycle repeats, over and over again.

In many people, particularly those who have battled with their cravings and/or their weight for most of their lives, or who find that triggers such as pregnancy, stress, stopping smoking, medications, and over-the-counter remedies make them start to crave carbohydrates and gain weight easily, this is the simple two-step process that occurs.

For others, however, these two steps are reversed. In these individuals we find that although they were normal-weight (or struggled only a little to maintain their weight) in their youth, the simple act of growing older appears to change their metabolism—making their bodies more insulin resistant. This is the first step in their two-step process. First, the insulin and blood sugar are channeled preferentially to the fat cells, and weight is gained far more easily than it was in younger days.

As the addiction moves into its second step, the body releases more and more insulin in an attempt to push through the resistance and force the insulin and the precious blood sugar to the muscles and organs that need it. The extra insulin leads to carbohydrate cravings, and with the eating of carbohydrate-rich foods even more insulin is released. In an attempt to protect itself from too many "insulin insults," the body becomes even more insulin resistant. Even the fat cells may "shut down" and the insulin, along with the sugar it accompanies, gets stuck in the bloodstream—and, in time, may lead to adult-onset diabetes.

In either case, whether carbo cravings or weight gain is the first sign, the cravings and the weight are symptoms of an underlying physical problem, which must be corrected if you are to live a slim and healthy life.

In addition, carbohydrate-rich snacks, which are eaten without the correct balance of protein and fiber, are more likely to set off an insulin imbalance than would fully balanced meals (which can help to maintain normal levels of insulin and blood sugar). You will begin to see that those "innocent" (even "healthy") little snacks of the past may have led you to crave more food, more intensely, and urged your body to take the energy needed by your muscles and organs and store it where you least wanted it—in your fat cells.

Some carbohydrate-rich foods, in particular the complex carbohydrates such as breads, pasta, rice, potatoes, and such, are essential to our diet. Others, including cakes and cookies, chocolate, ice cream, and donuts are important pleasures to many of us. On this program you can have all of them,* but, and here's the important "but," you must learn *how* to eat these foods so that they do not set off the excess release of insulin that has in the past led to your cravings and weight gain.

You can have the carbohydrate-rich foods you love and need and not set off your cravings and weight gain.

The Carbohydrate Addict's Basic Plan will provide you with three easy Guidelines that will help you to keep your cravings and your weight under *your control.* For now, just remember that all carbohydrate-rich foods, including starches, snack foods, and sweets (as well as fruits and fruit juices) and even some starchy vegetables, *when eaten frequently* and without balance, can trigger the loaded genetic gun that can make it very difficult for you to stay slim and healthy.

Sugar Substitutes

Sugar substitutes may "fool" the body calorie-wise but they cannot deceive the body's insulin response. Though they are short on calories they can, nevertheless, cause an excess release of insulin and the cravings and weight gain that usually follow.

The rule of thumb is this: if it tastes sweet, your body thinks it is getting sugar. If your body thinks that it is getting sugar, your body releases insulin, and if you are prone to releasing too much insulin, then anything that tastes sweet, no matter how "low-calorie" it is, can lead to increased cravings and weight gain.

---

*All foods are permitted on this program. If your physician recommends that you avoid or limit any of these or any other foods, however, your physician's advice has priority and should most certainly be followed.

> **If you think that diet sodas and "sugarless" gums, mints, and candies can give you a "free ride" on the road to weight loss, you are in for a bumpy ride to nowhere.**

If you think that diet sodas and "sugarless" gums, mints, and candies can give you a "free ride" on the road to weight loss, you are in for a bumpy ride to nowhere. Sugar substitutes may seem to cut calories at the *moment* you consume them, but if you are carbohydrate addicted, they can trigger a heightened insulin response that will soon drive you to high-carbohydrate, high-calorie foods.

Even if you are somehow able to successfully and repeatedly fight off your carbohydrate cravings, we have found that frequent intake of sugar substitutes may put your body in a fat-making mode, making it easier to gain and more difficult to lose weight. (You'll learn more about sugar substitutes in the coming chapters.)

Ounce for ounce, fructose (fruit sugars) and high-fructose sweeteners (which, despite their name, can be made from glucose) carry the same caloric value as table sugar and, when consumed often, appear to cause the same insulin response. The former Surgeon General of the United States has noted that for "carbohydrate-sensitive individuals" fructose may lead to increased health-related risks.

For now, be aware that anything that tastes sweet, high-calorie or low-, can set off your insulin trigger, but be assured that we will help you disarm this most powerfully loaded gun.

MSG

Monosodium glutamate (MSG) is a concentrated form of sodium that is usually extracted from grains or beets. As the authors of *The Joy of Cooking* note, MSG has long been known as the "magic powder of the East."

MSG is often added to foods because it intensifies flavors and is used in commercially processed foods such as canned soups, sauces, luncheon meats, bottled and dry salad dressings and dips, canned and frozen meats, fowl, and fish. It is the main ingredient in flavor enhancers and is added to hot dogs, bouillon cubes, chicken stock, jarred gefilte fish, and *many* other foods.

MSG has long been used in Chinese cooking, and although some people think that they are able to avoid its effects by requesting "no MSG" in their meals, they may be unaware that it is virtually impossible to avoid MSG in Chinese food because it is present in the bean curd and soy sauce so prevalent in this type of cooking.

MSG goes under many names. According to a recent report on the television show *60 Minutes,* MSG can be listed in *any* of the following ways: monsodium glutamate, MSG, hydrolyzed food starch, hydrolyzed plant protein, flavor enhancers, or natural flavors. A food that claims to contain natural flavors, then, can contain MSG without listing it as such.

**MSG is given by scientists to laboratory animals
to *make the laboratory animals fat.***

We are still learning about the ways in which MSG affects different people. Clearly, there are real variations. In some people, MSG's effects are much more pronounced than in others. After consuming the additive, some people experience one or more symptoms of an "MSG reaction," including intense headaches, disorientation, or leg swelling. Others may be unaware of any reaction whatsoever although the lack of symptoms does not mean that MSG is not taking its toll.

Although some carbohydrate addicts may be aware of weight gain, increased hunger or cravings, and/or water retention after consuming MSG, other carbohydrate addicts never make the connection between their intense enjoyment of Chinese food or their weight gain following the consumption of many processed or fast foods and the MSG that is so often present. In our research, carbohydrate addicts have documented all of the following reactions to MSG intake: substantial weight gain (2 to 4 pounds in one day), water retention, irritability, tiredness, lack of motivation, strong cravings for carbohydrate-rich foods in general or an intense and repeated desire for the same food that originally contained the MSG (Chinese food, for instance).

Very few people are aware that MSG is actually given by scientists to laboratory animals for research purposes, to *make the laboratory animals fat*. MSG appears to affect the hunger and weight-control centers of the brain, and while many scientists are still trying to clarify the mechanism behind its actions, we have little doubt that for the carbohydrate addict MSG—under any name and in any form—is a trigger for carbo cravings and weight gain.

While The Carbohydrate Addict's LifeSpan Program will help you to reduce the insulin response that may be part of MSG's powerful impact, in addition, if you are MSG-sensitive, you will probably find The MSG Easing Option, in Chapter 6, "Options for Life," very helpful.

Good Home Cooking: Marcelle's Story

"I always thought that I just loved Chinese food," Marcelle L.'s letter began. "I don't mean loved it, I mean *loved* it. When my husband was alive, I always cooked good regular meals for him. He didn't care for Chinese food so I didn't get to have it except on rare occasions. After he passed away, I figured, why not enjoy what I always wanted? Here I was, sixty-seven years old, and it wasn't worth cooking for myself. Within a month or two I realized I was ordering Chinese food delivered more often than not. I found myself eating it four or five times a week, more if you count leftovers as snacks. Nothing gave me the rush like that first bite, and as long as I kept it high in vegetables and protein and low in fats and sugars, I figured I was okay.

"You would have thought I would have gotten the idea that things weren't okay, though, because I kept gaining weight and gaining weight and the only thing that I really enjoyed was sitting down to my favorite meal."

Marcelle's letter went on to tell us that she suspected that she was "sensitive" to monosodium glutamate because, in the past, she often felt "out of sorts" after eating foods containing MSG but that until she heard us on TV she thought that she was avoiding the additive by making certain to request "no MSG" whenever she ordered Chinese food.

"When you said that MSG is found naturally in soy sauce and teriyaki, my mouth fell open," she wrote. "When you said that it can be found in up to one-third of all restaurant food, something clicked. Homemade food never gave me the punch that restaurant food or fast foods did, even when the restaurant food didn't actually taste that good. There's just something in it that satisfies me like nothing else and Chinese food is the worst (or best, depending on how you look at it)."

Marcelle went on to tell us that her cravings and her weight problems had escalated after her husband's death. "I had assumed that it was all 'psychological,' a way to make up for my loss, but now I realize that that was the time that I began eating out a lot and that a chemical, a chemical!, was making me hungry and addicted and miserable."

Although she did not have to give up her restaurant food, Marcelle reported that she chose to go back to cooking for herself. "I forgot what a good cook I was and how much I love cooking. I've lost over forty pounds and I look and feel like a new woman," she let us know a few months later. "So, feeling adventurous, I went on a 'cook's tour' and not only did I get the encouragement and great ideas I wanted but I found someone to share my good cooking and the good times to come as well."

Stress

When you experience stress of any kind, either good or bad, your body releases "stress hormones." Several of these hormones can trigger your body's tendency to overrelease insulin. Moderate levels of stress that continue for some time appear to cause different physical changes than short-term periods of acute stress, but both appear to result in higher levels of insulin and increased cravings and weight gain.

When you experience stress of any kind, either good or bad, your body releases "stress hormones."
These hormones, in turn, often trigger the release of insulin.

Extreme physical stressors, such as lack of sleep or intense exercise or physical exertion can, in addition, deplete the body of some of its chromium stores. Chromium is an essential element required for regulating blood sugar levels. With decreased chromium levels, the body may compensate by releasing extra insulin, with the result being greater or more frequent carbohydrate cravings. Similar responses may be experienced to the stress that comes from losing a loved one through death, divorce, or separation. Ironically, even "good" experiences that are enjoyable but intense may be perceived by your body as "stress" and lead to an increase in your carbohydrate cravings.

While you may never be aware of the impact of the stress on your insulin levels, it is likely that during, or some time after, a stressful event you will find yourself irresistibly drawn to carbohydrate-rich foods. You may tell yourself that eating will "make you feel better," and you are probably right, for the moment, but what you may not know is *why* the food makes you feel better and how you can feel better without gaining weight or losing control of your eating.

The Carbohydrate Addict's LifeSpan Program's Basic Plan and its Options for Life can help you change the way that stress impacts on your body so that you can feel better and stay better as well. The Basic Plan of The Carbohydrate Addict's LifeSpan Program will help disarm the stress trigger itself and many of the Options for Life (Chapter 6), in particular the Stress Reduction Option, may help you to control and limit the impact that stress can have on your body (and on your cravings and weight).

**Stress is a powerful insulin trigger
but you can greatly reduce its impact.**

For now, just start to become aware of the types of stress you may be experiencing: Is the stress in your life continual, at a low level? Is it intermittent but very strong? Are you under pressure and unable to speak about it openly? Do you feel helpless and unable to reduce the stress by anything you do?

There are subtle but important differences in the trigger we call "stress" and each of them can affect your body in a different way.

Remember, that while stress is a powerful trigger and one that is often difficult to control, you can make an important difference in the *impact* that stress has on *your* body.

Medications and Over-the-Counter Remedies

Many medications, whether purchased over the counter or by prescription, as well as over-the-counter remedies (stool softeners, antacid tablets or liquids, cough drops and syrups, for instance) may increase your insulin levels and as a result increase your carbohydrate cravings and your tendency to gain weight. You may take some medications or remedies on occasion only, as when you have a headache or backache, a flare-up of arthritis or such. Other medications, such as female hormone replacement therapy, or drugs to reduce high blood pressure or to lower blood cholesterol, may be taken on a regular basis.

It is important to understand that many medications and remedies can have a great impact on your cravings or on your weight or on both.

If you are carbohydrate addicted, it is important to recognize the potential impact of medications and over-the-counter remedies on your cravings and weight, so that you can identify what may have been an unknown source of increased hunger and weight, and, armed with this knowledge, you will be able to discuss these effects with your physician.

It is most likely that your physician will *not* change your medication or remedy recommendations based on concerns regarding its impact on your insulin levels, and indeed in all likelihood there is no real need to do so. Your physician will probably decide that the benefit of the medication or over-the-counter remedy outweighs its potential for insulin-related drawbacks and, happily, The Carbohydrate Addict's Basic Plan and its Options may help counterbalance many of the medication or remedy's insulin-increasing effects.

Most important, *never* stop nor reduce either prescribed or recommended medications or remedies because of concerns regarding your insulin levels, your cravings, or your weight. Your physician must guide you in all of these matters. Self-prescribing is clearly not the intent of this section. We want you to understand that these medications and remedies may raise your insulin levels and thereby affect your eating and your weight but we also want you to understand that The Carbohydrate Addict's LifeSpan Program can help offset many of the fat-storing effects of these drugs and the Over-the-Counter Remedy Timing Option (in Chapter 6) may help you reduce the insulin-raising power of many over-the-counter remedies.

The Carbohydrate Addict's LifeSpan Program can help offset the fat-storing effects of many medications and over-the-counter remedies.

Many medications and over-the-counter remedies may increase blood insulin levels by increasing the release of insulin or by making the body more insulin resistant or, in some cases, by doing both.

Following The Carbohydrate Addict's Basic Plan can help reduce your insulin levels so that you can offset or reduce the insulin-triggering effects of these medications and remedies. In Chapter 6, "Options for Life," you will discover an alternative way to take antacid tables, stool softeners, and other remedies that can also help reduce the cravings and weight gain that many over-the-counter remedies can stimulate.

Some Medications and Remedies That Can Trigger Your Cravings and/or Weight Gain*

Antacid pills and liquids (over-the-counter), used on occasion for:
   Heartburn, indigestion
Anti-inflammatory drugs (including aspirin, acetaminophen, ibuprofen, etc.), used on occasion to reduce or eliminate:
   Headache, backache, pain, and/or fever

Anti-inflammatory drugs (including aspirin, acetaminophen, ibuprofen, etc.), used regularly for:
  Arthritis symptom reduction
  Coronary-risk reduction†
  Pain management
Antihypertensive drugs, used regularly for:
  High blood pressure reduction
Beta blockers, used regularly for:
  High blood pressure reduction
Birth control pills, used regularly for:
  Birth control
  Menstrual regulation
(Cholesterol) lipid-lowering drugs, used regularly to:
  Reduce blood cholesterol levels
Cold and allergy lozenges, cough drops and syrups (over-the-counter), used on occasion to:
  Relieve sore throat and/or coughing
Corticosteroids (cortisones), used regularly or on occasion for:
  Inflammation reduction
  Healing facilitation
  Reduction or prevention of autoimmune reaction
Diuretics, used regularly or on occasion to:
  Reduce water retention
  Reduce high blood pressure
Female hormones, used regularly as:
  Replacement therapy during or after menopause
  Replacement therapy after total hysterectomy (or removal of ovaries)
Insulin replacement therapy and/or blood sugar regulators, used regularly to:
  Control blood sugar levels in adult-onset diabetics
Stool softeners, used regularly or on occasion
Vasodilators, used regularly for:
  Reduction of high blood pressure

*Never stop or reduce prescribed or recommended medications or remedies because of concerns regarding your insulin levels, your cravings, or your weight. Your physician must guide you in all of these matters. Self-prescribing is clearly not the intent of this chart.
†Aspirin, used for reducing coronary risk, is typically prescribed at dosages so low that they may or may not cause a significant insulin response.

Alcohol

Scientists have discovered that the body appears to metabolize the alcohol found in beer, wine, liquor, and mixed drinks in a similar way as it metabolizes carbohydrates. For the carbohydrate addict this means that prolonged consumption of alcohol or a simple round of drinks can lead to carbo cravings and/or weight gain.

In addition, when you consider the sugars that are often added to wines or mixed drinks and the snacks that usually accompany them, it is no mystery why we often refer to a man's paunch as his "beer belly."

On the other hand, on The Carbohydrate Addict's LifeSpan Program, a glass (or two) of wine, beer, liquor, or a mixed drink can be enjoyed without fear of rebound cravings or weight gain. The Basic Plan's Guidelines will help you learn how you can at times indulge, if you choose, without triggering an insulin overresponse, and the Options of the Program can help you keep your insulin levels on track.

Smoking Cessation

Without doubt, giving up smoking may be one of the best things you can do for your health. The very act of stopping smoking (cessation), however, can trigger intense and/or recurring cravings for sweets and other carbohydrate-rich foods as well an increased tendency to gain weight.

At this time, there is no complete understanding as to the changes in metabolism that take place when we start smoking or when we give up smoking, although some researchers are beginning to examine the changes that smokers, as well as those who give up smoking, experience.

When you start to smoke the body appears to respond to this change by releasing insulin as well as "stress" hormones, in the same way that it would respond to any stress or sudden change. As you continue to smoke, muscles and organs appear to become more insulin resistant and, in an attempt to override this resistance, the body may continue to overrelease insulin. When you give up smoking, another increase in insulin release may occur as the body once again experiences a sudden change or "stress."

If, then, insulin levels peak when we first begin to smoke as well as when we quit and they remain high in response to the body's smoking-related insulin resistance, why do we generally experience a decrease in cravings when we begin to smoke and increases in cravings and weight when we quit smoking?

Scientists are not quite sure how to explain these seeming contradictions, but answers are beginning to emerge. It now appears that many smoking-related processes may override insulin-related hunger and weight-gain changes. For instance, the nicotine absorbed with each cigarette temporarily increases the basal metabolic rate and so, for a time, the nicotine inhaled may override insulin's hunger- and fat-making abilities. If you continue to smoke, although these "insulin-countering" processes may be responsible for continuing to help keep your weight low (or at least lower than it might have been), insulin's negative impact may be silently and steadily damaging your health and, perhaps, shortening your life as well.

When you stop smoking, insulin levels jump once again and cravings and weight gain often return with a vengeance, for this time no smoking-related changes can compensate for the body's insulin onslaught. These cravings do not seem to be caused by "psychological factors," nor do they reflect the need for "oral satisfaction," as is common myth, but rather they appear to be a direct response to increases in insulin, the "hunger hormone."

While insulin-related cravings and weight gain may present some temporary challenges to the smoke-ender, the long-term health benefits of giving up smoking are virtually undeniable, and while many of the explanations of the underlying processes are still hypothetical, practitioners and researchers alike have found that there are effective and practical ways to counter the increases in cravings and weight that often go along with smoking cessation.

Elizabeth Bohorquez, R.N., of the Sarasota Hypnosis Institute and Center for Lifestyle Change has found that, among other techniques, a four-week plan that combines the Guidelines of this program along with the Chromium Option used *prior* to smoking cessation helps greatly reduce or eliminate the cravings associated with quitting smoking and may help smoke-enders begin to lose weight in a matter of days. Other researchers and practitioners have reported similar successes and ease as well.

The good news is that The Carbohydrate Addict's LifeSpan Program, both in its Basic Plan and its Options, in particular the Chromium Option, can help reduce the high insulin levels that often come from giving up smoking. As your insulin levels normalize, you will probably be happy to find a great reduction in the cravings and weight problems that you may have experienced when you stopped smoking; at the same time you will help your body to recover from the years of insulin-related damage that may have occurred. If you normalize your insulin levels before you actually stop smoking, you will probably greatly reduce or eliminate carbohydrate cravings and weight gain.

Antinutrients

Many people are aware of the term "empty calories," which applies to those foods that add nothing to a person's nutrition except calories that the body will later turn into fat. We often try to avoid or to limit these foods with the idea that the calories we take in should supply us with the vitamins or minerals we need as well.

Antinutrients actually reduce the vitamin or mineral reserves that we already have in our bodies.

Antinutrients can leave us "worse off" nutrition-wise than before we ate them.

What most people fail to realize, however, is that there are foods that are far worse for us than those with just "empty calories." Foods that act as *antinutrients* actually reduce the vitamin or mineral reserves we already have in our bodies, so that after eating them we not only have failed to add to our nutritional status but we have actually depleted it as well.

That's right. By draining your body's store of vitamins and minerals, these foods can, literally, leave you "worse off" nutrition-wise after you eat them than you would have been if you had not eaten them at all.

If you are carbohydrate addicted, your body may interpret this nutritional depletion as a "stress" and can release insulin which, in turn, can call you to eat more antinutrients. You can easily find yourself in a nutrition-depletion eating cycle that can virtually never be satisfied.

In their comprehensive text, *Understanding Vitamins and Minerals*, the editors of *Prevention* magazine looked at some of the most commonly consumed antinutrients, including, in particular, sugar-sweetened colas. These drinks, they reported, are not simply "empty calories" but, rather, deplete the body of thiamine. Without thiamine (vitamin B_1), the brain and nervous system cannot do their job. Even a slight deficiency of thiamine can lead to depression, poor memory, irritability, lack of initiative, insomnia, and the inability to concentrate.

Some antinutrients can lead to a thiamine deficiency and to a "Dr. Jekyll and Mr. Hyde" personality change.

And sugary colas are most certainly not the only thiamine bandit in your diet. Thiamine is used in the burning of carbohydrates and many researchers would agree with Dr. Derrick Lonsdale, whose practice regularly includes patients with thiamine deficiency. Dr. Lonsdale has found that many of his patients (some only in their teens) exhibit a variety of neurological symptoms, including depression, insomnia, and chronic fatigue, after consuming diets rich in snack foods and simple sugars. Dr. Lonsdale describes a "Dr. Jekyll and Mr. Hyde" personality change in which these patients become "sensitive to criticism, aggressive, or hostile." According to Dr. Lonsdale, symptoms may also include "irritability or acting out."

It is important to understand that thiamine, and all other nutritional supplementation, should be undertaken only under a physician's guidance. We simply want you to understand that many of the foods you eat may be robbing your body of its nutritional stores and that your body's appropriate and protective response may be the extra release of insulin.

In this way, like a man in a lifeboat on the ocean who drinks salty seawater in a attempt to quench his thirst and finds that the water itself makes his condition worse, you may come to realize that the very foods you are eating and the ways in which you are eating them have been making you *less* nourished—and hungrier—with every bite.

**The antinutrients that you are eating
may have been making you *less* nourished
—and hungrier—with every bite.**

Other antinutrients include additives and foods that are strong iron-blockers—interfering with your body's ability to take in this essential mineral. EDTA, a chemical preservative that is often used in commercially processed or canned foods, is a strong iron-blocker. But EDTA is not the only "guilty party." It has been estimated that more than 3,000 chemicals are used in the commercial foods we eat and that, in one way or another, many of them act as antinutrients— robbing our bodies of their storehouses of vitamin and minerals.

Phosphates that are added to ice cream, candy, beer, soft drinks, and baked goods are powerful iron-blockers, and many of our dairy products, while terrific sources of calcium, when consumed in large quantities, or, perhaps, too often, can interfere with our bodies' ability to absorb iron.

Eggs also contain an anti-iron factor and this iron-blocker binds not only with the iron in eggs themselves but with the iron in other foods that may be eaten *with* the eggs—with toast, for instance. A simple cup of tea can do the same thing, for tannic acid is a strong iron-blocker as well. Since iron is essential to the formation of red blood cells, the body's lifeline, the depletion of this precious mineral may be sensed by the body as a powerful stressor, with insulin— once again—being called into action.

**Do not be fooled by food labels that tell you that
foods are "fortified" with iron.
Much of the iron in them cannot be absorbed
and is practically useless.**

By the way, do not be fooled by food labels that tell you that foods are "fortified" with iron. The iron that is added to baked goods, for instance, is usually *ferric* iron—which is not absorbed by your body—instead of *ferrous* iron—which occurs naturally in the foods you eat and *is* absorbed. Chances are, the fortified form of iron you are eating in many "fortified foods" is practically useless.

It is important to understand that antinutrient actions are not confined to foods only. Many of the medications* and over-the-counter remedies we take, including sedatives, antacids, anticonvulsants, corticosteroids, diuretics, stool softeners, anti-inflammatories, cough and cold remedies, drugs to lower blood pressure, for Parkinson's disease, gout, and excess cholesterol as well as oral contraceptives and estrogens can rob us of a whole host of essential vitamins and minerals, including vitamins B_6, B_{12}, C, D, K, folic acid, iron, magnesium, niacin, and potassium. Depletion of these nutrients may, again, be perceived by your body as a "stress" and can, in turn, increase the release of "stress hormones," raising your body's release of insulin, followed by intense or recurring cravings for carbohydrate-rich foods.

Even high levels of noise, experienced by the body as stress, may rob us of our precious stores of magnesium, an essential nutrient for a healthy heart. And the louder the noise, the greater the magnesium depletion and, consequently, the greater the stress on the body.

**Caffeine can increase your carbohydrate cravings.
But you can have your cake—and
coffee—and lose weight, too.**

Caffeine

Caffeine, whether it is found in coffee, tea, colas, or other drinks, can increase your carbohydrate cravings in two different ways. First, acting as an antinutrient, caffeine appears to flush potassium and thiamine as well from your body. Research conducted in Switzerland by Dr. J. C. Somogyi and Dr. U. Nageli, and published

---

Never stop or reduce prescribed or recommended medications or remedies because of concerns regarding your insulin levels, your cravings, or your weight. Your physician must guide you in all these matters. Self-prescribing is clearly not the intent.

in the *International Journal of Vitamin and Nutrition Research*, reported that after consuming a single quart of coffee over a three-hour period, subjects appear to suffer up to a 50 percent loss in their ability to absorb thiamine.

Second, caffeine may lead to increased carbohydrate cravings as part of a less understood process in which caffeine may stimulate the sympathetic nervous system, which, in turn, can lead to increased insulin levels. While little research has yet been able to clarify the process, this increase in insulin may explain why so many of us have an inclination to reach for "something sweet" along with our coffee.

But don't worry! You can choose to continue enjoying caffeine in coffee, tea, cola, and the like if you prefer, or, as an alternative, you may select the Caffeine-Reducing Option as part of "Options for Life" (Chapter 6). In either case, The Carbohydrate Addict's Program's Basic Plan and the Chromium Option can help reduce many of the blood sugar fluctuations that caffeine may trigger and, should you choose, make decreasing your caffeine consumption a great deal easier.

Simple Sugars and the Chromium Drain

The most important antinutrient action, by far, seems to be the draining of the body's reserves of the essential nutrient chromium. Chromium is lost when we eat carbohydrate-rich foods, particularly simple sugars (table sugar, candy, cakes, cookies, soft drinks, fruits and fruit juices, and the like).

The type of chromium that your body requires to help insulin to do its jobs is called *Glucose Tolerance Factor chromium*, or GTF for short. Without enough of this type of chromium, your body will often overproduce insulin—leading you to crave the very foods that robbed it of its chromium stores in the first place. In addition to simple sugars, processed flour can also steal the chromium from your body and the phosphates in milk can bind up the chromium in your food and make it unusable.

**Even "healthy foods" like fruit, juice, and milk
can steal the chromium that
keeps your blood sugar in balance
and helps protect you from heart disease and diabetes.**

The importance of Glucose Tolerance Factor chromium is just beginning to be realized by scientists from around the world who are discovering, as Dr. Rebecca Riales reported in the *American Journal of Clinical Nutrition*, that chromium deficiency may raise insulin levels in the blood, increase the body's resistance to insulin, and add to other undesirable physical changes that can lead to atherosclerosis (that is, the narrowing of blood vessels that can contribute to heart attack or stroke).

Dr. Richard A. Anderson, of the United States Department of Agriculture's Human Nutrition Research Center, estimates that nine out of ten American diets are deficient in chromium. When you add the antinutrient chromium-depletion effect of simple sugars, you come to realize that you could very well be one of the millions of Americans who may, unknowingly, be suffering from a chromium deficiency—and the high insulin responses and cravings and weight gain that may follow.

You will learn how to short-circuit the chromium drain caused by sweets in your diet and reduce your health risks, all at the same time.

The good news is that The Carbohydrate Addict's Basic Plan and its Options for Life, in particular the Chromium Option, will help you get the *right kind of chromium you need for your body* and, in Your Health-Promoting Bonus chapter (Chapter 4), you will learn how Glucose Tolerance Factor chromium has been shown to decrease the risk factors associated with maturity-onset diabetes and cardiovascular disease, which comes from improving your insulin, cholesterol, and triglyceride levels. At the same time, you will learn how to short-circuit the chromium drain caused by the sweets and processed foods in your diet.

Time Bombs

The one thing that most insulin triggers have in common is that if they were avoided, we would be able to escape the cravings and weight gain that they bring with them. Some triggers, however, such as certain medications and quitting smoking, are quite valuable to other aspects of our health; other triggers, such as the foods we love that contain antinutrients, give us a great deal of pleasure. It would be ideal if we did not have to suffer cravings and weight gain in order to enjoy and to benefit from them, and, needless to say, we do not.

**Time bombs are inevitable but
we do *not* have to be their unwilling victims.**

In contrast to triggers, however, time bombs are inevitable. We cannot escape growing older, illness, menopause, and the like. We can, however, reduce the effects of these biological changes so that we are no longer the unwilling victims of their impact.

Aging

Each passing decade brings about changes in insulin levels and the way the body uses insulin. Many researchers, including Dr. S. Del Prato in his scientific report *Hyperinsulinemia: Causes and Mechanisms*, have concluded that, as part of the natural aging process, our bodies appear to grow more insulin resistant, keeping more insulin in the bloodstream or, as others observe, channeling food energy to the fat cells. Though scientists are not certain as to why these processes occur, some have speculated that in prehistoric times of feast and famine, channeling food energy to the fat cells may have meant the difference between life and death for those in their later years (which, at that time, may have meant those approaching forty). By closing down some of the passageways by which food energy entered the muscles and organs, blood sugar was channeled into the fat cells, for storage, until it was needed for survival during times of famine. Excess insulin in the blood helps keep the drive for food high as well.

Today, when hunger rears its ugly head, forty-, fifty-, sixty-, and seventy-year-olds need look no further than the nearest refrigerator for a quick snack or an easy meal; and so this same fat-making tendency has turned against us, making us overweight and unhealthy.

In addition to these physical changes, as they grow older, many people tend to eat smaller meals that are more carbohydrate-rich—and they tend to eat them more frequently as well. We may choose sandwiches in place of the large plates of food of our youth. We may prefer several light "snacks" throughout the day and, unfortunately, throughout the evening as well.

We may think that we are eating the same as we did in our younger days and wonder why we are gaining weight. In some cases we are, in fact, eating the same but because of higher insulin levels, the food we eat, particularly the carbohydrates, are being more readily transformed into fat. Some of us, on the other hand, are not eating any more food, but we are eating more carbohydrate-rich foods and we may be eating them more often. This practice helps raise insulin levels even higher, stimulating cravings and weight gain. And some of us are simply eating more and know it, though we find ourselves unable to stop. Again, the cravings and weight gain are a simple result of increased levels of the "hunger hormone" insulin.

Getting older no longer has to mean gaining weight.

In all cases, The Carbohydrate Addict's LifeSpan Program will help you correct the cause of what you may have labeled a "slower metabolism" so that getting older no longer has to mean gaining weight.

The Dwindling Chromium Bankbook

As we get older, our bodies seem to have an increased need for the nutrient chromium. Unfortunately, at this same time of life, our chromium reserves seem to be at their lowest. Like a bank account that is dwindling just when we need the money the most, our bodies most require the help of chromium as we grow older—when we have the least.

Remember that Glucose Tolerance Factor chromium is essential in helping insulin to do its jobs and that without enough chromium the body compensates by releasing extra insulin. The excess insulin, in turn, can increase your carbohydrate cravings and your tendency to gain weight. Often the very food that you crave will further decrease your chromium stores, continuing the low chromium–high insulin release–low chromium merry-go-round. This entire cycle seems to go faster and become stronger with each added decade.

But the increased need for chromium that comes with aging is one of the easiest time bombs to diffuse, and The Chromium Option that you find in Options for Life (Chapter 6) will guide you in choosing the correct amount and the right kind of chromium so that your body can stay rich in that essential nutrient—for life.

Inactivity

For some people, activity reduces insulin levels and, as would be expected, when they are inactive, their insulin levels (and their weight) go up. For carbohydrate addicts in particular, however, the latter seems to be most true, for while some carbohydrate addicts find that activity reduces their cravings and helps them to lose weight, others find that this is simply not the case. Some carbohydrate addicts report that exercise itself seems to stimulate their hunger.

While some carbohydrate addicts find that activity reduces their cravings and helps them to lose weight, others find that this is simply not the case.

Different reactions to activity is not as strange as it seems and appears to be related to differences in blood sugar levels and how well the body uses the insulin (and the sugar) in the blood—that is, how insulin resistant you are. But no matter how your particular body responds to activity, many carbohydrate addicts seem to agree that inactivity makes them crave carbohydrates more and most certainly puts weight on more easily.

Some people assume that if you have a greater tendency to gain weight when inactive, it comes from burning fewer calories. This does not appear to be the case. Calorie-burning represents just a small piece of the puzzle. Only about one-fifth of the calories we burn comes from "activity-related metabolism"; the remaining calories are burned during "resting metabolism." Resting metabolism, the other four-fifths of the calories you burn, may be directly related to your insulin levels, and when you are inactive, your insulin levels go up, putting you in a carbo-craving and fat-making mode. When you are inactive, you gain weight not simply because you are burning fewer calories but often because your insulin levels may be high as well.

The insulin connection to inactivity is very important, for when you cannot be active, due to an injury, illness, age, or other physical limitations or because of time constraints, The Carbohydrate Addict's LifeSpan Program can help keep your insulin levels—and consequently your cravings and your weight—under control.

When you are inactive, you gain weight *not* simply because you are burning fewer calories but mostly because your insulin levels may be high as well.

Being inactive does not have to mean being overweight.

Illness and Surgery

Illness and surgery create stresses on the body that many of us have been taught to ignore. Our bodies, however, do respond to these stresses and they often release high levels of insulin in response to signals from "stress hormones."

These hormones may have served an important purpose in prehistoric times when being ill meant that you were not able to go hunting. Putting food energy away in the form of fat may have, at that time, been the key to survival. Today, although illness no longer means being deprived of food, the body continues to hoard.

The Carbohydrate Addict's Basic Plan and its Options for Life can help you to reduce the triggering effects of illness or surgery that can lead to carbohydrate cravings and weight gain. As always, check with your physician and be guided by his/her recommendations.

Please note: If you are planning surgery, you may want to discuss choices that may minimize or avoid insulin responses, such as alternative choices in medications or the timing of over-the-counter remedies.* As in all things, what is best for your immediate well-being must take priority over weight concerns, but when a choice can be made, talk to your doctor about options that will not cause increased insulin release.

Seasonal Changes

If the coming of fall or winter seems to bring about changes in your emotions (sadness, feelings of loss, depression, even feelings of dread), you may be suffering from seasonal affective disorder (SAD), a physical imbalance that appears to be related to the shortening period of daylight that occurs as winter approaches.

Many of those who suffer from seasonal affective disorder tell us that, like animals anticipating hibernation, the coming winter seems to signal them to take in more carbohydrate-rich food. Even when they manage to keep their carbohydrate cravings under control, they say that their bodies just seem to store more fat in the winter.

Their perceptions are, in fact, right on target. For those with a genetic predisposition to a sensitivity to seasonal changes, the shortening daylight appears to trigger their body to go into a "conservation mode," driving them to take in more and more carbohydrate-rich foods and then quickly turning that incoming food into fat (for storage in the fat cells). For those with seasonal affective disorder, each coming winter is a time bomb, waiting to set off their cravings and their weight gain.

Not surprisingly, preliminary research ties seasonal affective disorder to an excess of insulin, and it has been our experience as well that since The Carbohydrate Addict's LifeSpan Program helps to reduce insulin levels, fall- and winter-related cravings and weight gain are often substantially reduced or, in many cases, eliminated. These effects have been so convincing that in his most recent book the researcher who first discovered SAD discusses the Guidelines of the Program as having special advantages for SAD-related carbohydrate cravings and weight gain.

---

*Never stop or reduce prescribed or recommended medications or remedies because of concerns regarding your insulin levels, your cravings, or your weight. Your physician must guide you in all of these matters. Self-prescribing is clearly not the intent. For suggestions on changing the insulin impact of many over-the-counter remedies, see "Options for Life" (Chapter 6).

So if the coming of winter has often meant the coming of weight, you may be happy to find that your seasonally related time bomb may automatically be "defused" as you continue to follow the Program.

Menopause and Past Pregnancies

Immediately before, during, and after menopause women experience many symptoms related to high insulin and/or low blood sugar levels. Many scientists, including Dr. Anthony J. Proudler of the Wynn Institute for Metabolic Research of London, U.K., have found that increased levels of insulin appear to be directly related to menopause and, as Dr. Proudler adds, "The hyperinsulinemia observed may contribute to the increased risk of cardiovascular disease seen in postmenopausal women." You will learn more about reducing your insulin-related health risks in Chapter 4, Your Health-Promoting Bonus, but for now it is important to understand that if you are a woman with a predisposition to high insulin levels, menopause may be a time bomb—literally waiting to go off—but, happily, one which we can help you to disarm.

Much of the tiredness, irritability, and anxiety that women think they should come to accept as they hit the "change of life" may actually be the result of insulin's powerful effect on their blood sugar.

Although pregnancy could be categorized as either a trigger or time bomb, we have included it in this section because it can cause the cravings and weight gain similar to those that accompany menopause. The hormonal changes may differ, the body's "reasons" may vary as well, but in both instances the insulin response is the same and the resulting hunger, weight gain, and feelings of dismay at watching the pounds mount are strikingly similar.

**The tendency to gain weight from both pregnancy and menopause are
often the result of *physical* changes, hormonal shifts,
that are neither your doing nor your fault.**

The tendency to gain weight from both pregnancy* and menopause are often the result of *physical* changes, hormonal shifts, that are neither your doing nor your fault. Some women who have gained a great deal of weight while pregnant or who were unable to take off (and keep off) their pregnancy-related weight find that menopause seems to repeat the process. With the first signs of menopause, or even before, many women find that their bodies seem to fight their attempts to maintain an acceptable (or even near-acceptable) weight level. Others tell us, with relief, that though they feared they might see the process repeat, menopause did not trigger the same fat-storing cycle they experienced when they were younger and pregnant. There does not seem to be any way to predict how menopause may affect your body's metabolic balance. Each of us is different; that's just the way it is.

The good news is, however, that if you are carbohydrate addicted and menopause triggers an increase in your hunger, cravings, weight, or low-blood-sugar–related tiredness or distress, this program can help stabilize your blood sugar levels and relieve much of the emotional discomfort, cravings, and weight gain so often associated with the prolonged period of time we call "menopause."

Even more important, as you will find in the Health-Promoting Bonus chapter that follows, in addition to its psychological and weight-loss benefits, this program can help you to lower your risk for many of the health problems that may follow menopause.

A Personal Note

If you are carbohydrate addicted, it is essential that you fully recognize that you are not to blame. You did not choose your family and your genetics and chances are that you have suffered more than your fair share for having inherited the right body in the wrong time.

*Although some of you who are reading this book may be past your child-bearing years, if you are not and if you are indeed pregnant or nursing, you should not be on this or any other weight-loss program other than one that your physician recommends and monitors. If, however, you are no longer pregnant or nursing, chances are, with your physician's okay, you will find that this program is ideal for losing the weight that was gained during past pregnancies.

But we have discovered a way out. Although you cannot change the fact that you may have inherited a body that sits poised—like a loaded gun ready to fire—you can keep the trigger from ever being pulled again and help to contain all of the time bombs that might otherwise be waiting.

CHAPTER 4

YOUR HEALTH-PROMOTING BONUS

Within the cause, lies the cure.

—Cicero, circa 70 B.C.

*I*magine, for a moment, that you are the parent of a child who has a fever. You are aware that the child has been exposed to a classmate who has chicken pox, and so as the fever rises, you look for the telltale skin eruptions that will confirm your diagnosis. As the eruptions begin to emerge, you may relax a bit, assured that the fever was simply the first sign that your child was indeed getting chicken pox.

Your logical approach to the fever comes, in part, from being aware that a virus caused both the rise in your child's temperature and the skin eruptions that followed.

But let us suppose for a moment that you lived hundreds of years ago. At that time, the cause of chicken pox was still a mystery. No one had ever heard of viruses or germs or the like and the mere thought that "invisible things" could cause disease was considered laughable at best and madness at worst.

People at that time were, however, aware that fever sometimes gave way to these eruptions and mothers were advised to wash their children in a variety of bathing solutions to rid their children's bodies of the fever. It was assumed, at the time, that the fever caused the eruptions and, consequently, if you rid the body of the fever, you could avoid the chicken pox itself.

Today, we are fully aware that fever is often a first sign that an infection has set in and that trying to "wash away" a fever will do nothing to change the course of the disease. We know this because we have come to recognize that viruses and germs are the "cause" of many infections and we understand that fever may be the earliest symptom to emerge; it is not in itself the cause of the disease.

On the other hand, even today, the causes of heart disease, high blood pressure, adult-onset diabetes, and the like have *not* yet been pinpointed, and while there may be many health risk factors that are known to coexist or to precede these diseases, that does not mean that these risk factors *cause* these diseases.

The health risk factor we call "overweight" appears to be *the first sign* that there is an emerging physical problem rather than the cause of the problem itself.

In particular, the health risk factor we call "overweight" appears, like fever, to be *the first sign* that there is an emerging physical problem rather than the cause of the problem itself.

Let us imagine that you have begun to put on some weight. You may find that you are eating a bit more, or more often, or that you crave more snack foods or sweets than you had in the past. You might not be eating any differently at all, but nevertheless you may find that you are putting on weight, pound after pound. Your doctor cautions you to lose weight, explaining that being overweight could "lead to high blood pressure" and, sure enough, after you have gained twenty or thirty pounds, your physician informs you that you do indeed have high blood pressure.

You accept the decree that you "caused" the high blood pressure by being overweight and, perhaps, you never question what caused the weight gain itself. Later on, if you develop undesirable blood-fat levels, gout, adult-onset diabetes, or even heart problems you may blame yourself even more for your "inability" to control your eating and/or your weight.

The assumption that the first of a sequence of symptoms (in this case weight gain) is the cause of other symptoms that follow (high blood pressure, for example) is what we call the "illusion of sequence." The illusion lies in the assumption that the first symptom of a physical problem is the cause of the other symptoms that follow.

If, like chicken pox, we could point to some physical problem or imbalance that was known to cause increased hunger, weight gain, *and* high blood pressure, we might more easily recognize that the weight gain did not cause the high blood pressure but, rather, that both the weight gain and the high blood pressure came from the same silent cause.

Literally hundreds of scientists are now reporting that an excess in insulin has been linked to nine of this country's top killer diseases and health risk factors.

In fact, literally hundreds of scientists are now reporting that an excess in insulin has been linked to high blood pressure, undesirable blood-fat levels and atherosclerosis, heart disease, stroke, adult-onset diabetes, gout, some forms of cancer, and more.

The power of excess insulin (also called *chronic hyperinsulinemia*) to help generate disease has led to its being given the name Profactor-H, meaning that it is the first factor, that is the underlying cause, in many of these diseases and disorders.

When an excess of insulin becomes the first factor, the underlying cause of weight gain, high blood pressure, undesirable blood-fat levels, heart disease, or adult-onset diabetes, it earns the name Profactor-H.

Exposing the Food Fat and Fiber Fallacy

About seventy-five years ago, in smaller cities and towns, it was an accepted truth that looking at a monkey when one was pregnant would result in giving birth to a child resembling the hairy primate. This kind of thinking is called "representative thinking"; it is a low-level logic that is often wrong and based on fears combined with the simple resemblance of things. It has little to do with the way things, or bodies, really work.

This kind of thinking is called "superstitious" when it is confined to a small group of the population or to those people we paternalistically call "primitive." When, however, this thinking is endorsed by our "wise men," that is, by our physicians, medical associations, and the media, it carries a strong and compelling message that is difficult to dispute—even when facts are on our side.

Scores of scientific studies, such as Dr. R. W. Stout's twenty-year review of the research, Dr. N. W. Flodin's report in the *Journal of the American College of Nutrition*, and Drs. Coulston, G. C. Liu, and G. M. Reaven's investigation into the relationship of diet to blood sugar, blood fat, and insulin, all overwhelmingly point to the key role that carbohydrate-rich diets and high insulin levels can play in raising your blood-fat levels. And, although major studies report that low-fat diets are failing to help most of us reduce our blood-fat levels, the media continues to act as if low fat is the answer.

**Big business appears to play a major role
in the low-fat cure-all push.**

Certainly, big business appears to play a major role in the low-fat cure-all push. Food manufacturers have found big sales in "healthy foods" that are full of artificial, and often cheaper, ingredients, and which offer poor taste but big promise. In addition to the considerable financial gain, the history of this newest of "crazes" may come from a simple misunderstanding.

> **The original research showed that diets that were low fat and *high fiber* reduced blood-fat levels— but high fiber may have been much harder to sell.**

The original research showed that reduced blood-fat levels came from diets which combined *high fiber* with low fat. Food manufacturers tried to sell high fiber to the public but were not too successful (remember the oat bran sell?). Low-fat foods were easier to sell than high fiber and, not so coincidentally, the essential high-fiber findings of the research results were dropped. Big sales followed, and although research report after research report has shown that low-fat diets *without high fiber* do not reduce blood fats and increase longevity, the media has almost totally failed to pass this information on to the public.

Indeed, in the back of this book, you will find among the reference list of research studies, many from the finest scientific and medical journals in the world, reports that conclude that not only do low-fat diets often fail to reduce blood-fat levels but that, for many people, the added carbohydrates in these diets strongly increase blood-fat levels and other risk factors as well.

The most prevalent form of undesirable blood-fat levels, by far, is called "Type IV" high blood-fat levels. This type of blood-fat problem has so strongly been shown to be related to dietary carbohydrates rather than to dietary fat that it has won the name "carbohydrate-induced" high blood-fat levels. And, even though it affects a far greater number of people than any other blood-fat problem, the American public is being duped into thinking that "food does not make fat, fat makes fat"; an out-and-out untruth. And so, many Americans are eating less and less fat and getting fatter and unhealthier by the day.

So how do we deal with all this conflicting information and who do we believe? We will tell you what has literally saved our own lives. Listen to your own body. If you are one of the millions of people in this country who are carbohydrate addicted, look at what happens when you eat so-called low-fat food (that, by the way, may be full of added sugar). Are your blood fats going down? Are you able to stay on your low-fat diet or are the sugars that have been added to so many of these "low-fat" foods stimulating you to eat more and to gain weight more easily?

Certainly, we urge you to talk this over with your personal physician. Take this book with you; show him or her the references in the back of the book.

> **One size, absolutely, positively, does *not* fit all.**

Remember, as in all things, one size does *not* fit all. If you are carbohydrate addicted, a low-fat, high-carbohydrate diet may be all wrong for you; as time goes by it may, literally, be increasing the very health risks that you have been trying so hard to eliminate.

> **If your physician prefers you to follow a low-fat diet,
> you will find special suggestions on page 214
> that will help you reduce your fat intake, your cravings,
> your weight, and health risk—all at the same time.**

While The Carbohydrate Addict's LifeSpan Program will help you reduce your risk for high levels of insulin and the blood-fat levels that often go along with it, if you and your doctor agree that a low-fat diet is preferable, you will find suggestions for decreasing your dietary fat *without* increasing your cravings, weight, or the health-risk rebound that most low-fat, high-carbohydrate diets can cause. For low-fat alternatives on The LifeSpan Program, see page 214.

Toppling Your High Blood Pressure Risks

Today, as many as 56 million people have been told that they have high blood pressure, or as it is technically named, *hypertension*, yet except for taking some medication and "kind of" watching their salt intake, people with high blood pressure pretty much get used to the idea that they have something that they have been told can be dangerous at "some future time." But that "future time" comes on without warning and too many come face to face with a heart attack or stroke when it is simply too late to do anything about it.

You, on the other hand, are about to learn what very few of those 58 million people know, or will learn for another twenty years, and the information could very well save your life. That vague disorder we call "high blood pressure" can be a pivotal, critical sign that your body is being flooded with high levels of insulin.

> **High blood pressure may be a vitally important, undeniable sign that abnormally high levels of insulin are silently damaging your body.**

In, and of itself, high blood pressure may or may not indicate that a silent insulin imbalance is making itself known but if you have high blood pressure in combination with recurring carbohydrate cravings, weight gain, *or* undesirable blood-fat levels, we have found it to be a vitally important second symptom—the second and often undeniable sign that a potentially health-endangering insulin imbalance is progressing in your body. It cannot be considered "just" high blood pressure; it is your body's cry for help and you must respond.

The most common form of high blood pressure has no clear or certain cause. Its medical name is *essential hypertension* and, if you have high blood pressure, the chances are 9 to 1 that you have essential hypertension. That means that, until now, most physicians were unable to pinpoint the *cause* of your high blood pressure. Your doctor might have told you to lose weight or to cut down on salt in your diet but these recommendations are not necessarily aimed at correcting the cause of the problem; rather, they may be simple attempts to reduce the symptoms.* And unless you remove the cause, you may be fighting the problem for the rest of your life.

Taken by themselves, excess weight and dietary salt intake may not be the *causes* of the high blood pressure. As we all know, many people who have perfectly normal blood pressure levels are overweight and/or consume great amounts of salt, and trying to control

Never stop or change your physician's recommendations because of concerns regarding your insulin levels, your cravings, or your weight. Work with your physician in all of these matters. Self-prescription is clearly not the intent of this text.

high blood pressure with low-salt or weight-loss diets may be likened to treating a fever with Tylenol; the medication may reduce the symptom for a while, but without correcting the cause of the underlying problem, the symptom is sure to return.

Today, scientists from around the world including, among so many others, Dr. E. Feraille and his colleagues from the College de France in Paris, Dr. A. M. Sharma and his colleagues from the Free University of Berlin, as well as Dr. K. Landin reporting in the *Journal of Internal Medicine*, and others are making astounding breakthroughs into the cause of high blood pressure. Once again the research reveals that the invisible villain appears to be excess levels of insulin, the result of both insulin overproduction as well as insulin resistance.

Excess levels of insulin can to lead to high blood pressure in three different and powerful ways.

Excess levels of insulin appear to lead to high blood pressure in three different ways. First, excess insulin can stimulate the sympathetic nervous system, which in turn can make your heart beat faster, blood vessels narrow, and blood pressure levels rise. If you have a family history of high blood pressure, high insulin levels could be causing a rise in your blood pressure in this way.

Second, insulin helps to regulate salt levels in the blood. The higher your insulin levels, the more salt is retained and the more water remains in your bloodstream. No matter how careful you are with your salt intake you may find that excess levels of insulin overpower all of your efforts. Since the salt helps retain fluid, more fluid flows through your arteries. More fluid through the same space causes greater pressure or, in this case, high blood pressure.

The third way in which high insulin levels can lead to high blood pressure is by narrowing the arteries through which your blood flows. Insulin has been shown to stimulate the production of cholesterol and the buildup of plaque in walls of arteries (you'll learn more about this in the "Healthy Hearts" section that follows). As the space for blood flow is decreased by the narrowing of arteries, blood pressure naturally rises.

The potent impact of insulin in action has led scientists to recognize that high blood pressure no longer appears to be an end state, not a physical disorder that stands by itself, but rather a *symptom*—a very important symptom—of a powerful underlying insulin imbalance. Not a problem to be simply controlled but rather one that—by correcting the underlying cause—can finally be eliminated.

Getting the Gout Out

Gout is a metabolic disease in which uric acid levels in the blood increase and form crystals in joint tissues, which leads to severe inflammation and the pain and swelling so frequently experienced by those with gout.

Until recently, the cause of gout was unknown. While many overweight people were known to suffer from gout, the underlying connection between gout and excess weight remained unclear. With the exception of increased consumption of beer by some, diet has not appeared to play a vital role in this disease, and although standard treatment has historically included the dietary restriction of foods high in purine content, such as anchovies, sardines, liver, kidney, and others, some researchers have concluded that dietary restriction is often not necessary (after, perhaps, finding that it did little good).

Exciting new research, however, is revealing important information about the cause of gout, and these revelations appear to explain both the obesity-gout connection as well as alcohol's role in this disorder.

Remember, for a moment, that excess levels of insulin (that come from either the overrelease of this hormone or from insulin resistance, or both) can lead to increased carbohydrate cravings and weight gain. And the findings of researchers such as Dr. F. Facchini and his colleagues, reporting in the *Journal of the American Medical Association*, who have found that insulin resistance leads to increased uric acid concentrations—the more insulin resistant, the more uric acid—or the work of other scientists, like Dr. C. H. Tseng and Dr. T. Y. Tai, who found in their three-year follow-up study that raised insulin levels themselves were linked to higher uric acid levels, and you begin to see that the same underlying insulin imbalance appears to be gout's common cause. No wonder overweight people are more likely to get gout; the same hormonal imbalance that can cause one can cause the other.

> **Until recently, the cause of gout was unknown but the latest scientific research shows a surprisingly strong insulin connection.**

Other scientists have clarified the role of diet in the development and advancement of gout. Not surprisingly, high-carbohydrate foods, like fruit or foods that are metabolized along carbohydrate-like pathways, like beer and other alcoholic beverages, have been shown to bring on gout attacks. These findings give even further support of insulin's role in this disease.

While reduction of high purine food is often said to be "wise," you may find that, with your doctor's guidance, this dietary restriction may no longer be necessary. Only 15 percent of uric acid comes from dietary sources, and trying to reduce uric acid by reducing the amount of end products of purine-rich foods may be an attempt to control the symptom rather than correct the cause.

As always, we urge you to work with your doctor. On The LifeSpan Program we believe you will discover a clear and significant decrease in your risk for gout and, should you already have this disorder, a welcome reduction of its impact on your body.

Beating Your Blood Sugar Blues: Hypoglycemia and Diabetes

Most of the things you do each day, you do without thinking. You walk to the bathroom, shower, eat breakfast, dress—and never consider the amount of judgment and coordination involved. You put yourself "on automatic" and trust your body to handle the tasks at hand.

In the same way, the regulation of many of your vital life functions, including regulation of your blood sugar levels, can usually be trusted to your body's unconscious control—that is, until something goes wrong.

When all goes well, as you begin to eat, your body releases insulin into your bloodstream in anticipation of the coming food energy. As some of the food energy is turned into a simple sugar (*glucose*) and released into the blood, the waiting insulin helps move the blood sugar to different parts of the body where it is used or stored away. Insulin "opens the doors" to these cells so that the blood sugar can enter freely. Insulin then signals the liver to store away any extra blood sugar for future use; the major portion is turned first into blood fat, then stored as fat in the fat cells.

Later, as blood sugar levels are slowly depleted, the stored energy (in the form of fats) can be used to fuel your body.

If too much insulin is present, however, this excellent balance can be put in jeopardy.

If you are carbohydrate addicted, after eating, your body releases too much insulin into your bloodstream. This excess of insulin can, in the early stages, sweep too much blood sugar out of the bloodstream, signaling your liver to turn it into fat and, most important, leaving you with too little blood sugar to supply your brain and other organs with the energy they need.

This condition is called *reactive hypoglycemia*, and it often occurs about two hours after eating. Your body "reacts" to the carbohydrate-rich foods that you have eaten by releasing too much insulin, which, in turn, helps sweep the energy out of your bloodstream, to be converted for storage in the liver and fat cells. Although you may have eaten only about two hours earlier, your blood sugar levels drop (reactive hypoglycemia).*

The more often they ate, the more their blood sugars fell and the hungrier, weaker, and less motivated they became.

In our research presented at the Annual Meeting of the American Institute of Nutrition, we reported findings that some carbohydrate addicts had such strong reactive hypoglycemic responses to carbohydrates that two hours after eating their blood sugar levels

---

*Fasting hypoglycemia (as opposed to reactive hypoglycemia) is an entirely different condition, stemming from an insufficient intake of energy that occurs when nourishment is absent for a prolonged period of time.

were almost half of what they had been after having fasted for ten hours.

We documented that, for these individuals, the more often they ate, the more their blood sugars fell until these levels "bottomed out." As these carbohydrate addicts' blood sugar levels rose then fell, they became hungrier, weaker, and less motivated—eating actually made some of them feel less "well" then they felt after fasting!

When these same people learned to balance the ways in which they ate carbohydrate-rich food using the Basic Plan and Options of The Carbohydrate Addict's LifeSpan Program, however, they found that they could eat the same carbohydrate-rich foods without the low blood sugar or the headaches, weakness, shakiness, irritability, loss of motivation, or hunger they had lived with for so long.

Low blood sugar is, unfortunately, often only the first stage of a progressive blood sugar imbalance, for as time goes by the fat cells begin to "resist" or to shut down to the onslaught of insulin. The organs and muscles remain "insulin resistant" as well and now, rather than blood sugar being swept out of the bloodstream too quickly, along with the insulin, it is "trapped" in the bloodstream; a condition known as adult-onset diabetes.*

Although statistics on diabetes are staggering (the incidence of adult-onset diabetes has increased by between 600 and 1,000 percent in the last sixty years; and every year diabetes claims 6 percent more people than the year before), statistics about reactive hypoglycemia are almost impossible to obtain. The American Diabetes Association and the Endocrine Society have issued a joint statement to the effect that hypoglycemia is probably often overdiagnosed and, following in their footsteps, some reports are calling the very existence of hypoglycemia into question.

Apparently, because some studies found that a small percentage of subjects had no hypoglycemic symptoms although they exhibited clinically low blood sugar levels, those who do experience low blood sugar symptoms are being told that the burden of proving their disorder has literally been placed on their shoulders.

*Juvenile diabetes, which usually affects the young, is an entirely different disease, stemming from the body's inability to produce insulin. In juvenile-onset diabetes the body does not produce enough insulin to remove glucose from the blood and take it to cells. In adult-onset diabetes, glucose becomes trapped in the bloodstream and cells do not get the nourishment they need to function normally.

> **The proof of a diagnosis of hypoglycemia has now been placed on the patient.**

Now, extremely low levels of blood sugar are no longer enough to qualify the problem as an "official" diagnosis of hypoglycemia. According to new standards, even though your blood sugar levels may drop rapidly and drastically, in order to be given an official diagnosis of hypoglycemia, laboratory technicians (during a five-hour blood testing procedure) must verify that your blood sugar levels drop to about half normal fasting levels *at exactly the same time* that you report experiencing the typical symptoms of low blood sugar (sweating, fatigue, headache, irritability, etc.).

The absurdity of placing the demand of proof on the patient can be likened to telling someone that they do not have high blood pressure unless they experience it at the same time as their physician notes that it is twice normal. Given the complex and demanding requirements for a diagnosis of hypoglycemia, it is no wonder that meaningful statistics on how many of us have hypoglycemia, and pinpointing those who regularly suffer from this disorder, are essentially unobtainable. No wonder that effective help for the hypoglycemic has been very hard if not sometimes almost impossible to find.

Signs of Reactive Hypoglycemia

An "official" diagnosis of insulin-related reactive hypoglycemia can call for a five-hour laboratory sampling of blood, but here are some simple signs to help you see if you may have this blood sugar imbalance.

Within approximately two hours after eating a full meal:

Do you feel weak?
Do you feel uncoordinated or somewhat confused?
Do you perspire without reason?
Do you get hungry or experience strong cravings?
Does eating make you feel better immediately and do you eat
   rapidly or consume great amounts of food?

Does your heart beat rapidly or start to pound?

Do you feel anxious; fearful without reason?

Do you feel irritable?

Do you feel restless or uneasy?

Do you lose energy, feel very tired, fatigued; lose motivation?

Do you get a headache?

Do you feel faint?

Do you feel drowsy?

Do you have a strange sense of altered awareness, almost a feeling of observing your own behavior?

If you sometimes have one or more of these signs after eating, the chances are you may have insulin-related reactive hypoglycemia.

While some carbohydrate addicts remain hypoglycemic all of their lives, never progressing to become diabetic, many scientists and physicians, from Dr. M. C. Linder in her medical textbook *Nutritional Biochemistry and Metabolism* to Dr. C. E. Koop, the former Surgeon General of the United States, in his *Report on Nutrition and Health* published by the U.S. Department of Health and Human Services, have reported that hypoglycemia may be only the first step in a far more serious sequence of medical problems that progress with each passing year, including adult-onset diabetes.

Many people think, mistakenly, that adult-onset diabetes is due to a *lack* of insulin. In the earlier stages of adult-onset diabetes, however, too much insulin is usually the problem. Muscles and organs resist "insulin insults" by "closing down"—not allowing the insulin, and the blood sugar it accompanies, into their cells. At first, the excess blood sugar (that is caught with the insulin in the bloodstream) is turned into blood fat and then stored preferentially in the fat cells. Early diabetics may notice fatigue as well as increased carbohydrate cravings along with a very easy weight gain at this point.

Later, as the diabetes progresses, the body tries to overcome the muscles' and organs' resistance by releasing extra insulin. Now, even the fat cells become resistant, and both the blood sugar and the insulin can remain "trapped" in the bloodstream. At this point, diabetics may notice an unexplained weight loss (the fat cells have closed down to the incoming energy), extreme lack of energy, and/or intense feelings of weakness or disorientation after eating. Over time, the pancreas can become "exhausted" in its fight to release more insulin and, although an excess of insulin had been the initial problem, the body is no longer able to produce enough of this vital hormone.

**The Carbohydrate Addict's LifeSpan Program
has been used with
great success to correct both hypoglycemia
and adult-onset diabetes
—without sacrifice.**

The Carbohydrate Addict's LifeSpan Program's Basic Plan, in particular in combination with the Chromium Option, has been used with success by adult-onset diabetics (with their physician's monitoring), especially in the disorder's early stages, because the Program appears to reduce both the excess levels of insulin as well as the resulting insulin resistance.

Because this program can quickly reduce your insulin levels and your body's resistance to insulin, however, it is important to note that for diabetics the need for oral and injectable medications may rapidly and drastically be reduced or eliminated; therefore if you are taking oral or injectable medications for the treatment of adult-onset diabetes, you must be closely monitored by your physician.

Healthy Hearts: Straight Talk

Too many people throw around too many terms, too easily, and when it comes to health, we need to set a few things straight. The heart is a muscle about the size of your fist and, like all muscles, it needs a steady flow of blood to stay healthy. Blood provides it with both nourishment and oxygen.

There are at least two different diseases that can be called "heart disease." The first is coronary *artery* disease, which involves damage to the arteries that lead out of the chambers of the heart and that feed the muscle of the wall of the heart. The second disorder is coronary *heart* disease, which involves damage to the heart muscle, itself.

Coronary artery disease is a term that is given to several different conditions that can narrow the coronary arteries and in so doing decrease or prevent the flow of blood to the heart muscle. When these arteries narrow from vessel injury and repair or from the accumulation of cholesterol and other fats (helping to form plaque), a person can be said to have *atherosclerosis* or *atherosclerotic changes.*

If the coronary arteries narrow enough from atherosclerosis, a blood clot has a greater chance to completely block the blood flow to the heart. Without the nourishment and oxygen that the blood provides, the heart (the muscle itself) may suffer permanent damage, that is, coronary artery disease.

A more generalized disorder, *cardiovascular disease*, involves the narrowing of the blood vessels throughout the body that feed the heart or provide it with oxygen. A blockage in one of these vessels can starve the heart of its needed blood supply or affect the brain (stroke).

Although other, healthier parts of the heart may help take over, once a heart is damaged the injury cannot be undone. Coronary artery disease and cardiovascular disease, however, may be preventable and in many cases may prove to be reversible as well.

Although the concept of insulin sensitivity and insulin resistance was first introduced into the medical literature over fifty years ago, as Dr. D. C. Simonson of Harvard's School of Medicine has noted, only during the past decade have the causes and the consequences of this imbalance begun to be clarified, especially in relation to the part they play in heart disease.

Today, research by some of the finest scientists and physicians from around the world (including Dr. H. Beck-Nielsen, Chief Physician of Odense University Hospital, Denmark; Dr. R. W. Stout of The Queens University of Belfast, Northern Ireland; Dr. S. Del Prato of the University of Padova, Italy; Dr. H. Lithell of Uppsala University, Sweden; and Dr. A. C. Grimaldi of the Service de Diabetologie of the Pitie-Salpetriere of Paris; as well as some of this country's most renowned researchers, including Dr. A. Garg and his associates of the Southwestern Medical Center in Dallas and Dr. R. A. De-Fronzo and Dr. E. Ferrannini of the Health Science Center of the

University of Texas) continue to confirm, validate, and verify the link between heart disease (and its risk factors) and excess insulin production and insulin resistance.

**Research from around the world continues to confirm the link between heart disease and excess insulin levels.
Reducing your insulin levels appears to be a most vital key to maintaining a strong and a healthy heart.**

While each person is different and the research continues to be compiled even as you read this page, scientist after scientist confirms the same message: reducing your insulin levels and insulin sensitivity appears to be a most vital key to maintaining a strong and a healthy heart.

The LifeSpan Program's Basic Plan and its Options have been designed with one goal in mind: to offer you a simple, rewarding, effective lifestyle plan that will help you normalize your insulin levels and reduce your insulin sensitivity—for life.

Cutting Cancer's Lifeline

There are several diseases that may be more destructive than cancer but none that seems to be more feared. That observation is not original (it was first voiced by Dr. Charles Mayo), but it undoubtedly echoes both our professional experience as well as our personal sentiment.

The truth is, nothing can guarantee that we will never get cancer, but there is a great deal that is known about how cancer grows and thrives and what can be done to help cut cancer's nutritional lifeline.

While there is great debate as to what "causes" cancer, there are probably as many "causes" as there are types of cancer. One day you read a report that says that high-fat diets increase your chance for breast cancer. The next day, another scientist, studying thousands of nurses over many years, finds that there appears to be no connection between high-fat diets and the incidence of breast cancer.

What's the answer? While the research continues, one truth

seems to be emerging: different people appear to respond to different carcinogens (cancer-causing agents) in different ways. For some, high fat may be the problem; for some, it may be sugar; for others it may be both—or something else altogether.

> **It is essential to learn how *your* body responds to foods, additives, and environmental influences that impact on *your* chances of developing cancer.**

It is essential, however, to learn how *your* body responds to foods, additives, and environmental influences that may impact on *your* chances of developing cancer.

For the carbohydrate addict, learning that high levels of insulin have been found to be a key stimulator for the growth of some types of cancer* is an essential first step. And discovering how to reduce these levels of insulin may make the difference between living in fear and knowing that you may have made essential, health-promoting choices.

Studies connecting high levels of insulin and growth of cancers of the breast, uterus, and ovary are just emerging but they are very powerful in their findings. As reported in the journal *Onkologie*, in 1990, Dr. P. Unterberger and his colleagues studied breast cancer in 752 patients. They found that although there was no relationship between the spread of breast cancer and blood-fat levels (among other risk factors), there was a strong relationship between high insulin levels and the spread of this disease.

Only two years later, two London cancer specialists, Dr. B. A. Stoll and Dr. G. Secreto, discovered new markers for increased risk of breast cancer. Excess levels of insulin, they reported, can cause hormonal imbalances that stimulated the growth of abnormal cells in the breast, in particular, cancer cells.

Other scientists, examining the spread of other cancers, reported similar findings. In 1990, Dr. Yoichi Sugiyama, a specialist in gynecological cancers, reported that in addition to excess insulin being

*High insulin levels have been found to correlate with increased growth of breast, endometrial, and ovarian cancers.

linked to excess weight, polycystic ovary disease, diabetes, and high blood pressure, all of which have been identified as risk factors for ovarian cancer and endometrial cancer of the uterus, patients with this type of cancer were found to have significantly higher food-related insulin levels.

The reports continue to accumulate. A recent article in the *International Journal of Cancer* by Dr. P. F. Bruning and his associates reported that high insulin levels and insulin resistance were a significant risk factor for breast cancer. Dr. D. M. Klurfeld of the Wistar Institute of Anatomy and Biology and others continue to explore and confirm these research reports.

In addition, researchers are now finding that the intake of simple sugars, including table sugar and fruit sugar (fructose), appear to stimulate the insulin rises that may then aid in the spread of some cancers. Dr. D. Yam and his colleagues, examining the insulin-tumor relationship, found that fructose, although it is "promoted as a healthy food additive," actually enhanced the growth of some tumors through the actions of excess insulin. Other researchers are reporting similar and even more startling findings. Dr. F. Kakar and his colleagues, in a report funded by the National Cancer Institute, noted that scientists had found rises in insulin levels, stimulated by the intake of dietary sugar, influence the growth of breast tumor cells. The report went on to note that these reports demonstrated that the correlation between consumption of dietary sugar and death from breast cancer became more pronounced with every decade of life.

> **". . . insulin also acts like a powerful fertilizer to tumor cells, greatly speeding up the growth of the harmful cells."**

C. Beverly, in a lay article that reviewed the hazards of sugary foods for those who have breast cancer, pointed out that insulin acts like "a powerful fertilizer to tumor cells, greatly speeding up the growth of the harmful cells."

The very good news is that on The Carbohydrate Addict's LifeSpan Program, you may be able to reduce both your high levels of insulin and, in doing so, your risk for the spread of these cancers. In addition, by choosing the Complex Carbo Option in Options for

Life (Chapter 6), you may be able to further reduce the potential impact of this "cancer fertilizer."

The Facts Can Set You Free

If before you began this book you had assumed (as you most probably had been told) that being overweight raised your risks for high blood pressure, undesirable blood fats, atherosclerosis, heart and vascular disease, stroke, gout, some forms of cancer, and adult-onset diabetes, you were probably surprised to find that so much of what you had been told might very well have been all wrong.

Now you know what so many scientists know—that the same imbalance that causes you to crave carbohydrates and to put weight on easily also increases your risk for these diseases. But now you can take heart knowing that, through The LifeSpan Program's Basic Plan and its Options, reducing your risk for this insulin imbalance can help reduce your cravings, your weight, and your risk for many of these killer diseases and risk factors, all at the same time.

PART II

THE CARBOHYDRATE ADDICT'S LIFESPAN PROGRAM:

FREEDOM FOREVER

CHAPTER 5

STEP ONE: THE BASIC PLAN

Thy path is plain and straight.

—Robert Southey, 1799

*I*n this chapter, you will learn about a weight-loss and health-promoting plan that is probably unlike any other you have ever encountered.

This program has been designed to fit your body's changing needs—for life. It consists of two essential parts that balance and complement each other, the Program's Basic Plan and its Options for Life.

If you are carbohydrate addicted and you have not been able to maintain success on other programs, your lack of success was not your fault! Chances are that the plan you attempted to follow was not designed to correct the *cause* of your weight gain and cravings.

In order for a program to help you lose weight *and* keep it off, it must correct the very cause of, and thus reduce, your cravings, weight, and many health-related risks. Feelings of deprivation, sacrifice, even the desire to cheat, are signs that a weight-loss plan has not corrected the *cause* of your eating or weight problems. On this program, instead of fighting your hunger—trying desperately to stick to impossible rules—you will find that the Guidelines will *help* you to move smoothly and easily along your path by literally changing the way in which *your* body responds to food.

The Program is simple—it involves no calorie counting, no measuring, no food exchanges.

To help ensure your success, you will find that The Carbohydrate Addict's LifeSpan Program includes four essential elements to success. It is

Simple. This program involves no calorie counting, no measuring, no food exchanges. Following the Guidelines will help to normalize the elevated blood insulin levels that led to your cravings and weight gain in the first place. On this Program you will not need to keep "track" of your eating because, as your insulin levels are reduced, your hunger and cravings will normalize as well.

Naturally slim people do not weigh or measure their food, nor do they count calories; they do not need to use excessive willpower to control their impulses, and, as your body comes into balance, neither will you. The Guidelines that follow will show you which foods you can eat at any time of the day and which foods should be saved for your daily Reward Meal®. Simple? You bet! And the best is yet to come.

To successfully and permanently lose weight, you must have a program that has been targeted to *your* needs.

Targeted. In order for any program to be successful, it must be personalized to fit *your* needs, *your* preferences, *your* lifestyle, and correct the cause of *your* weight problems; if it is to work for life, it must be designed to reverse the metabolic changes that come with each passing decade. Just as you would expect a physician to prescribe a medication that was meant to correct your particular medical problem, you have a right to expect a weight-loss and health-improvement program to do the same.

This program is targeted to the correction of the cause of your cravings, weight gain, and increased health risk. It focuses on the needs of the adult; for those of us in our forties, fifties, sixties, and beyond. The Guidelines and strategies that follow are designed to help you *stay* on your path—they will not, as so many programs do, present a daily obstacle course that you may be forced to try and navigate. The Options of the Program will allow *you* to choose which changes you want to make and when you want to make them.

You are an adult; we will not treat you like a child. We will help you and guide you—we have designed a program that will make weight-loss and health-risk reduction easier than you have ever imagined, but at the same time we respect the fact that you have preferences and challenges of your own and that in the end, in order for any program to be successful, it must be targeted to your lifestyle's needs and challenges as well.

After a while, most other programs can become impossibly demanding and rigid.

Adaptable. One of the most typical problems of commercial and traditional weight-loss programs is their rigidity. Certainly, they may say that they are customized and individualized, but in the end they almost always entail involved food manipulations and planning. Most of us have different eating preferences and patterns when we are on vacation or at parties, at family celebrations; even on weekends. Yet most other programs act as if we were robots who all eat in the same way every day. At best, on other programs you can "save up" for special occasions; at worst, you watch silently as your pleasures, and your life, seem to slip by.

**On this program, if you are hungry, you can eat more.
If you are busy, you can eat out.
If you are in the mood for an exquisite dessert,
you can have it
—without breaking your program and without guilt.**

The Carbohydrate Addict's LifeSpan Program will help you to adapt your plan to fit your life; vacations, holidays, celebrations, even weekends will no longer mean sacrifice or deprivation (neither will weekdays, as a matter of fact). If you are hungry, you can eat more. If you are busy, you can eat out. If you are in the mood for a splendid dinner and an exquisite dessert, you most certainly can have it—without breaking your program and without guilt.

You will find that this program is adaptable to restaurant eating or home cooking, to low-fat or vegetarian diets, if you prefer. It is, literally, your choice. By learning *how* to eat the food you love, you will find that you can be free to choose when, where, and what and how much you want to enjoy.

The Carbohydrate Addict's LifeSpan Program succeeds because it rewards you with both weight loss *and* the foods you love.

Rewarding. Most weight-loss programs have one reward and one reward only. You lose weight—for a time. And although when we begin any program that reward sounds good enough to us, after a while the promise somehow seems to lose its power. Sometimes the weight loss just doesn't seem to come fast enough. It starts off okay, but in time it dwindles or, even worse, comes to a standstill. Sometimes the weight loss is fast but for some reason it just doesn't seem to be worth all the sacrifice—certainly not for the rest of our lives.

When weight loss is your sole reward, with only the possible addition being some small or limited amounts of food exchanges as "special treats," you are almost bound for failure. Even when you succeed in taking off all the weight you wanted to lose, your daily reward will be nothing but maintaining that lost weight, hardly enough to stand up to the sight of some exceedingly tempting "goodie."

The Carbohydrate Addict's LifeSpan Program succeeds because it rewards you with both of the things you want: weight loss *and* the foods you love. On this program you are free to enjoy the foods you find most pleasurable everyday, and without restrictions on amounts.* The Program's Guidelines will help you balance the

---

*All foods are permitted on this program. If your physician recommends that you avoid or limit any of these or any other foods, however, your physician's advice has priority and should, most certainly, be followed. Suggestions for making low-fat or low-salt choices can be found on page 214.

meals you eat, but given that balance you *will* be able to eat the foods you love every day. We will show you *how* to eat the foods you enjoy so that you can truly have your cake and lose weight, too.

THE BASIC PLAN

The Carbohydrate Addict's LifeSpan Program consists of two parts: The Basic Plan and the Options for Life portion. Each of the Guidelines in The Basic Plan, as well as every Option of the Program, focus on reducing your insulin levels and, with them, your cravings, your weight, and your risk for health-related problems.

The Basic Plan consists of only three Guidelines.

The Basic Plan consists of three Guidelines. Each of the Guidelines is essential and the three together will immediately help you to reduce your cravings and weight. After two weeks on the Basic Plan, you can select an Option to add to your Program. While some people find that the Basic Plan is all they need initially to eliminate their carbohydrate cravings and to lose weight, the Basic Plan is intended as the first step, followed by the selection of Options, in a two-step plan for lifestyle change. A complete list of Options and personalized guidance in selecting and using the Options for Life section follows in the next chapter. For now, let's get started with your Basic Plan.

Directions

Follow all three easy Guidelines of the Basic Plan for two weeks. Within a matter of a few days you should notice a dramatic decrease in or elimination of your cravings. Be sure to weigh yourself each day and record your weight on Your Progress Chart (page 173). At the end of two weeks, you will be able to calculate your average weekly weight loss and, in addition, the weekly weight loss you can probably expect in the weeks to come (see Chapter 7, A Great Measure of Success).

After two weeks on the Basic Plan, you will be ready to move to the next chapter and select any Option of your choice.

The Three Guidelines

Guideline #1: Eat a Balanced Reward Meal®
Every Day

Once each day, eat a well-balanced Reward Meal. In addition to Carbohydrate-Rich foods, including the starches, snack foods, or sweets that you need and love, your Reward Meal should include salad as well as Craving-Reducing vegetables and protein. (Your other daily meals and snacks will be detailed in Guideline #3.)

You can choose any meal as your Reward Meal; dinner, luncheon, or breakfast. Most people find that they enjoy looking forward to the same meal each day as their Reward Meal and enjoy the freedom of changing the timing of their Reward Meal, now and then, depending on social engagements, vacations, and celebrations. The majority of our readers choose their evening meal as their Reward Meal, although some enjoy their Reward Meal at lunch; the choice is up to you. If you choose breakfast as your Reward Meal, remember that you must still maintain the recommendations for balancing the Reward Meals that follow. (We'll give you some useful balancing and timing hints in Chapter 8, "A Lifestyle Plan—A Plan for Life.")

Begin your Reward Meal with at least two cups of fresh salad* with lots of leafy green vegetables and, if you like, some dressing. The rest of your Reward Meal should consist of equal portions: $1/3$ Craving-Reducing protein, $1/3$ Craving-Reducing vegetables, and $1/3$ Carbohydrate-Rich foods (including dessert). *You do not need to weigh or measure* your food. Simply judge that the thirds are equal by looking at your portions. A good guide is to imagine a plate divided into thirds. Now, in your mind's eye, place the vegetables, the protein, and the carbohydrates (including dessert) in each of the thirds. They should look just about equal. Take average-sized portions first; you *can* go back for seconds.

---

*If you cannot or do not wish to eat salad, you can choose at least one cup of cooked Craving-Reducing vegetables instead. These vegetables take the place of salad only; continue to include additional Craving-Reducing vegetables in your main meal, as well. You may choose different Craving-Reducing vegetables or more of the same.

Reward Meal

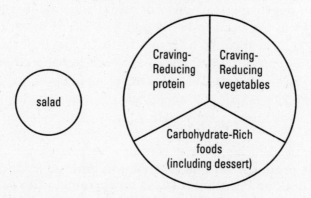

1/3 CRAVING-REDUCING PROTEIN (regular or low-fat varieties):
   all meats, poultry, fish, cheese, eggs, and tofu (full listing in the Craving-Reducing Foods List, pages 120–21).
1/3 CRAVING-REDUCING VEGETABLES:
   all non-starchy vegetables (full listing in the Craving-Reducing Foods List, pages 120–21).
1/3 CARBOHYDRATE-RICH FOODS (including dessert):
   all starches (breads, pasta, rice, etc.), starchy vegetables (potatoes, peas, corn, carrots, etc.), snack foods, fruits, juices, and sweets (full listing in the Carbohydrate-Rich Foods List, pages 122–23).

If, after you have finished all the food on your plate, you desire additional food, you are free to go back for more but make sure that, with the additional food you take, you still maintain the 1/3, 1/3, 1/3 portions. *Do not* go back for more Carbohydrate-Rich foods *only*. If you are hungry, you can have seconds, but (except for the salad, of which you can always have more) you *must* have seconds of everything (in equal portions). These seconds can be large, if you are very hungry, or small, if you just want a bit more, but all three portions must be equal. In the same way, if you are not hungry enough to eat all of your first plateful, eat less of *all* of the three portions; do not eat mostly Carbohydrate-Rich foods and leave most of the vegetables.

Balance is crucial in your Reward Meal. You need the salad for fiber, filler, and nutrition; you need the protein for the minerals it contains and to help stabilize your blood sugar levels; the vegetables are an important source of fiber and filler as well as nutrition, and you need the carbohydrates for energy, nutrition, and satisfaction.

Unbalanced Reward Meals will most certainly make the difference between losing weight or losing nothing at all and, in addition, they can have a negative impact on your health and well-being as well.

Most of us are used to being told how much to eat of any particular food. "Eat this much of this and that much of that," we are told. Or "$1/2$ cup of this equals one bread exchange." On this program, you will never again live by the numbers because The Carbohydrate Addict's LifeSpan Program has been designed to correct the source of your hunger and weight gain.

On this program, no one will need to limit your food intake. The LifeSpan Program focuses on correcting the *source* of your hunger so that you will not *want* to overeat.

Remember that your cravings and weight gain are regulated by the amount of insulin your body releases. The more *often* you eat Carbohydrate-Rich foods or heavily carbo-loaded meals, the higher your insulin levels. The higher your insulin levels, the more food you want. A single daily Reward Meal helps break the carbo-craving cycle by decreasing the *frequency* (not the amount) of Carbohydrate-Rich foods that are eaten every day. Although you still get the satisfaction of eating the foods you love, your insulin levels drop and with them your cravings, your tendency to gain weight, and your health risks as well.

When the intense drive to overeat or to snack frequently on Carbohydrate-Rich foods is lifted, no one will have to limit your food intake; you will not *want* to overeat. In addition, as you continue to follow the Program, your body should be better able to handle the carbohydrates that you do eat at your Reward Meal and be less prone to quickly convert it into fat, allowing you to use the food energy you take in and to burn what you have *in the past* already stored as fat.

Guideline #2: Complete Your Reward Meal Within One Hour

From start to finish, complete your Reward Meal within sixty minutes. This might seem like an odd recommendation. In the past, you have probably been given limits on what you can and cannot eat as well as restrictions on how much you can eat, but chances are you have never been given a maximum limit on *how long* you can eat. We are about to change all of that.

> **If you are eating too much or too often,**
> **don't blame yourself—**
> **you are simply exhibiting a powerful sign that**
> **your body is out of balance.**
> **A balanced body eats just enough, feels satisfied,**
> **then stops eating—naturally.**

When you are eating correctly for *your* body, there is no need to restrict the *quantities* of food you eat—a balanced body eats in balance, feels satisfied, then stops eating, naturally. If you are eating too much or too often, don't blame yourself—you are simply exhibiting a powerful sign that your body is out of balance.

When you eat carbohydrate-rich foods, your body releases insulin in two waves. This is called the *biphasic* release of insulin. The first wave, or phase, hits within a few minutes of seeing, smelling, tasting, or even thinking about food. The first wave of insulin is an on-off mechanism and the amount of insulin that your body releases in this first wave is preset, dependent on how much and how often you have eaten carbohydrate-rich foods in the past twelve to twenty hours.

If you have been eating lots of carbohydrate-rich foods, or you have been snacking on them frequently, or both, your body expects that each new meal or snack will also contain lots of carbos, and it releases lots of insulin to handle the carbohydrate-rich foods. You have probably experienced this first wave of insulin release when, after having taken a bite or two of food, you suddenly find that you are "hungrier than you thought you were." That increase in hunger, the intensified pleasure that that food gave you, is often evidence of your body's first wave of insulin.

In order to reduce this first insulin release (and the insulin resistance that follows), Guideline #1 confines all of your carbohydrate-rich foods to a once-a-day Reward Meal. In that way, because no recent meals have primed your "insulin regulator," your body does not expect more carbohydrate-rich food and it is "fooled" into releasing far less insulin. At all your meals, including your Reward Meal, you find that you are less hungry and far more satisfied—and that your body seems to store in the form of fat far less of the food energy that you do take in.

The second wave of insulin release is *not* a preset amount; it varies depending on how much carbohydrate-rich food you eat at that particular meal and it can make up for an unexpectedly carbohydrate-rich meal by releasing more insulin as it is needed.

You probably have experienced this second phase of insulin release when your meals have gone on for extended periods of time, at family celebrations or holidays, for example. At these meals, you may have eaten until you were satisfied but then found that as you continued to snack and nibble, you became *less* satisfied—even to the point where you felt that you might never feel finished (even though you might have eaten to the point of being uncomfortable). This is evidence of insulin's second wave; it reaches its peak at about sixty-five or seventy minutes after you start eating and it is the very reason that Guideline #2 is needed.

**Each of the three Guidelines of the Basic Plan
helps restore the carbohydrate addict's body
to its natural balance.**

By finishing your Reward Meal within sixty minutes, your insulin levels will probably remain far lower than if you had continued eating past the one-hour limit, because you have finished your meal *before* the second wave of insulin release has reached its peak. Because the meal is over, your body is then able to sense that no more insulin is needed and, with insulin levels remaining lower, you will feel far more satisfied, both at the meal as well as after.

Both phases of insulin release may have made a great deal of sense when we were prehistoric cavemen; they allowed us to eat great quantities when a rare find of grains or fruits were found, and the more we ate, the more our bodies stimulated us to keep eating—we had to consume great quantities then, while the food was there for the taking.

Today, with carbohydrate-rich foods available all day long, every day of the year, we can no longer afford to continuously signal our bodies that it is time to eat. Guidelines #1 and #2, in combination with Guideline #3 that follows, will help stop the "keep eating" signals that your body has been getting.

For now, just remember that all the foods you love and need are available every day in your Reward Meal (your other meals and snacks will be addressed in Guideline #3), but make sure you keep your well-balanced Reward Meal feast confined to one hour—from start to finish. (In addition, you will find some simple, real-life suggestions for keeping to your one-hour limit in Chapter 8, "A Lifestyle Plan—A Plan for Life".)

Guideline #3: Eat Only Craving-Reducing Foods at All Other Meals and Snacks

At all meals and snacks, other than at your Reward Meal, eat Craving-Reducing foods *only*. You will find a complete list on pages 120–21. In general, Craving-Reducing foods include high-fiber vegetables and protein-rich foods. Craving-Reducing Meals and Snacks should be well balanced and should include both high-fiber and protein-rich choices. The amount you eat is not critical as long as you include both protein and high-fiber vegetables at any Craving-Reducing Meal or Snack. Some people eat 1/2 protein, 1/2 vegetables; others choose less protein and more salad and vegetables. We generally recommend that you take "average-sized portions" and go back for more if you like but, in the end, the size and proportions are truly up to you.

Remember, on this program, you do not have to weigh or measure; as insulin levels normalize, your cravings will be dramatically reduced and most people find that, at times, they may literally "forget

---

**The size and proportions of your Craving-Reducing Meals
are up to you.**

---

to eat." We know that seems impossible to believe right now, but you are almost sure to see things quite differently after a short time or so on the program.

If you want to skip a meal because you simply are not hungry, you are free to do so as long as you feel well and your physician does not object. In the same way, if you want a snack, you are free to enjoy any of the Craving-Reducing foods you desire, as well.

By definition, a Craving-Reducing breakfast does not include the usual cereals, fruits, breads, or pastries that you may be used to having in the morning. On the other hand, those foods set in motion the insulin and carbohydrate-craving cycles that most likely have kept you battling your hunger and your weight.

Your choices for breakfast are many. You can choose to skip breakfast or have only a cup of coffee or tea (with milk or cream and sugar substitute, if you like). If you want to eat a small breakfast or prefer a full meal, you can choose from any of the Craving-Reducing foods on pages 120–21. In addition, we have included a wide variety of Craving-Reducing breakfast suggestions in the Meal Plans section (page 193) as well as some exciting special Craving-Reducing breakfast recipes for muffins, pancakes, a breakfast soufflé, a special cinnamon "bread," and a crustless quiche, all made from Craving-Reducing ingredients (beginning on page 120). You will also find useful hints for alternative Craving-Reducing breakfasts in Chapter 8, "A Lifestyle Plan—A Plan for Life."

A Vital Liquid Asset

You may have heard it before, but rest assured you will hear it again, here. As part of any weight-reducing, health-promoting program, be sure to drink 6 to 8 glasses of water every day.*

Taking in enough water may sound simple at first, but as your

---

*Unless otherwise directed by your physician.

cravings and general desire to eat decreases, you will find it easy to forget to take in enough liquid. So make your daily water quota available (get a large insulated mug, if you like) and desirable (we love cool spring water), but most of all, drink it!

Chewing Gum: A Sticky Business

When it comes to insulin release and the increase in cravings and weight gain that it can cause, it seems to make no difference whether your chewing gum is sweetened with sugar or with a sugar substitute (such as an artificial sweetener). No matter what they contain, chewing gums appear to increase insulin release in two ways.

First, their sweet taste falsely signals the body that a carbohydrate-rich meal is coming. In readiness, the body responds by releasing insulin to assist in getting the incoming food energy to the muscles and organs that may need it and to prepare to save any leftover energy in your fat cells. Since very little food energy is contained in the gum, an overabundance of insulin remains in the bloodstream, signaling you to take in more gum or, instead, other carbohydrate-rich foods. Each new fresh stick of gum is perceived as the beginning of yet another "sweet meal" and insulin levels rise higher and higher, increasing your cravings as well as your body's resistance to insulin (raising your tendency to store fat or develop adult-onset diabetes).

Chewing gum can also increase insulin release through a second "pathway," which we describe as a "neurological stimulation." In this way, the chewing or sucking itself simulates, or mimics, eating. The body thinks you are indeed taking in food and responds appropriately by releasing insulin. Then the same cycle of craving, insulin resistance, and weight gain can begin again.

On this program it is important to avoid all chewing gums. If this seems difficult at first, don't worry. Within a few days on the Program, as your insulin levels drop and your cravings start to disappear, you will notice your "need" for chewing gum slip away.

CRAVING-REDUCING FOODS LIST

NOTE: ANY FOOD *NOT* LISTED BELOW SHOULD BE CONSIDERED A CARBOHYDRATE-RICH FOOD.

PORTIONS DEPEND ON YOUR INDIVIDUAL NEEDS. UNLESS YOUR PHYSICIAN ADVISES OTHERWISE, CHOOSE "AVERAGE-SIZED" PORTIONS. GO BACK FOR MORE IF YOU LIKE. THERE IS NO NEED TO MEASURE OR WEIGH FOOD.

MEATS: ALL REGULAR AND LEAN MEATS, INCLUDING:

Bacon*	Beef	Corned beef
Ham	Hamburger	Hot dogs (all meat)
Lamb	Pastrami	Pork
Rabbit	Sausages (no added	Venison
Veal	sugar)*	

Most luncheon meats contain added sugars and fillers and those not listed in this meat section should be considered Carbohydrate-Rich foods and should be saved for Reward Meals only.

FOWL: LIGHT OR DARK VARIETIES, WITH OR WITHOUT SKIN, INCLUDING:

Capon Chicken Cornish hen Duck Goose Pheasant Quail Squab Turkey (ground or whole)

FISH AND SHELLFISH: ALL VARIETIES, CANNED, JARRED (NO SUGAR), OR COOKED (NO BREAD CRUMBS), INCLUDING:

Bass	Bluefish	Calamari	Clams	Cod
Crabmeat	Flounder	Haddock	Halibut	Lobster
Monkfish	Oysters	Perch	Salmon	Sardines
Scallops	Scrod	Shrimp	Smelt	Sole
Sturgeon	Swordfish	Trout	Tuna	

DAIRY AND NON-MEAT ALTERNATIVES: REGULAR OR LOW-FAT VARIETIES OF:

Eggs Egg substitutes* Cheese (all varieties except low-fat ricotta) Cream cheese Cottage cheese*

Milk, cream, or half-and-half (up to 2 ounces daily in one cup of coffee or tea or in cooking; *not* nondairy creamers) Sour cream Tofu (soybean curd)*

Vegetarian meat alternatives that contain 4 grams of carbohydrate or less per average serving

VEGETABLES: FRESH, STIR-FRIED, SAUTÉED (NO BREADING), STEAMED, OR BOILED NON-STARCHY VEGETABLES:

Alfalfa sprouts	Arugula	Asparagus
Bamboo shoots	Bean sprouts	Broccoli*
Brussels sprouts	Cabbage (all)	Cauliflower
Celery	Cucumbers	Endive
Green beans	Greens (all)	Kale
Kohlrabi	Lettuce	Mushrooms
Okra	Onions (as seasoning only)	Parsley
Peppers (green or red*)	Radishes	Scallions
Snap beans	Sorrel (sour grass)	Spinach
Tomatoes (raw, about 1/4 per meal)		Wax beans

OILS, FATS, AND DRESSINGS:

Butter or margarine, regular or low-fat substitutes

Mayonnaise: use regular only (not low-fat) in Craving-Reducing Meals. Low-fat mayonnaise can contain added sugar. See page 221 for an easy low-fat mayonnaise alternative.

Oils: all varieties including corn, olive, safflower, sesame, soybean, sunflower, vegetable, etc.

Salad dressings: all regular and low-fat varieties where sugar is not among first four ingredients.

EXTRAS:

Capers (for garnish only)	Dill pickles
Garlic (fresh or powdered)	Herbs
Horseradish	Juice (citrus, small
Ketchup (1 to 2 tablespoons only)	amounts, for cooking only)
Mustard	Mayonnaise (regular only)
Onion (fresh or powdered, for cooking only)	Olives (green or black; no pimientos)
Seeds (poppy or sesame, for cooking only)	Pepper or Salt
	Spices
Wine* (dry varieties, for cooking only)	Vinegar (white, all other varieties*)

BEVERAGES:

Carbonated water   Club soda (nonflavored)*   Coffee
Seltzer (nonflavored)   Tea

*If you are particularly sensitive to carbohydrates, you may find that these foods can cause rebound cravings or reduced weight loss. If so, or if you have concern, eliminate them or save them for Reward Meals only.

CARBOHYDRATE-RICH FOODS LIST

(TO BE COMBINED WITH CRAVING-REDUCING FOODS AT REWARD MEALS)

NOTE: HERE ARE *EXAMPLES* OF SOME OF THE MANY CARBO-HYDRATE-RICH FOODS YOU CAN COMBINE WITH CRAVING-REDUCING FOODS AT YOUR DAILY REWARD MEAL.

ALL FOODS THAT ARE NOT SPECIFICALLY LISTED ON THE COMPANION CHART (CRAVING-REDUCING FOODS) SHOULD BE CONSIDERED CARBOHYDRATE-RICH.

PORTIONS DEPEND ON YOUR INDIVIDUAL NEEDS. UNLESS YOUR PHYSICIAN ADVISES OTHERWISE, CHOOSE "AVERAGE-SIZED" PORTIONS. YOU CAN GO BACK FOR MORE IF YOU LIKE. THERE IS NO NEED TO MEASURE OR WEIGH FOOD. SEE PAGE 112 FOR BALANCING FOODS AT REWARD MEALS.

BREADS, GRAINS, CEREALS: ALL VARIETIES (REGULAR, LOW-FAT, LOW-SUGAR, WHOLE GRAIN, ETC.), INCLUDING:

Bagels	Biscuits	Breads	Pancakes
Breakfast bars	Cereals (hot	Cornmeal	Tempura
Couscous	or cold)	French toast	coating
Granola	Croissants	Tahini	Waffles
Tabbouleh	Grits	Stuffing	

DAIRY: REGULAR, FROZEN, AND LOW-FAT VARIETIES OF:

Breakfast drinks	Cream	Creamers (nondairy)
Ice cream	Half-and-half	Ice milk
Low-fat ricotta cheese	Milk	Yogurt

FRUIT AND JUICES: ALL FRUITS (COOKED, DRIED FRUIT, FRESH), FRUIT JUICES, OR VEGETABLE JUICES, INCLUDING:

Apples	Bananas	Carrot juice	Cantaloupe
Cherries	Dates	Figs	Grapefruit
Grapes	Kiwi fruit	Lemons, Limes	Mangoes
Oranges	Papaya	Peaches	Pears
Pineapple	Plums	V-8	

LEGUMES, SEEDS, NUTS AND NUT BUTTERS: ALL VARIETIES, INCLUDING:

Baked beans	Black beans	Cashews	Chestnuts
Chick peas	Hummus	Peanut butter	Kidney beans
(garbanzos)	Peanuts	Split Peas	Pistachios
Lentils	Sesame seeds	Water chestnuts	Walnuts
Pumpkin seeds			

LUNCHEON MEATS: ALL VARIETIES WHICH CONTAIN ADDED SUGARS, MSG, OR FILLERS

PASTA, NOODLES, AND RICE: ALL FRESH AND DRY VARIETIES, INCLUDING:

Pasta (all varieties including shells, rigatoni, spaghetti)	Chinese noodles	Rice (brown, pilaf, white, wild)
	Egg noodles	
	Spinach noodles	
		Tabbouleh

SNACK FOODS, SWEETS, AND EXTRAS: ALL VARIETIES OF SNACKS, INCLUDING THOSE SWEETENED WITH SUGAR *OR* SUGAR SUBSTITUTES, INCLUDING:

Cakes	Candies	Chips	Chocolate
Cookies	Crackers	Fructose	Gelatin desserts
Honey	Mints	Popcorn	Pretzels
Puddings	Rice cakes	Snack bars and mixes	Sugar

For sugar substitutes, see the "Carbohydrate Act-Alikes," section that follows, under "Sugar Substitutes."

VEGETABLES: ALL THOSE *NOT* LISTED AS CARBOHYDRATE-REDUCING VEGETABLES, INCLUDING:

FRESH, STIR-FRIED, SAUTÉED, WITH OR WITHOUT BREADING, STEAMED, OR BOILED VARIETIES:

Beets	Zucchini	Tomatoes (when more than $1/4$ per meal)	Peas
Squash	Corn		Potatoes
Carrots			

BEVERAGES:

All fruit juices and drinks   All sugar-sweetened drinks and soda
All beverages containing alcohol   All flavored seltzers and club sodas

For artificially-sweetened (diet) sodas, see the "Carbohydrate Act-Alikes", section that follows under "Sugar Substitutes."

CARBOHYDRATE ACT-ALIKES: ALTHOUGH THESE FOODS AND BEVERAGES ARE NOT NECESSARILY HIGH IN CARBOHYDRATES, MANY CARBOHYDRATE ADDICTS RESPOND WITH CRAVINGS AND/OR WEIGHT GAIN AS IF THE FOODS, INDEED, WERE CARBOHYDRATE-RICH. CAREFULLY READ RECOMMENDATIONS FOR EACH CATEGORY.

ALL ALCOHOLIC BEVERAGES, INCLUDING BEER, WINE, MIXED DRINKS, LIQUORS, ETC:
Treat these drinks as if they were carbohydrate-rich foods. Save them for your Reward Meal and, for ideal meal balance, consider them to be part of your $1/3$ portion of carbohydrates.

SUGAR SUBSTITUTES:
If you are particularly sensitive to carbohydrates, you may find that noncaloric sugar substitutes can cause increased cravings and/or reduced weight loss. If they do, or if you have concern, save them for Reward Meals only or eliminate them altogether (for more details, see Chapter 6, "Options for Life").

CHEWING GUM:
All chewing gum, whether sweetened with sugar or a sugar substitute, can act as a strong carbohydrate act-alike. See the note that immediately follows this chart for important details.

SOY BEANS (ROASTED OR BOILED), SOY SAUCE, TERIYAKI, MISO (SOYBEAN PASTE), TEMPEH:
These foods often cause increased hunger, cravings, or reduced weight loss. Save them for Reward Meals only (for more details, see Chapter 6, "Options for Life").
NOTE: SEE TOFU (SOY BEAN CURD) EXCEPTION BELOW.

TOFU (SOYBEAN CURD):
If you are particularly sensitive to monosodium glutamate, you may find that tofu can cause increased hunger, cravings, or reduced weight loss. If so, or if you have concern, eliminate it from all meals or save it for Reward Meals only (for more details, see Chapter 6, "Options for Life").

An Essential Addition: Moving On

While some individuals have lost weight and maintained their weight loss on the Basic Plan alone, to get the maximum benefit in craving elimination, weight loss, and health promotion, we strongly urge you to add Options (from the next chapter) to your Basic Plan.

> **With your cravings gone and your weight coming down, you may be tempted to not go any further, but true success is effortless and permanent and the Options that follow will help you in your victory.**

The initial reduction of cravings that you will experience by following the three Guidelines of the Basic Plan may be so great that you might very well be tempted to go no further. But we urge you to reconsider. The Basic Plan is like a suit of clothes that may at first seem to be just the right size, but in order to fit perfectly, it must be tailored to match your body's dimensions as well as your preferences.

The Basic Plan was designed to remove the overwhelming imbalance of insulin that drives your carbohydrate cravings and urges your body into a fat-making mode. The basic is the first step in a lifestyle change program. The Options portion of the Program, which follows, is meant to complement the Basic Plan and it focuses on helping you to continue to take the weight off and to keep it off for life—without struggle—while reducing your health risks at the same time.

The Options for Life portion of the Program will help you to literally tailor the Program to fit your particular body's responses and the challenges of your particular lifestyle; it will help you fine-tune the Program to your daily routine as well as to your personal needs and preferences.

Some people tell us that they are unsure as to whether to continue following the Basic Plan only or to move on and begin adding Options to their program. Others want to know when they "must" add Options. Here is how to make the right choice for you:

Follow only the three Guidelines of the Basic Plan for at least two weeks. After two weeks on the Basic Plan, if your carbohydrate cravings have been pretty much eliminated and you and your physician agree that you are losing weight at a satisfactory rate,* the choice is really up to you. You can stay with the Basic Plan as it is (although, as you know, we would always encourage you to add Options as described in the next chapter).

If, on the other hand, you sometimes still feel moderate twinges of cravings or are tempted to eat carbohydrates at times other than at your Reward Meal, or if your weight loss is not as steady as you would like or is going too slowly,* adding Options is an absolute must. Each Option will help you to reduce the insulin levels that may be stopping you from achieving absolute success.

Remember, "holding on" and trying to cope with hunger or cravings is not success; true success should be effortless and fun—and the Options that follow in the next chapter can greatly help you to achieve your long-sought victory.

*To increase the probability of permanent weight loss, most people should maintain a weekly average weight loss of between $1/2$ and 2 pounds per week. For more details, see Chapter 7, "A Great Measure of Success."

CHAPTER 6

STEP TWO: OPTIONS FOR LIFE

Choose which seems best and, in the doing, it will become agreeable and easy.
—Pythagoras, circa 550 B.C.

*A*fter at least two weeks on the Basic Plan, you can begin to add Options to your program. Each Option is designed to further reduce your insulin levels and your body's insulin resistance and, in doing so, help to secure your easy and permanent weight loss and an even greater decrease in your health risk factors.

> *You* choose which Option you want to add,
> as well as *when* and *in which way* you want to add it.

The Options are simple to follow, and they are targeted to the source of your cravings and weight gain and possible increased health risk; the powerful triggers and time bombs that may have, without your ever knowing it, influenced the direction of your life.

The Options that follow are adaptable to your lifestyle and to your preferences (*you* choose which Option you want to add, *when* and *in which way* you want to add it) and they will reward you with the twin goals of the food you truly enjoy along with a freedom from eating concerns and weight problems.

In addition, as we have seen over and over again, the freedom from guilt and from the fear of gaining back lost weight are welcome bonuses that seem to naturally go along with the Program and its Options.

First Option, First Choice

When you choose an Option you are, in essence, making a choice to continue to decrease your cravings, increase your rate of your weight loss, and maximize the health-promoting benefits of the Program.

At any time after you have been on the Basic Plan for at least two weeks, you can begin to add Options, one at a time. Do not be concerned if some time has passed since you first began the Program. As long as you have been maintaining your three Guidelines for the last two weeks, you can freely add any Option of your choice, at any time.

Select the Option that seems most appealing to *you*.

While continuing to follow all three Guidelines that make up the Basic Plan, select the Option that seems most appealing to you. Some choose the easiest Option, such as the Chromium Option or the Over-The-Counter Remedy Timing Option. Others choose an Option that describes a change that they "have been wanting to do, anyway"; such as the Activity and Movement Option or the Stress-Reduction Option. Others begin with those Options that will most powerfully influence their weight loss, such as the Food Frequency Reducing Option, and are often happily surprised at how easy and rewarding these Options turn out to be.

Choose any single Option that is most appealing to *you*. This Option will be your initial choice.

. Read through the Option carefully so that you totally understand what is expected. Think through your day and plan how you might best incorporate the Option into your routine (decide on a private place where you can do some of your Stress-Reduction exercises, for instance, or which time of day is best for you to add your Movement or Activity Options, or at which health food store you will buy the chromium that you will need for your Chromium Option).

Then, while continuing to follow the three Guidelines of your Basic Plan, add the Option of your choice to your routine.

If, when you first begin an Option, it fits comfortably into your life, then most certainly continue. On the other hand, if any particular Option does not feel right from the start or is far more demanding than you anticipated, if you find yourself resenting it or "cheating" quite often, then drop it. If an Option fits somewhere in between, if it feels new and you are not sure whether or not you want to continue it, give it a full two-week trial period. At the end of two weeks, make a decision whether to continue it or drop it.

**Your Option choice is not carved in stone;
it can change as your needs and preferences change.**

Your Option choice is not carved in stone; as time goes on, your Options can change as your needs and preferences change. You may choose an Option for a time, for instance, then find that as your lifestyle changes, as time demands grow heavier, a previously chosen Option is no longer workable for you. You are free to drop that Option, without guilt or self-recrimination. Remember that your Program must be livable to bring about a lifestyle change. This is not a contest of perfection but rather a program that is designed to endure.

After adding an Option for at least two weeks, or after deselecting an Option, you are free to add another, if you like. We certainly encourage you to add Option after Option, but we insist that you pay attention to your own thoughts and feelings. Add an Option when you want to increase your weight-loss rate, decrease your cravings, or increase the health-promoting benefits of the Program, but add the Options you want, when you want to.

Add the Options you want, when you want to but always continue following your Basic Plan.

Always, always, always, continue to follow the Basic Plan. The Options are meant to be an adjunct, a supplement to the Basic Plan; they are never meant to replace adhering to the three Guidelines of the Basic Plan.

Continue adding Options as you like, but no more often than once every two weeks. If you do not want to add any new Options, don't. If there are Options that you have tried in the past but dropped, we encourage you to try them again after a period of time.

As time goes by, the physical changes that come with staying on the Basic Plan, or from other Options, will often make a previously challenging Option far easier or more appealing than it might have been in the past. So, if you have tried an Option and decided not to continue it, don't consider it off-limits forever. Give it another chance at some later date and see if, in fact, it isn't far more appealing.

One last word of guidance. Some Options may advise that you make a change only when it feels desirable and comfortable. That is an important recommendation. Contrary to what you may have experienced on other programs, on this Program we do *not* need you to push yourself to perfection. It will only cause you to rebel in the future.

Give yourself the right to make changes at a comfortable pace; and as your body comes in balance, naturally, change will come easily. Remember that to succeed for life a program must be livable and satisfying, so allow yourself the rewards you deserve.

When things are easy, pleasurable, and give us what we want, we do not need to "motivate" ourselves to do them. In the same way, if you are caring and sensitive to yourself, you will find that you will be far more likely to stay on your Program indefinitely—without struggle. So, if an Option says, "Skip a meal or snack only when you don't really want it," take heed of the entire message—not just the first few words. If you take it naturally, that Option will move you in the right direction, at the right time, and without struggle. Give the Program your best, follow the Guidelines and choose appropriate Options but, at the same time, be realistic and considerate of yourself as well.

Nine Options for Life

The Chromium Option

A special form of the inexpensive and common nutrient, chromium,* available through virtually all health food stores, has been found to have significant effects on insulin levels and on the weight and health problems that an insulin imbalance can often bring.

The specific form of chromium that we have been using in our own research and which has been shown to be so effective is called *Glucose Tolerance Factor chromium* or GTF chromium, for short.†

Chromium occurs naturally in our foods, but research scientists are finding that as many as nine out of ten of us have diets that do *not* supply us with adequate amounts of chromium.

Studies by the U.S. Department of Agriculture have found that nine out of ten of us have diets that do *not* supply us with enough chromium.

To make matters worse, many of the foods that we eat regularly, including refined and processed foods, milk, sweets and sodas— even those foods which are often considered "healthy," such as fruits and juices—can literally rob us of our vital chromium stores. To add to this chromium piracy, emotional and physical stress can further deplete our bodies of this precious nutrient, and so, given

---

*Throughout this book, unless otherwise indicated, the term *chromium* can be assumed to mean the trivalent nutritional form of chromium.

†You may have heard a great deal about GTF chromium's "sister" nutrient, chromium picolinate, but chromium picolinate is still somewhat new and the research on Glucose Tolerance Factor chromium is, at this time and to our thinking, far more tested and compelling.

today's challenges, eating adequate amounts of chromium-rich foods may no longer be enough.

Chromium has been called the "essential cofactor" of insulin; it is insulin's partner, helping insulin to do its jobs. And, like partners working together, when one is unable to do his part, the second must compensate. So it is with insulin and chromium. When your body does not have enough chromium, it needs more insulin to do its work, and so your body meets its responsibilities by releasing additional insulin.

An entire domino effect of eating, weight, and health problems can begin with a simple deficiency of chromium.

An entire domino effect of eating, weight, and health problems can, in this way, begin with a simple but powerful deficiency of chromium.

Carbohydrate cravings increase as additional insulin is released. At the same time, your organs and muscles may become more resistant to insulin; first, channeling insulin and blood sugar into the fat cells (leading to weight gain and low blood sugar), and, later, as even the fat cells resist the onslaught of insulin, trapping insulin and blood sugar in the bloodstream (leading to adult-onset diabetes).

More than twenty years ago, Dr. K. N. Jeejeebhoy and his colleagues reported in the *American Journal of Clinical Nutrition* that chromium deficiency resulted in abnormal blood sugar levels, undesirable blood-fat levels, and slower metabolic rates. Over the past two decades, scientists like Dr. A. S. Kozlovsky and his colleagues, reporting in the scientific journal *Metabolism*, continued to confirm that chromium deficiency is common to heart disease and diabetes, and as researcher and author Dr. Richard A. Passwater reported, chromium deficiency "results in arterial plaque formation, which in turn can induce blood clotting, which causes a heart attack."

Each passing decade takes its toll on our chromium stores in two ways. First, the older we get the more our bodies appear to need chromium and, second, at the same time, the older we get the more likely it is that we are not taking in the chromium we need or that stress and other factors are robbing us of our vital chromium stores. When you look at both facts together, you realize that we are getting the least chromium just when we need it the most.

The good news is that correcting this problem appears both easy and inexpensive; in addition to its ability to help your body process carbohydrates and reverse the effects of stress hormones, supplementing your diet with chromium now appears to have a powerful effect on reversing and preventing many of the health problems and health risk factors that have long been associated with the "natural process of aging."

Chromium by Any Other Name

Natural food sources of chromium include brewer's yeast, black pepper, mushrooms, wine, beer, and other foods, and although we may vow to consume greater quantities of these foods, trying to include adequate amounts of chromium in our diets does *not* appear to be the practical approach to avoiding or correcting a chromium deficiency because of the depletion of this vital nutrient by so many other foods and environmental influences. We can eat only so much brewer's yeast and black pepper, and there is only so much beer or wine we should consume. In addition, while we can limit how many times each day we take in carbohydrates, the chromium depletion that follows the consumption of processed or refined foods, as well as the stresses we encounter daily, is virtually unavoidable.

We get the least chromium when we need it most. Supplementing your daily chromium intake with a single dose of chromium could be an essential aid in keeping your insulin and blood sugar levels in balance.

Though it is generally preferable to get the nutrients we need from the food we eat, supplementing your chromium intake with a single dose of a specific form of chromium may prove to be the most beneficial way for the carbohydrate addict to help keep insulin levels in balance.

There are many types of chromium that you can buy at your local health food store but only one that we would suggest at this time: Glucose Tolerance Factor chromium,* also called GTF chromium. GTF chromium tablets are made from brewer's yeast, so if you are "yeast sensitive" mention this fact to your physician. The label should say that it is "certified biologically active."

Several brands meet these guidelines; we, ourselves, use Solgar's GTF Chromium, which is certified biologically active. A word of caution: If you choose a different brand, be careful that you choose a brand that contains *only* Glucose Tolerance Factor chromium. Some manufacturers add extra niacin or other ingredients so that they can develop new patents; other companies try to attract the consumer with "added nutrients"; some may believe that added nutrients "help" chromium do its job. We strongly suggest that you choose GTF chromium and GTF chromium alone.

Solgar and other companies produce more than one kind of chromium, so read the label carefully.

Solgar and other companies produce more than one kind of chromium, including chromium picolinate as well as inorganic forms of chromium (which your body may not be able to use as well), so do not purchase by brand name only—look for the words "Glucose Tolerance Factor chromium."

Many people who are familiar with the more publicized type of chromium, chromium picolinate, ask us if picolinate is a fair substitute for GTF chromium. As compared with GTF chromium, chromium picolinate is still somewhat new and the research on Glucose Tolerance Factor chromium is, at this time and to our thinking, far more tested and compelling.

If your health food store does not have GTF chromium or you do not want the brand they carry, do not let them talk you into

---

*Individual health needs and concerns should be considered; therefore check with your physician before adding GTF chromium supplementation to your diet. GTF chromium may reduce the need for insulin; if GTF chromium is taken, diabetics should be closely monitored by a physician.

something else. Ask them to order the GTF you want. In general, it should cost approximately $9 to $10 or so for 100 tablets, each containing 200 micrograms (200 g) of GTF chromium.

The National Research Council says that 50 to 200 micrograms of trivalent chromium each day is the "safe and adequate" intake for adults. *Most* pills contain 200 micrograms, so one pill each day fulfills the "safe and adequate" daily intake recommendation. Not all brands contain 200 micrograms, so it is important to read the label.

Do *not* take your GTF chromium with food or with medications.

Take your GTF chromium at the same time every day, but do *not* take it with food or medications. Zinc, found in so many of your foods or in your vitamins or supplements, can interfere with the absorption of the chromium, so take your GTF with water and with nothing else.

The benefits of GTF chromium may take anywhere from one to several months to become observable, but long before *you* notice the difference, your body will already be responding to this most needed nutrient.

The Activity and Movement Option*

We have all been told that a strong exercise regimen is good for the cardiovascular system. We would most certainly agree with the fact that if you are able and willing to maintain such a regimen, your cardiovascular system may well benefit. Many of us, however, find that we do not have the time, are not physically able, or simply cannot maintain the motivation that is needed for the exacting commitment that intense exercise regimens require.

Many of us do not have the time, are not physically able, or simply cannot maintain the motivation needed for intense exercise regimens.

If you are able to maintain high levels of regular exercise, that may be beneficial to you, and, with your physician's guidance, we would encourage you to keep it up. If, on the other hand, you fall into the majority of the population who cannot or will not be able to sustain these high levels of activity, we have very good news for you.

In terms of weight loss, moderate or even mild activity levels (including lower-impact movement approaches) appear to be quite helpful in reducing insulin levels and decreasing the body's resistance to insulin. The result: less hunger, more "fat-burning," and greater health promotion—all without demanding time and energy commitments. The "burning" of calories no longer appears to be the most important component in exercise-related weight loss. Researchers are finding that the lowering of insulin levels may be fundamental in helping you to lose weight, and, in combination with the Basic Plan, even mild or moderate activity or movement choices can help you reduce your insulin levels and decrease your body's insulin resistance.

So when you select your Activity or Movement Choice within this Option, consider your own needs and limitations. Be realistic. Think about the following: How much time can you really commit

*Always check with your physician before beginning any new movement or activity program.

(on a regular basis)? How motivated are you likely to remain? Can you maintain your choice when the weather is bad? Consider physical limitations carefully. Do not make promises that you will later break and for which you will later blame yourself.

**Be realistic. Select an easy choice.
Do not make promises that you will later break
and for which you will later blame yourself.**

It is far better to select a choice that takes less time and effort and which you maintain than a far more rigorous one that you are forced to abandon because it is simply not right for you.

Start off with an "easier" commitment; as your insulin levels and weight decrease, and as your energy levels increase, you can always move to higher levels. It is far better to be consistent at an easier alternative than on-again-off-again with a more demanding choice.

Remember, always check with your physician before beginning any new movement or activity program.

Movement and Activity Choices*

Do any of the following kinds of activity (Light, Moderate, or
   Vigorous) for either:
A. 15 minutes, three times each week, or
B. 15 minutes every day or 30 minutes, three times a week, or
C. 30 minutes every day or 1 hour three times a week.

Light Activities

Walk: brisk but easy pace
Dance: bouncy but easy pace
StairMaster, NordicTrack, treadmills, etc.: very easy, even pace
Pool exercises: a wide variety of light, easy activities
Biking (regular or stationary): easy, even pace
Bowling
Golf (continued on page 138)

*Please select Options only as they do not conflict with your personal
physician's recommendations.

Moderate Activities

Walk: moderate pace
Dance: moderate pace
StairMaster, NordicTrack, treadmills, etc.: moderate, even
   pace
Pool exercises: moderate, fun activities
Biking (regular or stationary): moderate pace
Jogging: light, brisk running
Swimming: moderate, even pace
Rollerskating: easy, even pace
Rope jumping: light, even pace
Tennis, racquetball, volleyball: light, easy pace
Free weights: moderate pace, some rest time included
Skiing: (cross-country or downhill): light pace
Aerobics: light pace

Vigorous Activities

Walk: fast pace, without interruption
Dance: fast pace, without interruption.
StairMaster, NordicTrack, treadmills, etc.: fast pace
Pool exercise: brisk exercises, without interruption.
Biking (regular or stationary): fast pace
Jogging: moderate or intense running
Swimming: fast pace
Rollerskating: moderate or fast pace
Rope jumping: moderate pace
Tennis, racquetball, volleyball: moderate or fast pace
Free weights: intense workout
Skiing: (cross-country or downhill): moderate or fast pace
Aerobics: moderate or fast pace

The MSG Easing Option

In Chapter 3, Loaded Guns, Ready Triggers, and Time Bombs, we detailed some of the craving and weight problems that can come from consuming MSG (monosodium glutamate), and although we will not repeat the details here, it is important to remember that MSG is often used *to make laboratory animals fat*; in our experience, what it can do to those little animals it most certainly can do to you.

**What MSG can do to laboratory animals
it most certainly can do to you.**

Remember that you may not realize MSG is in your food; Chinese restaurants may state that their foods contain "no added MSG," but if a restaurant uses soy sauce or teriyaki in its cooking, MSG is naturally present. In the same way, MSG may be added to your foods under many other names (see the chart that follows), yet you may never suspect that you are consuming it—until you experience the hunger, cravings, weight gain, or other symptoms that are often associated with MSG consumption.

This Option entails two steps: (1) label reading to uncover "hidden" MSG, and (2) the easing of your MSG use. Since food manufacturers have made it difficult to easily assess whether or not foods contain MSG, we will tell you what to look for and where to look for it.

Fresh produce, meats, fish, poultry, and the like rarely contain MSG. Restaurant foods often contain MSG, but some foods are more likely to be MSG-laden than others, and in the list below you will learn which foods you should be wary of. Oriental foods that contain soy sauce or teriyaki contain natural MSG.

Packaged and canned foods often contain moderate-to-high quantities of MSG, but with some help you will be able to spot the culprit. To determine whether or not a packaged, frozen, processed, or canned food contains MSG, look at the *ingredients*—not the nutritional portion of the label but, rather, the list of ingredients.

According to law, MSG must be included in the list of ingredients,

Finding the "Hidden" MSG in Your Food

Check the ingredients of all foods. MSG can be listed in any of the following ways:

Hydrolyzed plant protein	Hydrolyzed food protein
Hydrolyzed food starch	Natural flavors
Monosodium glutamate	Vegetable protein

PACKAGED, FROZEN, PROCESSED, DRIED, OR CANNED FOODS:
Many packaged, frozen, processed, dried, or canned foods may contain MSG but those foods that most consistently contain MSG include:

Bouillons	Consommés	Dips
Fish and shellfish	Meats (canned)	Hot dogs
(canned, jarred)	Salad dressings	Miso (soybean paste)
Luncheon meats	Soups	Sauces
Poultry (canned)	Teriyaki sauce	Stocks
Soybeans (roasted	Soy sauce	Stews
or boiled)	Tempeh	

RESTAURANT FOODS:
The packaged, frozen, processed, dried, or canned foods listed above may also be served at restaurants.

In addition to those above, look out for following restaurant foods that most consistently contain MSG:

Cheese sauces	Sauces (on meats and	Hot dogs
Luncheon meats	poultry, in particular)	Oriental dishes
Soups	Stews	

DELI FOODS:
Many deli luncheon meats, flavored cream cheeses and dips, as well as cold deli salads (tuna, chicken, and others) contain MSG. To determine if a food has MSG, do not rely on the counter-person's opinion. Ask to see the label yourself.

If a food item is "homemade" by the deli, either get the information from a deli person who knows and whom you can trust or, as an alternative, simply assume the food does indeed contain MSG.

but—and this is a big but—it can be referred to by many names (see the list that follows). Multiple names for MSG can result in consumers being unaware that they are indeed consuming MSG.

Your first task will be to be able to identify the MSG that may be "hidden" in your foods. Later we will tell you how to ease your MSG intake for better weight loss and craving reduction.

After determining which of the foods you eat contain MSG, you are ready to begin the second part of your Option.

After determining which of the foods you eat contain MSG, you are ready to begin the second part of your Option. For *one week*—a week that will serve as a comparison period—eliminate all foods that contain MSG, or that you think *might* contain MSG, from *all* your meals. Do this for one week only.

During this week continue to keep track of your weight and be aware of your general levels of hunger and cravings as well. After one week, you are free to add MSG-rich foods to your one daily Reward Meal only. Do not add any MSG-rich foods to your Craving-Reducing Meals. If after adding MSG-rich foods to your Reward Meals for one week, you notice no increase in your hunger, cravings, or weight, you can continue having them at your Reward Meals only.

If, however, there is an increase in *either* your hunger, your cravings, or your weight, immediately decrease or eliminate your intake of MSG-rich foods altogether from all meals.

Whether or not you notice any increase in hunger, cravings, or weight after adding MSG-rich foods to your Reward Meals while following this Option, never include them in your Craving-Reducing Meals.

The One MSG Exception That Makes the Rule

Tofu (soybean curd) contains a small amount of MSG, yet for many people it does not seem to cause increased hunger, cravings, or weight gain. During the one-week comparison period described above, in addition to removing MSG-rich foods from all meals, also eliminate tofu from all meals.

After one week, you can add tofu (along with other MSG-rich

foods) to your Reward Meals. If there is an increase in hunger, crav-ings, or weight gain, eliminate only other MSG-rich foods from your Reward Meal first. If the hunger, cravings, or weight gain continue for another week, you will have to eliminate tofu from your Reward Meal as well.

If, on the other hand, you notice no increase in hunger, cravings, or weight after adding all the MSG-rich foods to your Reward Meal, or if eliminating other MSG-rich foods corrected the problem, you can continue enjoying tofu at your Reward Meal.

If tofu at your Reward Meal does not increase your hunger, crav-ings, or weight, you are free to try adding tofu to your Craving-Reducing Meals as well. If tofu seems to cause increased hunger, cravings, or weight gain when you add it to your Craving-Reducing Meals, enjoy it at your Reward Meals only.

While following this Option, tofu is the only MSG-rich food that should ever be included in Craving-Reducing Meals. If you are par-ticularly sensitive to monosodium glutamate, you may find that tofu can increase rebound hunger and cravings and reduce weight loss when added to all meals. If so, or if you have concern, eliminate it from all meals or save it for your Reward Meals only.

**Your body is telling you how the foods
you eat are affecting *you*.**

If you find at any point that you begin to crave carbohydrates or start to gain weight, listen to your body; it is telling you how the foods you have been eating are affecting *you*, especially those which contain MSG.

The Over-The-Counter Remedy Timing Option

What you consume is certainly important in determining your cravings, weight, and health risk, but *when* and *how* you consume it may be equally important.

In this Option, you will learn how to change the timing of many of your over-the-counter remedies so as to help reduce their ability to increase your insulin levels (and so, your body's resistance to insulin as well).

> **Taking an anti-inflammatory only
> a couple of times a day
> could be significantly
> contributing to your battle with your weight.**

There are basically two ways in which over-the-counter remedies can raise your insulin levels. The first is by a general metabolic change that "cools" or "slows" the body. Anti-inflammatories such as aspirin, ibuprofen, acetaminophen, and the like found in products like Bayer, Tylenol, Advil, and others fall into this category. These products may affect your insulin levels by changing your whole metabolism, and while in general their benefits may outweigh any possible weight- and craving-related disadvantages, The LifeSpan Program's Basic Plan and its Options will help your body better handle the rises in insulin these types of remedies can cause.

A second group of over-the-counter remedies seems to raise your insulin levels much more directly and can more easily be lessened or eliminated entirely. These remedies are perceived by your body as "sweet" and include, among others:

Antacid tablets and liquids (like Tums, Rolaids, Mylanta, and others)
Breath fresheners (liquid, mints, or tablets such as Binaca, etc.)
Cough drops, syrups, and lozenges (for cough or sore throat)
Stool-softeners (like Metamucil, Konsyl, and the like)

These are nonprescription remedies that almost always contain at least one kind of sugar or sugar substitute in their nonactive ingredients. Manufacturers tend to place the list of active ingredients in a far more obvious place on the label than the "nonactive" ingredients, so it takes a bit of persistence sometimes to locate the sugar or sugar substitute (if it is listed at all).

However, you do not even have to try and locate the "sweet" addition to the remedy, unless you are simply curious. For the purposes of this Option, just assume that, in all likelihood, all of these over-the-counter remedies must contain some sort of sweetening agent, for if they were ever made without a sweetening agent they would be intolerable to the taste—and would never be marketable.

To incorporate this Option into your Program, first try to eliminate as many *nonessential* over-the-counter remedies as possible. Never eliminate a remedy that your physician has recommended or that you think is important to your health or well-being, but do consider having a glass of cool water rather than unthinkingly popping a cough drop in your mouth, or take a minute to brush your teeth and tongue rather than using a commercial breath freshener.

Reserve for your Reward Meals as many of the remaining essential over-the-counter remedies as possible. Some of these remedies are relatively easy to save for your Reward Meal; stool-softeners, for instance. Many of our people tell us that it really does not seem to matter which time of day you take them and they find that the bonus of decreased cravings and increased weight loss are a welcome benefit.

On the other hand, other remedies, like antacids used for stomach upset and cough medications, may by their very nature require that they be taken at times other than Reward Meals. If you cannot combine them with your Reward Meal, try (if possible) to combine them with a Craving-Reducing Meal, in order to try and reduce their insulin impact. If you cannot combine these remedies with either a Reward Meal or a Craving-Reducing Meal, then you will simply have to take them at a more appropriate time. At least do be aware that any increase in cravings or a slow-down in weight that *might follow* is not your fault and that the Program's Basic Plan and other Options can help correct the insulin imbalance that these remedies can cause.

Try to correct the need for the remedy, if at all possible. If not, just hold on until the need for this remedy has passed.

The Over-the-Counter Remedy Timing Option:
Putting the Option to Work

Anti-inflammatories

Examples: Aspirin, Tylenol, Advil, etc.

Remedy's effects: May decrease your body's ability to "burn" calories. Can decrease weight loss.

What you can do: Continue all over-the-counter remedies recommended by your physician.
Eliminate any other remedies that are no longer needed.
If you need to continue some over-the-counter remedies, keep in mind that although your weight loss may be somewhat slowed, the Program's Basic Plan and Options will help you continue moving toward your goals.

Antacids, breath fresheners, cough and cold medications, stool-softeners

Examples: Tums, Rolaids, Mylanta, Binaca, cough drops of all kinds, Metamucil, Konsyl, etc.

Remedy's effects: Body may sense remedy as a "sweet food" and can cause increased insulin release, leading to increased cravings and weight gain.

What you can do: Continue all over-the-counter remedies recommended by your physician.
Correct the need for the remedy whenever possible.
When possible, include all remedies in Reward Meals.
Include with Craving-Reducing Meals those remedies that must be taken at times other than at Reward Meals. When a remedy cannot be included in a meal, relax and accept that while there may be an increase in cravings or a slowing of weight loss, the Program's Basic Plan and Options will help offset the insulin-increasing effects of the remedy.

The Stress-Reduction Option

We have all heard how harmful stress can be to our health (this news itself causes stress); we are repeatedly told to avoid it. Life is so complicated, however, and so much is outside our control that for most of us eliminating stress is an unattainable goal.

At most, we can hope to somewhat reduce the stress in our lives or, perhaps, to reduce the effect it has on our bodies. Stress reduction is even more critical to the carbohydrate addict, for stress hormones raise insulin levels (which explains why so many people turn to food while under, or immediately after, a stressful experience). Many carbohydrate addicts seem to be particularly sensitive to this response, and for them stress reduction is a valuable part of any weight-loss, health-promotion program.

By choosing this Option, you are making a commitment to focus on recognizing and learning which steps to take to limit or reverse the effects that stress can have on your life (and your cravings and your weight as well).

The ideal situation, of course, is to be able to avoid unnecessary stress, and, needless to say, when you can do so without compromising other priorities in your life, we urge you to consider a stress-free course of action. At the same time, we recognize that there are times when stress is simply unavoidable.

When you cannot avoid stress altogether, we have some suggestions for limiting and relieving stress's effects on your body.

Recognizing Stress When You See It (and Feel It)

Your first task is to become sensitive to your body's response to stress. Many of us fail to realize that we are feeling pressured or stressed until we simply cannot stand it anymore and retreat completely or, more likely, explode. We then get caught up in feeling guilty or angry or both and in so doing we put ourselves under even greater stress.

When, on the other hand, you are able to recognize your body's early responses to stress, much more of the control resides in your hands. Using some of the techniques that follow, you may find it far easier than you had thought to limit or avoid stress's insulin-releasing power (and avoid the stress eating that can often follow).

> **The key to becoming sensitive to your body's stress response comes from learning to trust yourself.**

The key to becoming sensitive to your body's stress response comes from learning to trust yourself. Rather than accommodating, pushing through negative thoughts and feelings as they begin to build within you, you must, instead, stop the process midstream, and focus on the very ideas and experiences that you are finding uncomfortable. Is the tightness in the back of your neck coming from tiredness or from the impossible demands that your boss is making on you? Is the funny feeling in the pit of your stomach related to going home and facing unfinished family business? Are you really hungry or will eating just make you feel "better" or perhaps give you an excuse to go to sleep and avoid the task that you don't want to do?

Commit the coming week to listening and learning about your body. You may find it better to work backwards; if you lose your temper or storm out or just retreat, try to recapture what you were feeling or thinking right before the emotional buildup. Make note of the thought or feeling but don't judge it; just be on the lookout for that feeling or that thought the next time it returns. Let it be your signal that *you* need to be attended to, that you are experiencing stress and that you need to take action to reduce stress's impact on your body.

Taking Action Against Stress

Once you become aware that you are under stress you basically have three choices: avoid escalation, limit the duration, or remove the impact.

Avoiding argument escalation involves refraining from the back-and-forth emotional acceleration that usually accompanies arguments—the screaming, fighting, crying, or fury that almost all of us have experienced. Avoiding these escalations does not necessarily involve "holding in" your feelings but, rather, not engaging in a useless verbal war. Check with a professional counselor, discuss alternatives with your friends, pick up a good book or audiotape by a favorite author. Do whatever you need to do to find the right "noncombatative" way to deal with highly charged conversations, but do plan an alternative action to help you avoid these argument escalations that can lead to "post-argument" carbohydrate hunger.

Limiting the duration of a stressful experience involves taking charge of the moment and giving up on "winning." By realizing that the real victory in any stressful moment involves taking care of your body and your health, you will find yourself able to calmly and effectively free yourself of the stressful situation.

Some people find that they can directly limit the duration of a stressful experience by forcefully stating their limits *before* the end points of time and emotion are reached. "I know it's important to come to some decision on this, but I can't think clearly right now. I don't want to walk out on this," they might add, "but I need time to let my feelings subside so I can think clearly." This example might be met with some resistance, if the other person is caught up in his or her emotions, but repeating the same point over and over will leave them with no other choice.

Other people find a more indirect approach better for them. It does not matter which tactics you employ in order to limit the duration of stress; what matters is finding the technique that is right for you, so that you remain focused on taking care of *your* self.

Removing the impact of a stress may mean removing yourself, physically or mentally, from the situation; it may mean actively focusing on yourself.

Removing the impact of a stress may mean removing yourself, physically or mentally, from a situation. Or you may find that you can remove a stress's impact by focusing on your own body through active exercises (such as jogging or dancing) or by stress-relieving exercises (like yoga or tai chi chuan). You may find a warm bath, a good nap, or fine companionship does the trick. Whatever works to relax you and remove the impact of stress (while staying on your program) should be planned for and incorporated into your life.

If you fail to plan for your own de-stressing choices, your body will, in the end, push you into less productive alternatives. Act as if you were your own honored guest; take the time and energy to treat yourself well and your body will show it.

Breaking The Sugar-Substitute Connection Option

NOTE: This Option applies to sugar substitutes that are often used to sweeten coffee, tea, "diet" sodas and drinks, or other "diet" foods. Packets of these sugar substitutes contain no caloric value (contain "zero" calories) or up to 3 calories each. For beverages that contain added juice or added flavors or all other beverages, see the Carbohydrate-Rich Foods list (page 122).

Many carbohydrate addicts consider sugar substitutes a "free ride," noncaloric "goodies" that can allow you to have "something sweet" with no weight-related repercussions. While many people continue to hold tightly to this belief, if they but kept an open mind, they would find that their real-life experiences often tell an entirely different story.

You may consider sugar substitutes a "free ride," but the sweet taste they provide may be keeping you in the yoyo diet cycle.

The sweetness of sugar substitutes can falsely signal your body that a sweet "meal" is coming and excess insulin may be released so as to handle the expected onslaught of high-caloric foods. When no carbohydrates are forthcoming, the high levels of insulin that remain can easily lead to increases in cravings, weight gain, and in health-related risks. (For more details, see Chapter 3, "Loaded Guns, Ready Triggers, and Time Bombs.")

Reducing or eliminating your intake of sugar substitutes can be one of the most important Options you can choose. First, decide if (1) you want to remove all sugar substitutes from your diet, or (2) if you want to confine them to your Reward Meal only, or (3) if you simply want to limit your intake throughout the day.

If you want to include sugar substitutes, we strongly recommend that you limit them to your Reward Meal only (these changes can really help guarantee a decrease in cravings along with your permanent weight-loss success), but, as always, the choice is really in your hands. But whether you eliminate or reduce your intake of sugar substitutes or confine them to your Reward Meal, be clear about which choice you are making. Be specific.

Don't say: "I'll just try and cut down on my intake of sugar substitutes." With something that can be as addictive as diet sodas or artificially sweetened coffee or tea you need to be far more specific.

Do say: "Other than at my Reward Meals, I will have only one diet soda or one cup of coffee with a sugar substitute during the day," or "I will have sugar substitutes at my Reward Meals only," or "I will not have any sugar substitutes at all."

**Watch how easy it can be to break
your sugar-substitute connection.**

It is *essential* that, whichever your choice, you remember that on this program cutting down or eliminating sugar substitutes may be far easier than you ever anticipated. Have lots of cold water or unflavored seltzer around, and as your cravings quickly diminish and your weight drops, watch how easy it can be to break your sugar-substitute connection.

The Complex Carbo Option

All carbohydrate-rich foods, of course, contain carbohydrates. In addition, they may contain fat and/or protein as well, but when dealing with carbohydrate addiction, it appears that the impact of carbohydrates on the body is the most important factor in weight loss and health promotion.

In general, the carbohydrates in carbohydrate-rich foods fall into two categories, simple sugars and complex carbohydrates. Some typical examples of simple sugars include table sugar, honey, fruit sugar (fructose), lactose (milk sugar), corn syrup, and high fructose corn syrup. Foods containing these simple sugars are often themselves referred to as "simple sugars" and include fruit and fruit juice, candy (including chocolate), cookies, ice cream, sugar-sweetened soda, etc.

Complex carbohydrates are those foods which are rich in starches. Some examples of typical complex carbohydrates include such grain and grain products as breads and crackers, rice, pasta, and such starchy vegetables as potatoes and corn.

Many carbohydrate addicts find their cravings and weight drop when they replace simple sugars with complex carbohydrates as part of their Reward Meal.

Although the body releases insulin whenever any carbohydrate-rich foods are eaten, either those containing simple sugars or those containing complex carbohydrates, many carbohydrate addicts find their cravings and weight remain lower when they eat primarily complex carbohydrates, as opposed to simple sugars, for the carbohydrate portion of their Reward Meal. Their experience is backed up by research that indicates that both the frequency of consumption as well as the type of carbohydrate consumed can strongly affect insulin responses.

This Option entails replacing simple sugars with complex carbohydrates for the carbohydrate portion of your daily Reward Meal.

To fulfill this Option, simply read over the Complex Carbo

Option Chart that follows. For your Reward Meal, as much as possible choose foods from the left-hand column (the complex carbohydrates) rather than the simple sugars in the right-hand column for the 1/3 carbohydrate portion of your Reward Meal.

Certainly there will be times when you want a special treat, and once in a while an "indulgence" is certainly to be expected.

Certainly there will be times when you want a special treat, even though it does contain simple sugars, and once in a while an "indulgence" is certainly to be expected. Just remember that to fulfill this Option you should choose complex carbohydrates rather than simple sugars as much as possible at your Reward Meal.

Also remember to keep your Reward Meal balanced; the sum total of all carbohydrates (complex and simple) in that meal should equal 1/3 and should be balanced with 1/3 protein and 1/3 Craving-Reducing vegetables in addition to a pre-meal salad. (For more details on balancing your Reward Meal, see Chapter 5, "The Basic Plan," page 107.)

In the chart that follows, you may notice that fruits and fruit juices are not listed. Although both fruit and fruit juice contain *simple sugars* (they are *not* complex carbohydrates), fruit also contains a great amount of fiber, which may help lessen the insulin-releasing impact of the simple sugar it contains. The verdict, then, is still out on fruit in your Reward Meal. Watch how your body responds to it. If you find that you want more and more fruit, or that your cravings or weight are not lessening as they should, discuss with your physician the possibility of replacing fruit with a high-fiber complex carbohydrate. Also look at the other foods you eat and the vitamins you take to make sure you are receiving all the nutrients that fruit might otherwise provide.

As opposed to fruit, fruit juice does not contain a high-fiber balance to its high-sugar content. Unless otherwise instructed by your physician, it may be best to replace all fruit juice with the whole fruit from which it was made. In any case, always include fruit (and fruit juice, if you have it) as part of the carbohydrate portion of your Reward Meal.

The Complex Carbo Option Chart

Choose any of the following foods containing complex carbohydrates:	Instead of any of these foods that contain simple sugars:
Bagels and other breads (preferably whole-grain)	Cake
Beans (legumes)	Candy
Chips (low-fat* or regular)	Chocolate
Corn	Cookies
Crackers	Donuts
Nuts* and seeds (low-fat or regular)	Fruited yogurt, regular or frozen
Pasta	Ice cream or ice milk
Peas	Pie
Popcorn	Pudding
Potatoes	Sherbet
Pretzels	Snack bars
Rice	

*Always follow your physician's guidance regarding low-fat alternatives.

The Caffeine Reducing Option

In the area of caffeine research, scientists seem to report widely varying findings. Researchers such as Dr. D. Robertson and his colleagues, reporting in the *New England Journal of Medicine*, have noted that caffeine can lead to rises in blood pressure as well as an increase of neurotransmitters (biochemicals in the body that communicate with the sympathetic and central nervous systems). Other researchers have reported that the body "adjusts" to caffeine intake and that long-term consumption of caffeine can decrease the probability of caffeine-induced high blood pressure.

Still other researchers have reported that caffeine consumption can lead to heart palpitations, tremors, nervousness, and insomnia. Withdrawal of caffeine has been found to cause headaches, and excessive intake of caffeine has been found to result in gastrointestinal problems, including diarrhea.

Of most importance to the carbohydrate addict, however, are such research findings as those by Dr. T. W. Uhde and his colleagues at the National Institute of Mental Health who report that caffeine consumption can lead to increases in the "stress hormone" cortisol by up to 500 percent! That's five times the normal amount of this insulin-releasing hormone.

You may not notice the insulin impact of caffeine, however. It can be hidden by the temporary stimulant effect of this substance (sometimes referred to as a "drug"). Because caffeine may make you feel "better" temporarily, you may not realize that the slump you hit two hours later can be the result of low blood sugar levels—coming from a caffeine-induced insulin release channeling your blood sugar into your fat cells. You may simply sense that you need another "cup of coffee" and reach for one, only to begin the cycle again.

**The Basic Plan and Options in this chapter
(especially the Chromium Option) may strongly
help reduce symptoms of "caffeine withdrawal."**

Many of our carbohydrate addicts report remarkable changes when they reduce or eliminate the caffeine in their diet. The initial headaches and feelings of tiredness that some attribute to "caffeine withdrawal" before beginning the Program are completely eliminated or minimized while on this program by the Program's Basic Plan as well as by the other Options (especially the Chromium Option) found in this chapter.

In any case, the decrease in cravings and increase in the rate of weight loss that so many carbohydrate addicts have reported after selecting the Caffeine Reducing Option seems to more than compensate for a temporary and reduced need for a caffeine "fix."

To select this Option, simply look over the list of foods, beverages, and remedies that follow. Whenever possible and when appropriate, choose noncaffeine alternatives for these items or avoid them altogether. On food and beverage labels, look over lists of ingredients carefully, and for over-the-counter remedies, read both the active as well as the nonactive ingredients lists.

Caffeine-Rich Foods, Beverages, and Over-the-Counter Remedies

Choose decaffeinated or noncaffeine alternatives or, if appropriate, eliminate:

Coffee
Colas and other soft drinks
Tea (regular and some herb teas)
Chocolate
Cough, cold, and flu remedies
Over-the-counter "diet" pills
Pain relievers (some aspirins and other anti-inflammatories)

The Food Frequency Reducing Option

Your body is amazingly adaptable. And although our research findings have documented that the more often carbohydrate addicts consume carbohydrates, the more they want them, you have probably suspected this "scientific finding" all along.

As The Program's Basic Plan and Options work to reduce your insulin levels, you have probably experienced a significant decrease of cravings and hunger along the way. You may *not*, however, have changed your basic eating pattern of three meals (and additional snacks) each day.

Some carbohydrate addicts find that the more they eat, the more they want.
They have trained themselves to "eat by the clock," allowing themselves food only when it's "time to eat."

Carbohydrate addicts have often been trained to eat "by the clock"—allowing themselves food at "acceptable" times. This is especially true for those of us who have felt that if we were allowed we could virtually eat all of the time.

On this Program, however, the reduction in cravings and the increase in control you experience will probably allow you to respond to your body's true hunger.

This Option asks you to respond to your body's *need* for food rather than old rules that may have dictated when you should eat. Stop eating by the clock. If it is "time" for a Craving-Reducing Meal and you are simply not hungry, put it off—or skip it altogether. You may choose to have it later in the day or during the evening. You may choose to have a smaller meal made up of Craving-Reducing foods (which would constitute a Craving-Reducing Snack) instead. In any case, do not eat if you are not hungry.*

The one exception to skipping meals relates to your Reward Meal. If you are not hungry when it is time for your Reward Meal, do *not* skip it altogether. You may choose to postpone your Reward

---

*Unless otherwise directed by your physician.

Meal for a while, but do remember that carbohydrates are important to your health and satisfaction and should be enjoyed every day. Eat a smaller meal if you are really not hungry (still balanced in smaller portions of salad, carbohydrates, protein, and Craving-Reducing vegetables), but do not skip your Reward Meal altogether.

If you want to skip or reduce any Craving-Reducing Meals or Snacks, you most certainly can. Some carbohydrate addicts assume that they will feel weak or get a headache from not eating, but their expectations are based on a time when they were eating carbohydrates often throughout the day—when their insulin levels may have been high and their blood sugar levels low. While we do not recommend that you do without food until you feel faint, we do offer you the choice to skip a meal when you aren't really hungry. You will probably be very surprised at how little you miss it.

Many of our readers find that breakfast is an easy meal to skip or to put off. You can have a cup of coffee or tea (decaffeinated if you like) with milk (only once at times other than Reward Meals) instead of breakfast. You may feel very comfortable and able to hold off until lunch at that time. Or, you may choose to postpone your breakfast until midmorning (11:00 A.M., for instance) and combine your breakfast and lunch. You may choose to skip one meal or another during weekdays and not on weekends, or vice versa.

Stay focused on your body and your hunger. Do not push yourself. Give yourself "permission" to skip or delay a Craving-Reducing Meal. Do not demand it. It will come naturally as your cravings are reduced.

Once your cravings are greatly reduced or eliminated, do notice if you are eating out of habit or because you are truly hungry, and if you eliminate or delay any meal, make sure you give yourself a "pleasure break" instead—that is, pleasurable activities other than food during your mealtimes.

Remind yourself that you do not have to eat in order to have a reason to leave your desk or to take a break. Bring headphones to work and during the time you would normally be eating, listen to some music you enjoy. Bring a book on tape to listen to or a favorite book to read. Bring some knitting. Take a walk or a nap. Choose any alternative, but do take the time that would have been used to consume a meal and "give" it to yourself in the form of some other

Birthday Blues: PJ's Story

PJ's letter was short but powerful. "It was my fifty-seventh birthday," he began. "We were supposed to go out with friends for dinner and celebrate(!) and when I went to put on my suit, that was the last straw. I couldn't button the jacket, and if I stuffed myself into the pants, I knew I was going to be miserable. I felt old and fat! I hated the people we were having dinner with, I hated my wife for agreeing to the dinner, and, most of all, I hated myself."

PJ went on to tell us that the summer before he had developed a stress injury from jogging and that because he could no longer exercise, he had "profoundly" lost his battle with his weight that he had been "holding at bay [no pun intended], for years."

"Within a few months, I started wondering if anyone noticed that I had put on weight, but now, with me bursting out of my suit, I had to face the truth. I swear I was not eating much more than I always did, but now it all just seemed to turn into fat.

"After my birthday snit-fit, my wife went out and bought your book. It's a wonder she didn't throw it at me. Anyway, I started your program right away and the guidelines were simple. I started losing weight and I felt terrific. Then, after a few weeks, it all slowed down. The cravings were gone but the weight wasn't coming off like it had been.

"I was about to weigh myself one morning, steeling myself for the latest verdict, when I heard that you were coming on the Today Show. I stopped, mid-weigh. There you were, talking about how diet soda can make some people hungry and even interfere with their losing weight. I had just bought a case of liter bottles of my favorite flavor, diet raspberry ginger ale. In the few weeks I had been on the diet, I had tripled my intake of diet soda and it paid to buy it by the case. I watched the interview and it was like you were talking right to me. You talked about chromium and how important it was, especially as we got older. It all made sense.

"Well, the long and the short of it is this: I added GTF and cut out all the diet sodas. My cravings were gone. I found myself 'forgetting' to eat lunch and rarely, if ever, wanting snacks (I used to be the Snack King of my family). The weight dropped. No effort. And has continued to drop. Today I am slim and my doctor swears I'm doing something very right. If I had stopped with just the guidelines, I would still be fat. Those 'options' weren't options, they changed my life."

But PJ added one final postscript. "P.S. By the way, my fifty-eighth birthday was last month and I still couldn't wear that suit. This time, though, it was three sizes too big, so I went out and bought two new ones instead."

pleasurable activity. (Doing errands or making phone calls are not acceptable substitutes unless you *really* want to do them.)

During your "lunch hour," you might want to take the phone off the hook or put it on voice mail or activate the answering machine during these times. If you work at home, get away from your duties and take the time for yourself.

If you make it a choice between food and work, you know what will be most likely to win.

Give yourself the choice either to eat or to not eat in combination with other pleasures. Don't make it a choice between food and work; you know what will be most likely to win then.

Two "No-No's" and an "Always"

Never skip meal after meal after meal. Don't eat Craving-Reducing Meals if you are not hungry, but always have at least one Reward Meal each day. Don't skip Craving-Reducing Meals if that leaves you feeling weak or with a headache or showing other signs of low blood sugar, or if you tend to get so hungry that you may go off your Program. This Option should spring from an easy non-hunger; it should never be a struggle. And, as always, do check with your physician.

PART III

PERSONALIZING YOUR PROGRAM:

SUCCESS FOR LIFE

CHAPTER 7

A GREAT MEASURE OF SUCCESS

The secret of success is constancy to purpose.
—Benjamin Disraeli, 1870

*O*ne of the greatest mistakes that most people make in any weight-loss program is their erratic approach to weighing themselves. Motivated far more by their years of fears than by logical thinking, some dieters pop on and off the scale more often than they open the refrigerator door. They weigh themselves at any time of day that might give them a low weight: after going to the bathroom, when feeling particularly slim, or after being "good" for an especially long period, all in hopes of tangible confirmation and proof of their sacrifices. On the other hand, dieters are equally known to weigh themselves after having "cheated" to see if "it shows" or in hopes of "getting away with it."

> **Motivated more by years of fears than by logical thinking, some dieters pop on and off the scale more often than they open the refrigerator door.**

Some dieters weigh themselves daily, every morning, and find that their attitude toward the coming day—and themselves—is determined by the numbers which appear before them. Traditionally, commercial programs and physicians weigh dieters once a week and from that weight determine a full week's success—or failure.

Yet all these ways of determining weight-loss progress have two things in common: they can lead to devastatingly powerful self-judgments based on a momentary measurement and, even worse, they are notoriously inaccurate in measuring *real* weight loss.

Your body is not a machine, and no matter what anyone has told you, you are far more than a simple mathematical formula which says that at any moment your body's weight is equal to the difference between calories consumed and calories used. Even machines don't work with that sort of perfection.

> **Your body is not a machine; calories in do not always equal calories out.**

Chances are, you have seen it firsthand yourself. You work hard on a diet, sacrificing, following the rules, and you simply do not lose the weight you "should have." Or you cheat a bit, eating forbidden food, perhaps a great deal of it, and just when you thought the scale would condemn you, it barely shows a gain.

You may have been told that 3,500 calories equal a pound of fat but almost all of us have had the experience of gaining several pounds overnight *without* the benefit of all those added calories. "Water weight," we conclude; a generalized catch-all term that sums up the fact that at times our scale seems to have a mind of its own.

We may try to coax our scale to become more predictable by practicing a sort of "scale ballet," balancing ourselves this way and that or moving the scale on that portion of the floor where it is most likely to give us the "best" weight, perhaps in hopes of finding a place in the room where the earth's gravity is least powerful.

Avoiding weighing yourself does not work.
You need a sane, sensible way to keep track of your progress
without pain or blame.

Some of us, brutalized by the self-blame that can come from trying to control this unfeeling opponent, end up avoiding weighing ourselves altogether, and try to convince ourselves that our clothes will adequately indicate our gains or losses.

But whether you tend to be scale-addicted, scale-phobic, or both, we have a sane and scientific way to evaluate your progress without the pain and frustration you may have experienced in the past.

This Way Out

Given that home bathroom scales are notoriously inaccurate (if a scale varies by as little as 1 percent and you weigh 150 pounds, you can expect it to be "in error" from one weighing to the next by $1^{1}/_{2}$ pounds in *either* direction), and given that our bodies' responses to the salt and additives in foods can add pounds to any particular weighing, it makes no sense to expect that any single weighing can be relied upon.

If your scale has only a 1 percent error,
it can easily vary from one weight to another
by 1 to 2 pounds in *either* direction.

Avoiding weighing yourself does not any make sense either. You need to be able to gauge your success on the Program, for motivation purposes as well as helping you to decide when to add another Option. If you are avoiding the scale, you most likely have been brutalized by its unfair declarations in the past and you need to free yourself of its, others', and your own judgments so that you can best use the information without abusing it.

We have an easy and effective way out. By using a series of daily weighings and finding your average weight (simple directions follow), you will avoid the ups and downs that often come with water retention and scale inaccuracies. You will be able to figure your "average" weekly weight loss and adjust your Program to keep your weight loss steady. Most of all, you will be able to stay motivated without feeling like you are at the scale's mercy.

Averaging Your Weight

Weigh yourself each day at about the same time and under the same conditions. It need not be at the same hour. If you sleep late on weekends, for instance, you can weigh yourself later than you would on weekdays; just do make certain that your weighing takes place in the same sequence of your day—after going to the bathroom but before breakfast, for instance. Weigh yourself while wearing the same kind of clothing; no clothing is best, and always, always, write down your weight on Your Progress Chart (page 173).

Weigh yourself every single day, even days when you feel "heavy"; your weekly average will compensate for daily differences. After one week you will be ready to average your weight.

How to Average One Week's Weight:

1. Add up all the daily weights for one week.
2. Divide that total by the *number* of weighings for that week (usually 7).
3. This gives you that week's average weight.

Example: Your weights for a week were as follows:

Week Beginning (date)	MON. (weight)	TUES. (weight)	WED. (weight)	THURS. (weight)	FRI. (weight)	SAT. (weight)	SUN. (weight)	Average Weight for Week
8/4/97	151	152	151	152	150	149	150	151

When you add up all the weighings, you get a total of 1055.

Now divide by the number of weighings (7). You can use a calculator if you like.

Dividing the total 1055 by 7 gives you 150.7 (rounded off to 151 lbs.).

This gives you your average weight for the week.

If, for any reason, you miss a weighing or two during a week (perhaps you were away), simply add all the weights that you do have, then divide the total by the number of weighings for that week (5 or 6 weighings, for instance).

At the end of your second week of weighing, simply subtract the second week's average from the first week's average. This will tell you how much weight you have lost, without the ups and downs of daily fluctuations.

Example: Your first week's average was 151 pounds; your second week's average was 149 pounds. On the average, you lost 2 pounds.

Your average weight loss can help guide you as you continue on the Program. In general, and with some exceptions noted below, you should continue to lose weight at the same rate as that which you calculated when you subtracted the second week's average from the first week's average. If you find that this weight loss (on the average) slows, adding Options (Chapter 6) should help keep you moving.

If you have been eating out a great deal during any particular week, a slowdown in weight loss or even some minimal weight gain should be expected (no more than 1 to 1½ pounds on the average). Wait one week only for the weight loss to resume, and if it does not, add an Option to your program. Also see Chapter 8, A Lifestyle Plan—A Plan for Life, for some additional guidance. You will find that it includes some surprising and useful hints.

It is essential that you leave old expectations behind. Be realistic, and learn to be content with a *healthy* weight-loss rate. Studies have shown repeatedly that those who lose their weight at a rate of no more than $1/2$ to 2 pounds per week are more likely to keep the weight off than those who lose weight rapidly. That may seem a bit slow to those of us who have been through a whole gamut of "fad diets" and "quick weight-loss plans" but $1/2$ to 2 pounds a week must become your expected weight-loss goal. Remember, this Program is all about breaking that yo-yo dieting cycle, for good!

The two of us together have lost more than 200 pounds at a slow and sensible rate, and we have kept it off for far more than a decade. We have helped others do it in the same way and we know what works. You cannot expect to lose ten pounds in a week, remain healthy, and keep it off. This is a lifestyle and lifelong program, a lifespan program; it will reward you every day with the food you love as well as a steady, sensible, and deprivation-free weight loss.

Some Important "Know's"

To stay on track, it is very helpful to concentrate on several "know's."

Know Your Goal

Decide on your goal weight. Do not pick a number out of the air and in general don't use some anonymous "ideal" weight chart. Consult with your doctor and be realistic (don't set a goal ideal for someone ten or twenty years your junior). Choose a weight that will help you stay healthy *and* happy.

Base your goal weight on your age and your particular body build, with a realistic eye towards your lifestyle and health needs.

**Choose a goal weight that will help you
stay healthy *and* happy.**

Know Your Body

Some of us have special weight-gain triggers. For the two of us, although we stay well within the confines of our respective programs, restaurant meals make our daily weights rise by several pounds. Added salt and unavoidable MSG seem to be the culprit. A generally richer type of cooking or some unknown factor may be the problem—we are not always sure of the exact cause—but whatever the source, we can be sure that when we eat our meals at restaurants while on vacation or business trips, our daily weights (and our weekly averages) will jump.

We have seen this happen repeatedly for over a decade and we neither panic nor react. We know as well that when we get home, the "restaurant weight" will disappear within a matter of days.

> **When you look at your average weekly weight loss, take into account *your* body's reactions, changes, and responses.**

Most menstruating and premenstrual women find their weights rise by 3 to 5 pounds even though their daily intake of food has not changed. The weights of men and postmenopausal women will naturally vary by several pounds as well, so it is essential that you do not react to your daily weights. Average your weekly weight, and, after calculating the change from your previous week's average, remember to take into account *your* body's reactions, changes, and responses.

Know Your Mind

Weigh yourself, write it down on Your Progress Chart (page 173), and let it go. Stay focused on your goal of sticking to the Program and letting the weight take care of itself. If your weight is not decreasing by $1/2$ to 2 pounds per week, read over the helpful hints in Chapter 5 and consider adding an Option (Chapter 6).

> **Reacting to daily weights can completely throw you off track. Stay focused on your program and your weight will take care of itself.**

Reacting to daily weights can completely throw you off track. If your weight goes up (from water retention or scale inaccuracy), you can rationalize that the Program is not working. If your weight remains the same as the day before, you can likewise convince yourself to "cheat" because you are not making enough daily progress. If the scale shows a particularly low daily weight, you can convince yourself that you can spare a "treat" and again rationalize going off your program. Whatever the reality, if you have a mind to, daily weights can be used as an excuse to lose sight of your goal.

Stay focused. Weigh yourself and make yourself leave all judgments behind. You are no more responsible for your daily weights than you are the numbers a laboratory technician might get from your blood tests.

Write down your daily weights, then use them in calculating your average weekly weight. Stay focused on following your Program; if you want to increase your weight-loss rate, simply add any Option as you desire.

The Blessed Sound Of Silence: Ginny's Story

"I can barely believe I'm talking about this in public," Ginny A. began, "but I want you to know what happened and I can't seem to put it down in writing."

The book-signing table was crowded with people who came to meet us and stayed to share their stories. "When you said that I had to average my weight, I just kind of skimmed over that. I mean, I wasn't ignoring what you said, I just didn't think it was *crucial* or anything. Besides, I had such terrible experiences with being weighed that I just couldn't bear the thought of getting on a scale every day and facing the voices in my head. It was as if my entire self-worth was being determined in that moment on the scale. So I figured that, although I would follow your other advice, I would stick to my way of weighing myself—once a week on Sunday morning."

Others around the table gathered closer, smiling sympathetically, as Ginny described the power that getting on the scale held for so many. "So I started your diet—I can't really call it a diet," she added parenthetically, "and it was easy, just like you said. And Sunday morning weigh-ins showed that I was losing weight, just like you said," she confirmed. "And the voices in my head congratulated me and I felt fine."

"Then something happened." The crowd around us grew quiet and listened. "I started living for my Sunday mornings; to prove to the voices in my head that I was 'good,' that I hadn't cheated. I started eating less on Saturdays so that I would show more of a weight loss and even considered taking a laxative to speed it up. I used to do it whenever I went on a diet and wanted to lose weight fast and I hated it; I became obsessed with my weight and everything I was became centered around that number. And no matter what else was happening in my life, the voices in my head, commenting on my weight loss, became the ultimate judge; telling me if I had succeeded or not.

"So I came to see you two years ago when you were on tour. You were signing books right here. I don't know if you remember," she went on, "but you yelled at me!"

We waited and so did all the others.

"You yelled at me. You said that no matter what I had to stop judging myself by my weight and that it was important to remember that if I was sticking to my program, I was succeeding. You said that even if I wasn't staying on my program 100 percent, I wasn't failing; I simply had to find out what was triggering my need to go off. You said that chances were it was something I was eating or that was hidden in my food. And most of all, you said that I had to average my weight, that I had to force myself to understand that daily weight changes were feeding my obsession."

Ginny went on to share that concentrating on her program, rather than her weight, lifted a burden of guilt that had been on her shoulders "for so long I never even noticed it anymore." By determining her weight based on weekly averages, Ginny found that a single weight's fluctuation could no longer throw her "off base." She found herself able to think more clearly, she told us, and if her weight didn't drop "dramatically each week," she was still able to stay calm and realistically plan changes for the week to come. Important changes that brought with them the success she had waited for so long.

"Besides losing sixty-five pounds"—she smiled, looking shy and proud at the same time—"I've lost the feeling that I'm being judged and yelled at all the time—not because I'm succeeding at losing weight but because I'm concentrating on me and my program—in the long run. I'm forty-one years old and for the first time in my life I don't feel like I'm always on trial any more. Now, instead of voices that demand that I prove that I'm all right, there is a blessed sound of silence."

YOUR PROGRESS CHART

Record your weight every day.

To see if you are losing weight, compare your weekly averages only.

(To get your weekly average, add up all the weights in that week, then divide by the number of weighings.)

Week Beginning (date)	MON. (weight)	TUES. (weight)	WED. (weight)	THURS. (weight)	FRI. (weight)	SAT. (weight)	SUN. (weight)	Average Weight for Week

CHAPTER 8

A LIFESTYLE PLAN—
A PLAN FOR LIFE

He who prepares for tomorrow, prepares for life.
—Ovid, circa 10 B.C.

*Y*ou have learned all about the Guidelines and Options that make up The Carbohydrate Addict's LifeSpan Program, and now it is time to adapt the Program to fit your particular lifestyle, preferences, challenges, and needs.

This chapter will help you customize your program so that you can stay with it, and enjoy it, for life.

The first section in this chapter, Planning Your Choices, will help you in broadening your Basic Guideline and Option alternatives. It includes advice on how to switch your Reward Meal timing, enhance your eating enjoyment at celebrations, parties, and vacations; Reward Meal timing tips; where to get a delicious fast-food Craving-Reducing Meal; saving time and money on the Program, and delicious Craving-Reducing breakfast alternatives.

The second section, Trouble Shooting, will help you pinpoint mistakes that can interfere with your weight loss or cause you to crave carbohydrates. In addition, it offers special advice on increasing your weight-loss rate with our easy substitution tips.

Planning Your Choices

Switching Your Reward Meal Timing

While most people enjoy their Reward Meal in the evening, there is no reason why you cannot enjoy a Reward Meal lunch or breakfast instead of a Reward Meal dinner. The only considerations that should be kept in mind in relation to changing your Reward Meal timing are that (1) in addition to your Craving-Reducing Meals you should only have one Reward Meal a day, (2) that your Reward Meal should always be concluded within one hour, and (3) that, whenever you have it, your Reward Meal should still be balanced and include salad, followed by protein, Craving-Reducing vegetables, and carbohydrates in equal portions.

Most people do not have trouble with the first two considerations, and while including vegetables and salad in a lunchtime Reward Meal does not usually present a problem, the very nature of typical breakfast foods makes the inclusion of salad and vegetables in a breakfast Reward Meal a bit more of a challenge.

**You can enjoy
a Reward Meal lunch
or a special Reward Meal breakfast treat.**

So, chances are, you will not hit any snags in switching your Reward Meal dinner to a Reward Meal lunch, but if you are considering switching to a Reward Meal breakfast, here is what we would suggest: Since your Reward Meal breakfast will not be ideal, do not plan to have it on a regular basis. Unless you intend to have salad and vegetables as part of a regular Reward Meal breakfast, save your Reward Meal breakfasts for special occasions. Then, on an *infrequent* basis, as long as your weight permits, you can enjoy the special treat of a somewhat less balanced Reward Meal breakfast.

Make sure that you include lots of protein in your Reward Meal breakfast, however, and if it is possible to include some Craving-

Reducing vegetables, that would certainly be a good idea. Do not make your Reward Meal breakfast a "carbo feast." Still, if you keep your Reward Meal breakfast as a special treat, you can probably "get away" with it being a bit out of balance, *once in a while*.

Most people really enjoy a Reward Meal breakfast on vacation or as part of a special celebration. Remember that if you are having a Reward Meal breakfast, your evening meal for that day should now include only Craving-Reducing foods.

The next day, when you return to your usual Reward Meal time, you may need an extra Craving-Reducing Snack to help get you back into your rhythm, but within a day you'll be back on schedule. Do not be concerned if your daily weight jumps a bit; extra carbohydrates (often taken in at Reward Meal breakfasts) can hold water. Just return to your usual Reward Meal timing *and* balance and your weight loss should resume.

Do not switch your Reward Meal timing on impulse. Do not suddenly decide, for instance, that pancakes sound good for breakfast and spontaneously change your eating pattern. Plan any change ahead of time and make it a special treat. (If those pancakes sound good, have them as part of a balanced Reward Meal dinner—for dessert, for instance.)

Parties, Celebrations, and Vacations

Here are some great ways to enjoy parties, celebrations, and vacations *without going off your program*. Switching your Reward Meal time is an easy way to get in on the fun without the guilt (see above).

You can also sequence a Reward Meal with a Craving-Reducing Meal to get you through a prolonged feast. Let's say you have been invited to a wedding celebration that includes a cocktail and hors d'oeuvres hour followed a bit later by a sit-down dinner. If you call ahead and find that the dinner includes all the foods you need for a Craving-Reducing dinner (salad, protein, and Craving-Reducing vegetables), you can feel safe in enjoying the cocktail and hors d'oeuvres hour as your Reward Meal, knowing that your Craving-Reducing Meal will follow.

Try to include some Craving-Reducing vegetables (from a crûdité platter of celery, cauliflower, and mushrooms and dip, for instance) and some protein (cheese and shrimp, for example). Enjoy your cocktails at the same time. Then, after a good hour or so in between, enjoy a dinner that includes only Craving-Reducing foods (for example, salad, asparagus, and steak). You probably will not be tempted by the dessert (you will have already had a Reward Meal cocktail hour and a Craving-Reducing Meal), but if the dessert looks good, remember that you can always take home some wedding cake and save it for tomorrow's Reward Meal.

Cruises and other vacations, family celebrations, and parties can be handled in the same way. Think of your Reward Meal as your "wild card" and your Craving-Reducing proteins and vegetables as your basic fare. Plan ahead, then enjoy.

The Magic Hour: Reward Meal Timing Tips

In addition to becoming lax on balancing Reward Meals, failing to complete a Reward Meal within one hour is one of the most typical reasons for a slowed or stopped weight loss. Keeping your one-hour Reward Meal is very important, and with a little planning and a bit of assertiveness it is more than doable.

Most people do not have any difficulty maintaining the sixty-minute Reward Meal time limit when eating at home; dining at a restaurant or at other people's houses, however, usually presents more of a challenge. Here are some helpful do's and don'ts for enjoying your Reward Meal within one hour:

Reward Meal Hour Don'ts

- Don't trust that you will "somehow" be able to get the food you need within the one-hour Reward Meal time limit. That can be a setup in which you end up in a compromising situation where you either have to fight for your meal or give up on trying to comply with this very important Program Guideline.
- Do not be shy, unassertive, or afraid of "being a bother." If you are dining at a friend's home, they almost certainly want to make your meal most pleasurable (if not, reconsider eating there altogether). If you are dining at a restaurant, don't wait for the waiter to wander by to tell him what you need. Explain what you need and when you need it. When we eat out, as the

waiter places the main course before us, we tell him to bring our dessert immediately. With this prodding, we just about get our dessert within our hour limit. Do not be intimidated by a waiter or maître d'. Remember that your pleasure is their business, literally.

Reward Meal Hour Do's

- Phone ahead. Either call the restaurant or home of your host and explain your Reward Meal time limit. Inform them that timing is essential to maintaining your eating program (many of our people simply say they have a "medical condition" which requires a time limitation).
- If you hit resistance, make alternative plans. Choose a different restaurant or tell your host that you will come for "coffee" after the meal (then have your Reward Meal on your own and join the party after you have taken care of yourself).
- Upon arriving, do remind your host or maître d' of your needs. Ask for their help but do not apologize. If you required medication, you would insure your ability to get what you needed—your eating program is no less important.
- Pack a portable dessert. In your jacket or pocketbook, hide a "goodie" that you can count on if dessert is late in coming. Even the most well-intentioned host can forget promises made prior to the pressures of entertaining. While meals are often served within the one-hour time limit, desserts can be put off until everyone has finished the meal and the plates are cleared away. With a dessert "up your sleeve," you are free to pull it out or excuse yourself and enjoy the final pleasure of your meal without compromising your Program's guidelines.

Fast Food, Good Food, and "Legal," Too

From time to time you may find that you crave a "special" Craving-Reducing Meal or you may find yourself in need of a fast Craving-Reducing Meal or snack. Good food at the nearest fast-food restaurant can serve either or both purposes.

New menu additions have made fast-food restaurants a legitimate choice for some Craving-Reducing Meals. The chicken breast sandwich (broiled and without the bun) combined with a large side salad (remove the carrot shreds) can offer you the change of taste or quick Craving-Reducing Meal you seek.

A few words of caution, though. Whether you choose the broiled chicken breast or a lean burger, pass when it comes to the added toppings (including the pickles and dressing) and throw away the bun immediately. Enjoy a salad or two, but discard the carrots. Read the salad dressing labels (they often contain MSG) and make certain that the iced tea contains no sugar (or sugar substitute if you have chosen that Option).

Do not make a fast-food menu your everyday fare. Use fast-food restaurants as a once-in-a-while alternative; you may have to choose carefully among their wide range of tempting treats, but with the above cautions in mind, they can provide fast and fun food when you most need it.

Saving Time and Money

Craving-Reducing proteins and vegetables can be prepared easily and less expensively if you get involved in a Buying Bonanza and a Cooking Celebration. Once a week, or every two weeks, make a major supermarket visit a Buying Bonanza. Bring a list of your favorite Craving-Reducing foods. Purchase great quantities of Craving-Reducing protein (whole or quartered chickens, turkey, roasts, chops, ground meat or turkey, fish, shellfish, etc.), a profusion of fresh Craving-Reducing vegetables (a large cauliflower, cucumbers, celery stalks, cabbage and lettuce heads, green beans, asparagus, etc.),* as well as some of your favorite Carbohydrate-Rich foods (breads, pastas, some special "goodies", etc.) for your Reward Meals.

Take your bounty home and start your Cooking Celebration. Season your poultry, fish, and meat and place them in the oven or broiler. Crank up the grill if you have one. While your protein roasts, bakes, or broils, turn on some good music or a good video tape and start cutting up your veggies. Leave your lettuce whole. Cook some cabbage if you like, and cut up enough cauliflower, mushrooms, green beans, and cucumber for the next two to three days.

Stick the rest of the celery, and the asparagus, in a few inches of

*Given your own financial and storage limitations.

water and place all the vegetables in the refrigerator. Cut-up celery does best if kept in cold water (change the water every day). By the time your vegetables are cut, your protein will be ready. Keep a two days' supply of protein in the refrigerator and package the remaining in meal-size labeled freezer bags. (We keep a list of the freezer meals on the side of the refrigerator.)

This bit of planning and efficient preparation will keep you in Craving-Reducing foods for an entire week; you will be eating what you enjoy and enjoying what you eat—without "making do" or putting up with last-minute meals that do not really satisfy you.

Craving-Reducing Breakfast Alternatives

Chances are, choosing a salad, protein, and some Craving-Reducing vegetables for lunch does not present much of a problem. Getting used to Craving-Reducing breakfast choices, on the other hand, may take a bit of planning and reconsideration, so we have included the following tips:

First, remember that whether or not you eat breakfast is truly *your* choice. You may prefer to have a cup of coffee or tea and wait to enjoy your first meal at lunchtime, or have a brunch (a combined breakfast and lunch) at 10:30 or 11:00 A.M.

You may choose to replace your missed meal with a Craving-Reducing Meal that takes place later in the day (in the evening, for instance) or skip the meal altogether. Many of our readers find that skipping breakfast comes easily and naturally and they tell us that, in the past, they only included breakfast because they thought they "had to." Research does not support this old wives' tale that has, unfortunately, been taken up in TV ads by food producers who have a vested interest in having you believe you must eat a "good" breakfast—one that just happens to include their product—every day.

Many of our people find that as they continue on their Program and no longer experience hypoglycemic (low blood sugar) responses, breakfast becomes an option rather than a necessity. So keep in mind that if you would like to skip breakfast and if you feel well doing so, you are free at any time to skip or postpone your first meal of the day. As always, check with your physician.

If, on the other hand, you enjoy and prefer to have breakfast, consider many of the choices listed in the Meal Plans and Recipe chapters that follow. These chapters include Craving-Reducing recipes for muffins, pancakes, a breakfast soufflé, cinnamon "bread," and crustless quiche. Enjoy them if you like, but be certain that you do not substitute traditional Carbohydrate-Rich forms of these recipes during Craving-Reducing Meals. You can always enjoy these "breakfast" foods as part of your balanced Reward Meal every night.

For those who want a quick, easy, and tasty Craving-Reducing breakfast, we recommend that you broaden your usual breakfast choices as you look over the Craving-Reducing foods list (page 120). Besides the typical eggs (and egg substitutes), cheese, and cottage cheese, consider some steak (lean, if you like) with your eggs or all by itself. Enjoy some chicken salad or some cold homemade chicken or roast beef. We love chicken or roast beef rolled up in lettuce leaves with a little mustard. Fill celery with some cream cheese (this is pretty rich so don't do it every day) or consider some cold poached or smoked fish. Add some cucumber slices for crunch. Look over many of the Craving-Reducing recipes in the Appetizer and Dips section beginning on page 222 for lots of great ideas.

Craving-Reducing breakfast choices are only as limited as your own imagination. With your Craving-Reducing foods list in hand, look over the foods in your refrigerator and in your cabinets. Check out the recipes in this book or your favorite cookbook. Don't limit yourself to typical American choices. The British enjoy fish (kippers) and kidneys, and even if these choices do not appeal to you, consider the following: Americans will eat sausages for breakfast but not hot dogs, ham but not pork, steak and eggs but not steak alone, and smoked fish but not grilled or baked or broiled fish. Open up your mind and you will be surprised at how you open up your options.

Troubleshooting

Craving Correctives

Within a few days on The Carbohydrate Addict's LifeSpan Program, by following the three Basic Guidelines, almost all carbohydrate addicts experience a significant decrease in carbohydrate cravings. Some of our readers notice a substantial reduction in cravings within a day or two; others swear that after a "couple of days" on the Program, they barely feel like eating at all. Individual responses vary a bit in intensity and time, but the one consistent experience is the "amazing" drop in cravings that takes place, at most, within the first week.

If you are still experiencing cravings after following the Basic Plan's three Guidelines for a full week, first make certain that you are not "misinterpreting" your cravings; some carbohydrate addicts find that tiredness or thirst can, at first, make them feel as if they want to snack. If you are neither tired nor thirsty, and you are still experiencing cravings after seven days on the Program, chances are you are unintentionally consuming Carbohydrate-Rich foods during your Craving-Reducing Meals.

You may not be aware of the hidden carbos; you may have "assumed" the foods you were eating did not contain carbohydrates, or you may have even been given false information regarding the contents of your food (at a restaurant or deli, for instance), but be assured that continued cravings almost always point to carbohydrates being consumed outside of the Reward Meal.

For three days, write down everything you eat and the times you eat it. It is best to include two work days and one day off, if that kind of schedule applies to you. On the same paper, note any experiences of cravings and the times you first become aware of them. Do not rely on your memory; you need the facts. With your three-day food and craving diary in front of you, look through your record and note the times when you experienced cravings. Now look to see which foods you ate about 1½ to 2 hours before you experienced the cravings. Chances are, one *or more* of these foods contain hidden carbohydrates.

Track down the information you need on these foods by more carefully examining their ingredients or checking with the deli or restaurant that sold them to you. These foods may contain hidden carbohydrates in the form of fillers (bread filler, rice, or other low-cost filler are often added to store-bought tuna salad, chicken salad, or shrimp salad) and all types of sugars (including dextrose, fructose, glucose, honey, corn syrup, high fructose corn syrup, brown sugar, fruit flavoring of any kind) can be added to many foods, especially so-called diet foods and luncheon meats. If you cannot isolate which food appears to be the craving-causing culprit, eliminate all suspected foods for a day or two and see if the cravings disappear. Then add them back, one at a time.

Be persistent. Reread the Program's three Guidelines (pages 112–24) and the lists of Craving-Reducing foods as well (page 120). Make certain that you are not including Carbohydrate-Rich foods in your Craving-Reducing Meals without realizing it or that you have not started to push some of the Program's limits, allowing yourself more than one cup of coffee with milk or cream outside of your Reward Meal, for instance, or carbo-drifting at your Reward Meal (that is, eating less Craving-Reducing vegetables or protein at your Reward Meal and more Carbohydrate-Rich foods in their stead).

If, after *very carefully* checking for hidden carbos in your Craving-Reducing Meals and making certain that you are clearly following the Guidelines and staying within the limits of the Program, you still experience carbohydrate cravings, consider some of the Options in Chapter 6, especially the MSG Easing Option, the Breaking the Sugar Substitute Connection Option, or the Food Frequency Reducing Option. These Options can help eliminate the cause of your cravings and help make your Program struggle-free, as it was meant to be.

Weight-Loss Boosters

On other programs, most dieters experience slow-downs and plateaus in their weight loss. On The Carbohydrate Addict's LifeSpan Program, a steady weight loss is far more typical. While no one's body can be expected to lose weight according to plan, if you are not losing an average $1/2$ to 2 pounds a week while following the Guidelines, in addition to adding Options from Chapter 6, we would recommend you explore some of the following alternatives.

1. Even though you may not experience strong cravings, follow the Craving Correctives suggestions above as a check for hidden carbohydrates and other obstacles to a steady weight loss.
2. Failing to balance Reward Meal portions and exceeding the one-hour Reward Meal time limit can slow, stop, or even reverse your weight loss. Keep your Program tight. Balance your Reward Meals and keep faithful to your

one-hour time limit. Reread the Basic Plan's Guidelines (page 111)—they are a mainstay of your Program.

3. Many people find that going the "extra yard" will make a significant difference in increasing their weight-loss rate, and the three suggestions that follow have been shown to work wonders. First, consider reducing your intake of "borderline foods" at Craving-Reducing Meals. These foods are marked with an asterisk on the Craving-Reducing Foods list (page 120) and could be slowing your weight loss. You can certainly still include these foods in your Reward Meals but always keep the balance in mind. You may also be able to increase your weight-loss rate by reducing your intake of cheese at all meals. Instead of cheese, choose other sources of protein, including poultry, fish, or meat, during Craving-Reducing Meals and go light on cheese even at your Reward Meals. To go the extra yard, you may also want to consider adding extra Craving-Reducing vegetables to your Reward Meals. This addition will make the vegetable $1/3$ of your Reward Meal heavier than the protein or carbohydrate portions. You can select more than one vegetable if you like to make this portion "heavier." This choice seems to help many people increase their weight-loss rate and, if you make the vegetables tasty, provides an easy "push" to keep your weight loss moving. At all times, make sure that you continue to drink 6 to 8 glasses of water each day.*

4. Consider adding one or more of the following Options to your Program: the MSG Easing Option, the Breaking the Sugar Substitute Connection Option, or the Food Frequency Reducing Option. These Options, as well as others in Chapter 6, can help to greatly increase your weight-loss rate.

*Unless otherwise directed by your physician.

Program First-Aid

Every once in a while we get a letter relating a familiar experience: one of our readers inadvertently ate some Carbohydrate-Rich food during a Craving-Reducing Meal and needs some advice on what to do in such a situation. They tell us of the deli person who assured them that the tuna salad contained no filler or of the restaurant chef who added sugar to a sauce, despite the waitress's assurance that he would not. Certainly, you want to be vigilant and avoid the situation whenever possible, but if you ever find yourself face-to-face with a Carbohydrate-Rich food sneaking into your Craving-Reducing Meal, it's important to know (1) how to recognize the signs of hidden carbos, and (2) what to do to counteract the "hidden" carbohydrate's effects.

Recognizing the signs of hidden carbos: Once you have been on the Program for a short time, and have experienced the lack of cravings and the rise in energy that often accompany it, you will almost certainly be struck by the powerful impact of hidden carbohydrates in Craving-Reducing Meals.

The first and most noticeable change is usually a tremendous increase in the intensity and frequency of carbohydrate cravings. We do not use the word "tremendous" lightly; many readers have referred to the change in the cravings as "astounding" or "amazing" or "overpowering." And the change often takes place within two to three hours after the hidden carbohydrate has been consumed, sometimes even sooner. In most cases, there will be no doubt in your mind as to whether or not something different has occurred; it will hit you "like a two-ton truck."

You may find yourself tired or anxious or both; some people describe the experience as feeling "fretful" or "irritable." Others tell us that they simply feel extremely fatigued or unmotivated. But in any case, the overwhelming experience is the rush of powerful cravings.

What to do: First of all, do not panic. Remember that the cravings you are experiencing are only temporary and that within 24 to 48 hours you will be right back on track. Your cravings are only a sign that your body is, once again, out of balance, just as it was before you began the Program.

It may *seem* to you that the cravings are more intense than you remember, but that is because now, on the Program, you know what it's like to be craving-free while in the past you had come to accept and accommodate to a semiconstant battle with your cravings. In contrast to the physical peace you have come to anticipate, the intensity of your renewed cravings seems even greater. So relax, don't blame or chastise yourself. Understand that the changes you are feeling right now will soon subside; use this experience as a powerful reminder of what used to be your daily experience and utilize it as a reinforcer, strengthening your awareness of how much better you feel because of your Program.

To counteract the physical effects of Carbohydrate-Rich foods consumed during a Craving-Reducing Meal, we have found that protein works wonders. If you like, for one or two days, add extra snacks of Craving-Reducing protein to your regular program. The protein-rich snacks are meant to help your body release glucagon, an "insulin-opposing" hormone, and they should help to greatly reduce your cravings and your hunger.

It is important to have available the food you need for your Craving-Reducing Snacks. For example, have some canned tuna or homemade tuna salad or chicken or lean beef on hand. Cheese or eggs can be helpful in an emergency, and if you are a vegetarian, you may need to rely on tofu, but meat or fish or poultry are your best choices.

Add some Craving-Reducing vegetables to your snacks as well (crunchy vegetables such as celery and green pepper are often the most satisfying) and lots of cool water or unflavored seltzer. Enjoy these snacks when you feel strong urges for carbohydrates. Don't scrimp on the snacks right now. Your job is to help "right" your body's balance, and if your daily weight goes up for a couple of days, it will drop down again soon and you will once again be "on your way." Be absolutely certain, however, that the proteins you eat during these Craving-Reducing Snacks do not themselves contain more "hidden" carbos; the last thing you want to do is to create more of an insulin imbalance.

So if you suddenly find yourself craving carbohydrates with an intensity that you have not experienced since before you began the Program, don't panic. It is simply a sign that your body is responding to an insulin "rush," and within a little time and with the help of some protein, you will soon be well on your way once again.

A Final Word

The suggestions that you find in this chapter are meant to provide you the benefit of our experience and that of thousands of our readers. They are not intended as guidelines but rather are recommendations that have worked for us and for others. Pick and choose those suggestions that look appropriate to you. Try on any suggestion for "size." If it fits, use it; if it does not, there are many others that you will, most likely, find far more appropriate.

The three Guidelines of this Program and its Options, as well as the suggestions in this chapter, are meant to provide you with the building blocks you need to make the life you want. The Guidelines are essential basics; the Options for Life and the suggestions in this chapter offer alternatives that can help you along the way, so that you, too, can enjoy freedom from carbohydrate addiction—for life.

CHAPTER 9

A DREAM COMES TRUE

Dreams grow holy when put into action.
—Adelaide Ann Proctor, 1859

*R*achael's Wish:

As a child and young teen, the last request in my prayers each night was the fervent wish that I wake up thin. As television made its way into my consciousness, I believed in the Walt Disney theme that beckoned me to wish upon a star so that all of my dreams would come true.

As the years passed and neither deity nor stars seemed to be forthcoming with my singular request, and as the pain of being rejected and teased, humiliated and abused tore at my very soul, I closed my mind and my heart to the belief that I would ever be free from my hunger, my ugliness, and my shame.

But God and life and—because of Richard—love, all worked in mysterious ways. After almost four decades of pain and self-blame my dreams did indeed come true. And the only thing that makes my joy even greater, makes my happiness complete, is knowing that the truths and freedoms that Richard and I have discovered are being used and shared and enjoyed by others.

Our greatest wish is that you may feel the strength and love that these pages enfold and bring to you.

PART IV

RECIPES AND MEAL PLANS:

EATING YOUR WAY TO FREEDOM

CHAPTER 10

SAMPLE DAILY MEAL PLANS

*T*he Carbohydrate Addict's LifeSpan Program has been designed to be an enjoyable, livable program that meets the needs of the meat-eater as well as the vegetarian, for the gourmet cook as well as the kitchen-phobic.

You can enjoy your meals at restaurants or on the go, at pleasurable feasts in the privacy of your own home or in the finest company. And no one ever need know you are on a weight-loss program. After a short while, as the Program becomes an easy way of life, even you are likely to forget that this is not the way you have always eaten.

The sample Meal Plans that follow are not meant to be used as a short-cut or substitute for a complete understanding of The Carbohydrate Addict's LifeSpan Program. Always follow the Program's Guidelines and Options; they have been designed to provide you with a wide variety of choices and a full grasp of the Program.

The Meal Plans that follow can be used as a model to guide you in the selection of choices for your two daily Craving-Reducing Meals and your one Reward Meal. If you are a vegetarian, a special non-meat alternative Meal Plan section also follows.

The sample Meal Plans in this section are meant only as suggestions, examples of the wide range of foods you can enjoy on the Program. In most cases, they include a far greater number of items and a wider variety than you will generally include on a daily basis, especially in respect to Reward Meals. Should you include all of these items at any one meal, make sure to adjust your quantities to reflect somewhat smaller portions given the greater number of items (if you want more, you can always go back for seconds), and, as always, remember to balance your Reward Meals (page 112).

Recipes for many of the dishes that are featured in our Meal Plans can be found beginning on page 219. Add your own favorite specialties or take some ideas from just about any cookbook you like. The choices are literally unlimited. Just remember that your Craving-Reducing Meals should include Craving-Reducing vegetables and protein only and that your Reward Meals should include a balance of salad, Craving-Reducing vegetables and protein, as well as Carbohydrate-Rich foods.

One important note: The Meal Plans that follow assume that breakfast and lunch are your designated Craving-Reducing Meals and that you enjoy your Reward Meal at dinner. If you need some suggestions on Reward Meal time-swapping, see Chapter 8.

Incorporating Low-fat, Low-salt, and Other Dietary Recommendations into Your Program

Dietary recommendations for Americans have been issued by the U.S. Department of Agriculture, the Department of Health and Human Services, the American Heart Association, and the Surgeon General of the United States.

These well-respected agencies offer these guidelines as an aid in the prevention of cardiovascular diseases, high blood pressure, stroke, cancer, obesity, adult-onset diabetes, and osteoporosis. Recommendations contained in these reports* are completely compatible with, and easily included into, The Carbohydrate Addict's LifeSpan Program.

Suggestions for incorporating these dietary guidelines into your program can be found in Health Agency Recommendations on page 214.

Before including any recommendation into your eating plan, be certain to consult with your doctor as to which of the Health Agency dietary guidelines are appropriate for you.

*The U.S. Surgeon General's *Report on Nutrition and Health*; the U.S. Department of Agriculture and the Department of Health and Human Services' *Report on Dietary Guidelines for Americans*; the American Heart Association's *Eating Plan for Healthy Americans*, and the American Cancer Society's *Eat to Live*.

Meal Plans

DAY ONE

Craving-Reducing Breakfast
Smooth and Cheesy-Good Omelet (page 236)
Canadian Bacon (or low-fat or low-salt substitute)
Iced or Hot Coffee or Tea

Craving-Reducing Lunch
Caesar Salad (page 269)
Garlic and Green Beans (page 286)
Hamburgers with Dill (page 259)
Water, Unflavored Seltzer or Club Soda,
Iced or Hot Coffee or Tea, or Diet Soda

Reward Meal Dinner
Green Goddess Cucumber Salad (page 383)
Herby Green Beans (page 394)
Black Peppercorn Tuna (page 350)
Crescent Rolls
Butter (or low-fat substitute)
Crème Brûlée (page 336)
Fruit of Choice
Beverage(s) of Choice

DAY TWO

Craving-Reducing Breakfast
Mushroom Crustless Breakfast Quiche* (page 237)
Iced or Hot Coffee or Tea

Craving-Reducing Lunch
Chef's Salad† (page 276)
Green Garden Mayonnaise (page 282)
Steamed Asparagus
Water, Unflavored Seltzer or Club Soda,
Iced or Hot Coffee or Tea, or Diet Soda

Reward Meal Dinner
Spicy Garden Salad with Dressing (page 385)
Broccoli-Cauliflower Sweet Delight (page 397)
Skewered Spicy Lamb (page 374)
White, Brown, or Wild Rice
Key Lime Pie (page 338)
Beverage(s) of Choice

*This is a special Craving-Reducing variation. Do not substitute a standard carbohydrate-rich recipe.
†Do not include any luncheon meats or poultry that contain fillers, sugars, or MSG. Best choices: cheese, roast beef, corned beef, or *homemade* turkey or ham.

DAY THREE

Craving-Reducing Breakfast
Cottage Cheese Muffins* (page 238)
Iced or Hot Coffee or Tea

Craving-Reducing Lunch
Oregano Chicken Salad with Dressing (page 271)
Savory Spinach (page 287)
Chicken in Olive Sauce (page 251)
Water, Unflavored Seltzer or Club Soda,
Iced or Hot Coffee or Tea

Reward Meal Dinner
Cucumber-Tomato Triumph Salad with Dressing (page 391)
Green Beans Amandine
Broiled Lamb Chops (page 369)
Warm Egg Noodles with Butter (or low-fat substitute)
Butter (or low-fat substitute)
Fresh Pears in Wine (page 339)
Beverage(s) of Choice

*This is a special Craving-Reducing variation. Do not substitute a standard carbohydrate-rich recipe.

DAY FOUR

Craving-Reducing Breakfast
Cinnamon "Bread"* (page 239)
Iced or Hot Coffee or Tea

Craving-Reducing Lunch
Tossed Green Salad (page 273)
with Creamy Herbal Dressing (page 283)
Steamed Cauliflower and Cheese (page 285)
Sultry Lemon Chicken (page 253)
Water, Unflavored Seltzer or Club Soda,
Iced or Hot Coffee or Tea, or Diet Soda

Reward Meal Dinner
Caesar Salad Roman-Style with Dressing (page 388)
French Onion Soup (page 411)
Sautéed Mushrooms with Green Peppers
Chicken Breasts Napoleon (page 357)
Bread Sticks
Butter (or low-fat substitute)
Iced Lemon Soufflé (page 332)
Beverage(s) of Choice

*This is a special Craving-Reducing variation. Do not substitute a standard carbohydrate-rich recipe.

DAY FIVE

Craving-Reducing Breakfast
Cottage Cheese Soufflé* (page 240)
Sausage (regular, low-fat, or low-salt)
Iced or Hot Coffee or Tea

Craving-Reducing Lunch
Cucumber Salad with Dressing* (page 270)
Steamed Asparagus
Shrimp with an Oriental Twist (page 248)
Water, Unflavored Seltzer or Club Soda,
Iced or Hot Coffee or Tea, or Diet Soda

Reward Meal Dinner
Tossed Green Salad (page 273)
with Lemon Mayonnaise Dressing (page 392)
Mexican Soup (page 413)
Garlic and Green Beans (page 286)
Yogurt Chicken Breasts (page 359)
Warm Onion Bread
Butter (or low-fat substitute)
Apple Cream Pie (page 346)
Beverage(s) of Choice

*This is a special Craving-Reducing variation. Do not substitute a standard carbohydrate-rich recipe.

DAY SIX

Craving-Reducing Breakfast
Western Omelet (page 241)
Bacon (or low-fat substitute)
Iced or Hot Coffee or Tea

Craving-Reducing Lunch
Spinach Salad with Dressing (page 278)
Steamed Green Beans or Broccoli
Saucy Sirloin Steak (page 254)
Water, Unflavored Seltzer or Club Soda,
Iced or Hot Coffee or Tea, or Diet Soda

Reward Meal Dinner
Popeye's Deluxe Spinach Salad with Dressing (page 387)
Steamed Cauliflower and Cheese (page 285)
Stuffed Pork Chops (page 377)
Simply Gingerbread (page 340)
Fresh Fruit of Choice
Beverage(s) of Choice

DAY SEVEN

Craving-Reducing Breakfast
Breakfast Pancakes* (page 242)
Iced or Hot Coffee or Tea

Craving-Reducing Lunch
Shrimp Salad with Dressing (page 275)
Tangy Cabbage (page 288)
Grilled Salmon Steak
Water, Unflavored Seltzer or Club Soda,
Iced or Hot Coffee or Tea, or Diet Soda

Reward Meal Dinner
Italian Salad with Dressing (page 396)
Minestrone Soup (page 414)
Veal with Peppers (page 381)
Steamed Asparagus
Hot Garlic Bread
Creamy Fudge Cake (page 334) à la Mode
Beverage(s) of Choice

*This is a special Craving-Reducing variation. Do not substitute a standard car-
bohydrate-rich recipe.

Vegetarian Meal Plans

DAY ONE

Vegetarian Craving-Reducing Breakfast
Breakfast Tofu Stir Fry, Western Style (page 289)
Iced or Hot Coffee or Tea

Vegetarian Craving-Reducing Lunch
Italian Salad with Dressing (page 386)
Garlic and Green Beans (page 286)
Vegetarian "Steaklet" Delight* (page 303)
Water, Unflavored Seltzer or Club Soda,
Iced or Hot Coffee or Tea

Vegetarian Reward Meal Dinner
Spicy Garden Salad with Dressing (page 385)
Broccoli-Cauliflower Sweet Delight (page 397)
Vegetarian Pacific Island "Chicken" (page 422)
White, Brown, or Wild Rice
Sponge Heaven (page 343) and Fresh Strawberries
Beverage(s) of Choice

*Check nutritional labels. At Craving-Reducing Meals and Snacks, all "vegetarian" meat alternatives should contain 4 grams or less of carbohydrate per average serving.

DAY TWO

Vegetarian Craving-Reducing Breakfast
Breakfast Pancakes* (page 242)
Vegetarian "Bacon"†
Iced or Hot Coffee or Tea

Vegetarian Craving-Reducing Lunch
Finger Salad (Celery Sticks, Cucumber Slices, Mushroom Caps,
Green Beans) with Green Salsa Dip (page 230)
Tangy Cabbage (page 288)
Tofu Oriental (page 291)
Couscous or White, Brown, or Wild Rice
Water, Unflavored Seltzer or Club Soda,
Iced or Hot Coffee or Tea

Vegetarian Reward Meal Dinner
Italian Salad with Dressing (page 386)
Green Beans Amandine
Vegetarian "Sausage" with Avocados and Fettuccine (page 420)
Carob Cake and Tofu "Ice Cream"
Fruit of Choice
Beverage(s) of Choice

*This is a special Craving-Reducing variation. Do not substitute a standard carbohydrate-rich recipe.
†Check nutritional labels. At Craving-Reducing Meals and Snacks, all "vegetarian" meat alternatives should contain 4 grams or less of carbohydrate per average serving.

DAY THREE

Vegetarian Craving-Reducing Breakfast
Cinnamon "Bread"* (page 239)
Iced or Hot Coffee or Tea

Vegetarian Craving-Reducing Lunch
Tossed Green Salad (page 273)
with Mustard Garlic Vinaigrette (page 284)
Savory Spinach (page 287)
Marinated "Burgers," Vegetarian Style† (page 297)
Water, Unflavored Seltzer or Club Soda,
Iced or Hot Coffee or Tea

Vegetarian Reward Meal Dinner
Popeye's Deluxe Spinach Salad with Dressing (page 387)
French Onion Soup (page 411)
"Seafood" Vegetable Triumph (page 426)
Sesame Flat Bread
Butter (or low-fat, nondairy substitute)
Banana Fritters (page 342)
Beverage(s) of Choice

*This is a special Craving-Reducing variation. Do not substitute a standard carbohydrate-rich recipe.
†Check nutritional labels. At Craving-Reducing Meals and Snacks, all "vegetarian" meat alternatives should contain 4 grams or less of carbohydrate per average serving.

DAY FOUR

Vegetarian Craving-Reducing Breakfast
Breakfast "Salami" and Tofu Stir Fry* (page 290)
Iced or Hot Coffee or Tea

Vegetarian Craving-Reducing Lunch
Italian Mozzarella Salad with Dressing (page 277)
Stir-fry Green Beans
Vegetarian Gingered "Steak"* (page 301)
Water, Unflavored Seltzer or Club Soda,
Iced or Hot Coffee or Tea

Vegetarian Reward Meal Dinner
Green Goddess Cucumber Salad (page 383)
Mexican Soup (page 413)
Sautéed Mushrooms with Green Peppers
Consummate Vegetarian "Burger" (page 418)
Couscous with Butter (or low-fat, nondairy substitute)
Key Lime Pie (page 338)
Beverage(s) of Choice

*Check nutritional labels. At Craving-Reducing Meals and Snacks, all "vegetarian" meat alternatives should contain 4 grams or less of carbohydrate per average serving.

DAY FIVE

Vegetarian Craving-Reducing Breakfast
Mushroom Crustless Breakfast Quiche* (page 237)
Iced or Hot Coffee or Tea

Vegetarian Craving-Reducing Lunch
Caesar Salad (page 269)
Steamed Asparagus with Cauliflower-Basil Dip (page 231)
Spicy Tofu Stir-fry (page 292)
Water, Unflavored Seltzer or Club Soda,
Iced or Hot Coffee or Tea

Vegetarian Reward Meal Dinner
Caesar Salad Roman Style (page 388)
Vegetable Delight (page 429)
Warm Pumpernickel Raisin Bread
Butter (or low-fat, nondairy substitute)
Simply Gingerbread (page 340)
Fruit of Choice
Beverage(s) of Choice

*This is a special Craving-Reducing variation. Do not substitute a standard carbohydrate-rich recipe.

DAY SIX

Vegetarian Craving-Reducing Breakfast
Celery Sticks and Cucumber Slices
Poached Salmon Steak, cold (page 246)
Iced or Hot Coffee or Tea

Vegetarian Craving-Reducing Lunch
Tossed Green Salad with Dressing (page 273)
Steamed Green Beans with Hot Spinach Dip (page 232)
Vegetarian Oriental "Burger" Casserole* (page 296)
Water, Unflavored Seltzer or Club Soda,
Iced or Hot Coffee or Tea

Vegetarian Reward Meal Dinner
Tossed Green Salad with Lemon Mayonnaise (page 392)
Steamed Asparagus
Tofu Oriental (page 291)
White, Brown, or Wild Rice
Fresh Fruit Salad and Sorbet
Beverage(s) of Choice

*Check nutritional labels. At Craving-Reducing Meals and Snacks, all "vegetarian" meat alternatives should contain 4 grams or less of carbohydrate per average serving.

DAY SEVEN

Vegetarian Craving-Reducing Breakfast
Scrambled Eggs (or egg substitute*)
Vegetarian "Sausage"†
Iced or Hot Coffee or Tea

Vegetarian Craving-Reducing Lunch
Bean Sprout Salad with Dressing (page 280)
Marinated Green Olives (page 225)
Vegetarian Parsley-Butter "Burgers"† (page 294)
Water, Unflavored Seltzer or Club Soda,
Iced or Hot Coffee or Tea

Vegetarian Reward Meal Dinner
Cucumber-Tomato Triumph with Dressing (page 391)
Potato and Garlic Soup (page 412)
Garlic and Green Beans (page 286)
Vegetarian "Sausage" Loaf (page 421)
Old-fashioned Rice Pudding (page 330)
Beverage(s) of Choice

*This is a special Craving-Reducing variation. Do not substitute a standard carbohydrate-rich recipe.
†Check nutritional labels. At Craving-Reducing Meals and Snacks, all "vegetarian" meat alternatives should contain 4 grams or less of carbohydrate per average serving.

BUYING INTO THE GOOD LIFE:

Where to Shop for Soy Flour and Vegetarian Choices

Soy, Oh Boy!

Almost all health food stores carry soy flour as part of their regular stock. If they are out of stock, you may want to ask the store manager to order a bag for you. In case you cannot locate a friendly and helpful store near you, we provide an address below that may be able to help you track down the store nearest you that carries soy flour. Soy flour is far lower in carbohydrates than wheat flour and for that reason we use it in many of our Craving-Reducing breakfast recipes.

For help in finding the nearest store that sells soy flour, write to:
Arrowhead Mills
Box 2059
Hereford, TX 79045

Vegetarian Alternatives: The Good News

A wide variety of non-meat alternatives for meat, poultry, and fish are currently available at supermarket and health food stores. New items are arriving on a regular basis and even as we list them they are being added to market shelves.

Here is a sampling of the many vegetarian (non-meat) alternatives on the market, although not all products are available at all stores. If you do not see the product you want, ask the store manager to order it for you. If the store manager cannot help you, you can write or call the distributors and manufacturers listed below for the name of the store nearest you; you can also check your business telephone directory for listings.

Some items qualify as Craving-Reducing foods (those with 0 to 4 grams of carbohydrates per average serving). Other items qualify as Carbohydrate-Rich foods (those with 5 grams or more of carbohydrates per average serving) and should be saved for Reward Meals only. Check labels for carbohydrate levels.

Vegetarian Meat Alternatives

Grillers (Morningstar Farms)
Okara Pattie (Natural Touch)
Garden Vege Patties (Morningstar Farms and Natural Touch)
Prime Patties (Morningstar Farms)
Better'n Burgers (Morningstar Farms)
Granburger (Worthington Foods)
Redi-Burger (Morningstar Farms)
Vegetarian Burger (Worthington Foods)
Vegan Burgers (Worthington Foods and Natural Foods)
Vege Burgers (Natural Touch and Loma Linda)
Vita-Burger (Loma Linda)
Sizzle Burgers (Loma Linda)
Fri-Pats (Worthington Foods)
Ground Meatless Burger (Worthington Foods)
Choplets (Worthington Foods)
Cutlets (Worthington Foods)
Multigrain Cutlets (Worthington Foods)
Patty Mix (Loma Linda)
Vegetarian Steaks (Worthington Foods)
Prime Stakes (Worthington Foods)
Swiss Stake with Gravy (Loma Linda)
Stakelets (Worthington Foods)
Vegetable Stakes (Worthington Foods)
Griddle Steaks (Loma Linda)
Dinner Roast (Worthington Foods)
Savory Dinner Loaf (Loma Linda)
Dinner Cuts (Worthington Foods)
Dinner Entrée (Natural Touch)
Country Stew (Worthington Foods)
Savory Slices (Worthington Foods)
Prosage, patties and links (Worthington Foods)
Deli Franks (Morningstar Farms)
Vege Franks (Natural Touch)
Leanies (Worthington Foods)
Big Franks (Loma Linda)

Linkettes (Loma Linda)
Big Franks (Loma Linda)
Veja-links (Worthington Foods)
Superlinks (Worthington Foods)
Little Links (Loma Linda)
Saucettes (Morningstar Farms)
Breakfast Links (Morningstar Farms)
Breakfast Strips (Morningstar Farms)
Ground Meatless Sausage (Worthington Foods)
Breakfast Patties (Morningstar Farms)
Stripples (Worthington Foods)
Sandwich Spread (Loma Linda)
Corned Beef (Worthington Foods)
Smoked Beef (Worthington Foods)
Bologno (Worthington Foods)
Salami (Worthington Foods)
Wham (Worthington Foods)
Veelets (Worthington Foods)
Pot Pie—Beef-Style (Worthington Foods)

Vegetarian Poultry Alternatives

Chick Patties (Morningstar Farms)
Sliced Chik (Worthington Foods)
Diced Chik (Worthington Foods)
FriChik (Worthington Foods)
Turkee Slices (Worthington Foods)
Smoked Turkey (Worthington Foods)
ChikStiks (Worthington Foods)
Crispy Chik Patties (Worthington Foods)
Golden Croquettes (Worthington Foods)
Pot Pie—Chicken-Style (Worthington Foods)
Chic-ketts (Worthington Foods)
Chicken Supreme (Loma Linda)
Fried Chicken with Gravy (Loma Linda)
Chik-Nuggets (Loma Linda)
Golden Croquettes (Worthington Foods)

Vegetarian Fish Alternatives

Vegetable Skallops (Worthington Foods)
Fillets (Worthington Foods)
Tuno (Worthington Foods)
Ocean Platter (Loma Linda)

For more information on vegetarian alternatives, you can write for the name of the store nearest you by writing to Morningstar Farms, Natural Touch, or Worthington Foods, all at:

Consumer Affairs
900 Proprietors Road
Worthington OH 43085

or call the Tree of Life Distributors:
    Midwest Division: (800) 999-4200
    Northeast Division: (800) 735-5175
    Northwest Division: (800) 366-3986
    Southeast Division: (800) 874-0851
    Southwest Division: (800) 800-2175
    Western Division: (800) 827-2803

LOW-FAT, LOW-SALT, AND OTHER HEALTH AGENCY DIETARY RECOMMENDATIONS*

and the Carbohydrate Addict's LifeSpan Program

Before incorporating any dietary guideline into your program, consult your physician. Only your doctor can determine which recommendations are appropriate to your individual needs.

HEALTH AGENCY RECOMMENDATION #1:

Eat a variety of foods.

TO INCLUDE RECOMMENDATION #1 INTO YOUR PROGRAM:

Vary your Craving-Reducing foods by choosing from an assortment of salad items, vegetables, proteins, and dairy items. In addition to Craving-Reducing foods, your Reward Meals should contain a variety of Carbohydrate-Rich foods, including grains, starches, additional dairy choices, fruits, juices, and "healthy" desserts.

HEALTH AGENCY RECOMMENDATION #2:

Reduce consumption of fat (especially saturated fat) and cholesterol.

TO INCLUDE RECOMMENDATION #2 INTO YOUR PROGRAM:

When appropriate, as directed by your physician, replace eggs with egg substitutes and use low-cholesterol margarine and cooking sprays in place of butter. You may choose low-fat or skim milk, low-fat or low-cholesterol cheeses, sour cream, cream cheese and

*Adapted from the U.S. Surgeon General's *Report on Nutrition and Health*; the U.S. Department of Agriculture and the Department of Health and Human Services' *Report on Dietary Guidelines for Americans*; the American Heart Association's *Eating Plan for Healthy Americans*, and The American Cancer Society's *Eat to Live*.

whipped cream substitutes. Instead of higher fat meats, select fish or chicken or turkey without skin, or choose very lean cuts of meat, trimmed of all fat. Substitute turkey for beef and pork in burgers and sausage. Use low-cholesterol mayonnaise. When you use oil, choose olive oil instead of heavy tropical or other saturated oils.

For information on the surprising facts about the impact of dietary fat on your cravings, your weight, and your health, see "Exposing the Food Fat and Fiber Fallacy" in Your Health-Promoting Bonus (Chapter 4).

HEALTH AGENCY RECOMMENDATION #3:

Add foods rich in vitamins A and C.

TO INCLUDE RECOMMENDATION # 3 INTO YOUR PROGRAM:

At your Reward Meals, choose a carbohydrate balance that includes citrus fruits and juices, strawberries, and cantaloupe as well as tomatoes.

At all appropriate meals include dark-green leafy vegetables as well as cruciferous vegetables (from the cabbage family). Select foods such as bok choy, broccoli, Brussels sprouts, cabbage, cauliflower, collard greens, kale, kohlrabi, mustard greens, rutabagas, turnips and their greens.

HEALTH AGENCY RECOMMENDATION #4:

Achieve and maintain a desirable body weight.

TO INCLUDE RECOMMENDATION #4 INTO YOUR PROGRAM:

By choosing The Carbohydrate Addict's LifeSpan Program and following its Guidelines and selecting appropriate Options for you, you will be well on your way to your ideal weight level and, in doing so, reducing many of the health risks often associated with excess weight.

HEALTH AGENCY RECOMMENDATION #5:

Increase consumption of complex carbohydrates and fiber by choosing whole-grain foods and cereal products, vegetables, and fruits. Avoid too much sugar.

TO INCORPORATE RECOMMENDATION #5 INTO YOUR PROGRAM:

At your Reward Meals, select as your balance of Carbohydrate-Rich foods whole-grain breads, cereal products, rice, pasta, fruits, potatoes and other starchy vegetables. At all meals, include lots of fiber-rich Craving-Reducing vegetables. At your Reward Meals, keep your intake of sugar low by choosing desserts made of complex carbohydrates or low-fat whole-grain snacks rather than candy.

HEALTH AGENCY RECOMMENDATION #6:

Limit the amount of salt-cured, smoked, and nitrate-cured foods.

TO INCLUDE RECOMMENDATION #6 INTO YOUR PROGRAM:

Choose ham, bacon, hot dogs, sausages, pastrami, corned beef, salami and other cold cuts on rare and special occasions.

HEALTH AGENCY RECOMMENDATION #7:

Reduce intake of sodium by choosing foods relatively low in sodium and by limiting the amount of salt added in food preparation and at the table.

TO INCLUDE RECOMMENDATION #7 INTO YOUR PROGRAM:

Limit the amount of salt you add while cooking or at the table. At all meals, choose low-salt varieties of canned and packaged foods as well as low-salt cheese and other dairy products. At restaurants, ask for low-salt alternatives. When possible, avoid smoked and salted products.

HEALTH AGENCY RECOMMENDATION #8:

If you drink alcoholic beverages, do so in moderation.

TO INCLUDE RECOMMENDATION #8 INTO YOUR PROGRAM:

On The Carbohydrate Addict's LifeSpan Program, alcoholic beverages are designated as "carbohydrate act-alikes" and confined to your Reward Meal times only. Balancing them (as part of your carbohydrate-rich choices) with the Craving-Reducing foods in your Reward Meal will naturally keep your intake to a moderate level. In addition, we have found that many of the Options you may choose may naturally help reduce strong cravings for alcoholic beverages and allow you to enjoy them in moderation, if you choose.

HEALTH AGENCY RECOMMENDATION #9:

Women should increase consumption of foods high in calcium, including low-fat dairy products. Women of child-bearing age should consume foods that are good sources of iron.

TO INCLUDE RECOMMENDATION #9 INTO YOUR PROGRAM:

At any meal feel free to include calcium-rich canned fish (such as mackerel, salmon, sardines, and water-pack tuna) as well as spinach and greens, oysters, tofu and low-fat cheeses along with iron-rich foods such as lamb, chicken, turkey, green beans, and mushrooms. At your Reward Meal you can choose to include Carbohydrate-Rich foods (such as iron-rich popcorn, potatoes, pasta, rice, and fresh and dried fruits, especially raisins).

If you are including dried fruits as part of the Carbohydrate-Rich balance of your Reward Meal, consider the fruit's proportion to the meal as if it were fresh and, along with any other Carbohydrate-Rich foods, balance it with equal portions of protein and Craving-Reducing vegetables.

To our knowledge, no scientific relationship has been established between osteoporosis or calcium depletion and carbohydrate addiction or hyperinsulinemia. Be certain to address any questions related to this problem or any other medical concerns to your physician.

CHAPTER 11

STARRING RECIPES:

A WORLD OF CRAVING-REDUCING CHOICES

*I*n earlier chapters you discovered that The Carbohydrate Addict's LifeSpan Program has been designed to reduce your release of insulin and, in doing so, reduce your cravings and your weight and cut your risk for many of this country's most prevalent and devastating illnesses.

Once each day, at your Reward Meal, you enjoy a balance of both Carbohydrate-Rich foods and Craving-Reducing foods. All of your other daily meals and snacks are made up of Craving-Reducing foods only. In this way you will be able to enjoy all the food you need and love while still reducing your insulin release as well as your cravings, weight, and health risk.

The first section that follows includes some examples of Craving-Reducing food recipes. Remember that only Craving-Reducing foods should be included in your Craving-Reducing Meals or Snacks. In addition, Craving-Reducing foods should be part of your Reward Meals as well, when you combine them with Carbohydrate-Rich foods for balance.

Craving-Reducing Recipes are offered only as examples of some of the Craving-Reducing foods available. Many other Craving-Reducing foods can be found in the Craving-Reducing foods List on page 119. For other suggestions, consult the sample menus section (page 196). When you plan your Craving-Reducing Meals, remember to choose only those items found in the Craving-Reducing foods List on page 000.

Craving-Reducing foods are low in carbohydrates (sugars and starches) so they can help keep your insulin release (and insulin resistance) low while reducing your cravings and your tendency to gain weight as well.

In this chapter you will find some of our favorite Craving-Reducing Recipes for:

Appetizers and Dips	page 222
Breakfast Choices	page 236
Seafood and Poultry	page 243
Meats (Beef, Pork, Lamb, and Veal)	page 254
Salads, Dressings, and Vegetables	page 269
Vegetarian (Non-meat) Alternatives	page 289

All Craving-Reducing foods may be baked, boiled, broiled, poached, roasted, fried, or sautéed, but during Craving-Reducing Meals, use no breading or batter of any kind. As always, keep your physician's recommendations in mind.

We have included low-fat and low-cholesterol alternatives for those who have concern about fat in their diets. For suggestions on incorporating low-fat, low-salt, and other dietary recommendations into The Carbohydrate Addict's LifeSpan Program's three basic dietary Guidelines, see page 214.

Recipes may be adjusted to account for desired changes in the number of servings. If, for example, you are cooking for yourself or for only one other, you may wish to reduce a recipe by $1/2$ or by $3/4$, or you may choose to make the full recipe and refrigerate the remainder for the next day or freeze the leftovers for future meals.

Keep in mind that the Craving-Reducing Recipes that follow provide examples not only for your Craving-Reducing Meals and Snacks but, when balanced with Carbohydrate-Rich foods, can be enjoyed at your Reward Meals as well.

A (Far Too) Sweet Addition

If you include mayonnaise at Craving-Reducing Meals, choose "regular" varieties only; do not use "low-fat" varieties. Low-fat varieties of mayonnaise often contain several forms of sugar in place of the fat that has been removed. These added sugars can increase your cravings and slow your weight loss.

To turn "regular" mayonnaise into a lower fat alternative, simply thin "regular" mayonnaise with a little water. By adding water, a little at a time, and mixing well, you can reduce the fat content of regular mayonnaise by 1/4 to 1/3 without adding any sugar. And you will be surprised at how little effect it has on the consistency of the mayonnaise.

A Modern Convenience for Old-Fashioned Cooking

The microwave oven can be a real blessing to those who love good cooking but are short on time. Use your microwave to warm up your refrigerated or frozen leftovers at home or at work and enjoy a wonderful homemade treat. (We even know one woman who "invested" in a purchase of a microwave oven for work. She swears that by no longer needing to order in from the local restaurant, she made up the cost within a few weeks and "eats like a queen" while losing weight at the same time.)

Craving-Reducing Appetizers and Spreads

Lemon Shrimp and Vegetables   *serves 2*

A citrus treat that is always a hit.

8 to 10 large parboiled
  shrimp, shelled and
  deveined
1 medium green
  pepper, cut into strips
4 stalks celery, split and
  cut into 2-inch sections

$\frac{1}{4}$ cup lemon juice
$\frac{1}{4}$ cup water
1 tablespoon butter
  (or low-fat substitute)
  Garlic salt, to taste
$\frac{1}{2}$ cup freshly grated
  Parmesan cheese

Place the shrimp and vegetables in a large bowl.

Mix the lemon juice and water and pour over the shrimp and vegetables. Let soak for 1 hour. Toss ingredients several times.

Drain the shrimp and vegetables (discard lemon water) and then sauté them in the butter until just cooked (about 2 to 4 minutes).

Transfer the shrimp to a broiler pan and sprinkle with garlic salt and cheese. Place under the broiler for 4 minutes.

Serve warm.

Stuffed Mushrooms   *serves 4*

A marvelous appetizer or snack that can be easily prepared the day before.

8 medium-sized fresh mushrooms	1/2 teaspoon minced fresh chives
1 tablespoon butter (or low-fat substitute)	1/2 teaspoon lemon juice
2 ounces cream cheese (or low-fat substitute)	1/4 teaspoon salt (or salt substitute)
1/2 tablespoon heavy cream (or milk)	Ground black pepper, to taste
	Paprika
	Parsley for garnish

Preheat the oven to 350°F. Remove the mushroom stems and discard them, wash the caps and dry them.

Put the butter in a shallow baking pan, and place in the oven to melt.

Combine the cream cheese, milk, chives, lemon juice, salt, and black pepper to taste.

Using a fork, mix until smooth.

Spoon a generous amount of the mixture into each inverted mushroom cap and sprinkle lightly with paprika.

Place the mushroom caps in a shallow baking dish coated with butter and return to the oven to bake for 10 to 15 minutes.

Place on a serving tray, garnish with parsley, and provide toothpicks.

Zesty Creamy Cheese Celery   *serves 2 to 4*

A special treat that can be thrown together as a snack or luncheon starter.

4 large celery stalks
4 ounces cream cheese
   (or low-fat substitute),
   at room temperature

1 teaspoon capers, minced
1 teaspoon fresh chives, minced
$1/4$ teaspoon dry mustard

Wash and let dry 4 large celery stalks. Cut them into 4-inch sections (do not split stalks lengthwise).

In a small bowl, combine the cream cheese, capers, chives, and mustard and fill celery with mixture.

Serve immediately or chill for 2 hours.

Marinated Green Olives
serves 2 to 4

This surprisingly tasty appetizer will quickly disappear from the serving plate. Serve it chilled and keep it coming.

$2/3$ cup tarragon, white, or wine vinegar
$1/2$ cup water
1 medium clove garlic, coarsely chopped

$1/4$ teaspoon dried basil
Dash of salt (or salt substitute)
1 can (8 ounces) pitted green olives, drained

Combine the vinegar, water, garlic, basil, and salt.

Drain the olives, place in a bowl with the mixture, cover, and marinate in the refrigerator overnight. Drain before serving.

Deviled Eggs   *serves 6*

This old family standard still works as a spicy and tasty snack or appetizer.

12 eggs*   2 tablespoons mild prepared
1/4 cup mayonnaise†   mustard
2 tablespoons chopped   2 teaspoons paprika
    green pepper

Hard-cook the eggs (10 minutes in boiling water), remove the shells, and slice the eggs in half lengthwise.

Scoop out and mash the yolks. In a mixing bowl, combine the mashed yolks with the mayonnaise, green pepper, and mustard.

When blended thoroughly, spoon the mixture into the egg white halves. Sprinkle with paprika and serve on a bed of lettuce.

*In this recipe, low-fat substitutes cannot be used in place of this item. Always follow your physician's recommendations.
†Do not use low-fat mayonnaise for Craving-Reducing Meals or Snacks as low-fat varieties of mayonnaise often contain added sugars. For an easy low-fat Craving-Reducing mayonnaise alternative, thin "regular" mayonnaise with a little water at a time and mix well.

Liver Mushrooms   *serves 2 to 4*

An unusual twist on a savory appetizer or snack that is best prepared the day before.

1 pound fresh, large mushrooms	2 ounces cream cheese (or low-fat substitute), at room temperature
3 tablespoons butter (or low-fat substitute)	$\frac{1}{2}$ teaspoon dried basil
$\frac{1}{4}$ pound chicken livers	Salt, to taste
$\frac{1}{2}$ tablespoon minced onion	Ground black pepper, to taste

Remove the mushroom stems and chop them well. Wash the caps. Melt 1 tablespoon of the butter in a skillet.

Add the washed mushroom caps and sauté (turning frequently) for 5 minutes. Remove and set aside.

Melt the remaining butter in the heated skillet, add the livers, mushroom stems, and onion. Sauté until the livers are browned.

Chop the liver-vegetable mixture finely and set aside to cool.

Combine the cream cheese with the liver-vegetable mixture. Add basil and salt and pepper to taste.

Spoon the mixture into the mushroom caps. Place on a bed of lettuce. Chill well before serving.

Cream Cheese and Herbs   *serves 3 to 4*

A delectable appetizer or snack that remains exciting.

1   clove garlic, minced
1/2 tablespoon minced onion
1/8 teaspoon salt
    (or salt substitute)
1/4 teaspoon dry mustard,
    or to taste
4   ounces cream cheese
    (or low-fat substitute)
1/4 cup mayonnaise*
1   tablespoon
    lemon juice

1/2 tablespoon pitted green
    olives, chopped
1/2 tablespoon pitted black
    olives, chopped
1/4 teaspoon dried sweet
    basil
Ground black pepper,
    to taste
Chopped fresh chives (or
    scallions or parsley)
Craving-Reducing vegetables

In a medium mixing bowl blend the garlic, onion, and salt. Add dry mustard to taste. Add the cream cheese and mix until smooth.

Next add the mayonnaise, lemon juice, olives (green and black), basil, and black pepper to taste. Blend well.

Place in a serving bowl, sprinkle with the chopped chives, and serve chilled with raw Craving-Reducing vegetables, including cauliflower, mushrooms, celery stalks, and green pepper slices.

*Do not use low-fat mayonnaise for Craving-Reducing Meals or Snacks as low-fat varieties of mayonnaise often contain added sugars. For an easy low-fat Craving-Reducing mayonnaise alternative, thin "regular" mayonnaise with a little water at a time and mix well.

Celery à la Egg   *serves 2*

A delicious appetizer or snack that is simple and satisfying.

3 hard-cooked eggs*	4 teaspoons mayonnaise[†]
6 large stalks celery	1 tablespoon mild prepared
½ cup finely chopped	mustard
green pepper	Chopped parsley for garnish
	(optional)

Chop the eggs finely.

Trim and wash the celery stalks.

In a medium mixing bowl, combine the eggs, green pepper, mayonnaise, and mustard.

Using a serving knife, spread the mixture into the hollows of the celery stalks and garnish, if desired, with chopped parsley.

*In this recipe, low-fat substitutes cannot be used in place of this item. Always follow your physician's recommendations.

[†]Do not use low-fat mayonnaise for Craving-Reducing Meals or Snacks as low-fat varieties of mayonnaise often contain added sugars. For an easy low-fat Craving-Reducing mayonnaise alternative, thin "regular" mayonnaise with a little water at a time and mix well.

Green Salsa

makes about 1 cup

Spicy and exciting but not "too" hot.

3 tablespoons vinegar
1/2 cup olive oil
1 teaspoon prepared
   spicy mustard
1 tablespoon chopped
   parsley

1 tablespoon chopped
   scallion
1 tablespoon chopped
   spinach
1 medium green or red
   pepper, finely diced

In a small bowl, combine the vinegar, oil, mustard, parsley, scallion, spinach, and green or red pepper.

Refrigerate until thoroughly chilled.

Cauliflower-Basil Dip   *serves 2 to 4*

This creamy dip will get your party off on the right foot. Serve the dip in a bowl surrounded with crisp, fresh Craving-Reducing vegetables, such as celery, cucumber sticks, green peppers, green beans, and raw mushroom slices.

½ medium head fresh cauliflower	2 tablespoons chopped fresh basil
½ cup cottage cheese (or low-fat substitute)	½ teaspoon salt (or salt substitute)
1 teaspoon white or wine vinegar	¼ teaspoon garlic powder
¼ cup plain sour cream (or low-fat substitute)	Spicy (hot) paprika, to taste
	Ground black pepper, to taste

Rinse the cauliflower, coarsely chop it, and set it aside.

In a blender or food processor, blend the cottage cheese with the vinegar. Add the cauliflower, sour cream, basil, salt, garlic, and black pepper to taste; blend until mixed.

Cover and chill overnight.

Hot Spinach Dip   *serves 6*

A real delight that is served piping hot and can be a wonderful sign of things to come.

1 package (10 ounces) frozen, chopped spinach	1/4 cup sour cream (or low-fat substitute)
1 tablespoon chopped chives	1/4 teaspoon ground black pepper
2 tablespoons butter (or low-fat substitute)	1/2 teaspoon garlic powder
	1/4 cup spinach water
3 ounces hot pepper cheese (jalapeño), grated	1/4 teaspoon celery salt

Cook the spinach according to the package directions, drain, and retain the water.

In a medium saucepan, sauté the chives in butter until the chives are flaccid.

Add the spinach, cheese, sour cream, pepper, garlic, spinach water, and celery salt and heat over low heat, stirring occasionally, until the cheese is melted and the mixture is creamy.

Hungarian Cheese Dip and Spread   *serves 6*

A spicy taste tickler as a prelude for the wonderful meal to follow.

4 ounces cream cheese (or low-fat substitute)	2 tablespoons dried basil
1/4 cup (4 tablespoons) butter (or low-fat substitute)	1 teaspoon spicy (hot) paprika
4 tablespoons sour cream (or low-fat substitute)	1 teaspoon poppy seeds
4 ounces feta cheese, crumbled	1/4 teaspoon salt (or salt substitute)
1 teaspoon prepared mustard	1/2 teaspoon capers
	Green pepper strips, celery chunks, and cauliflower florets

Mix together the cream cheese and butter. Add the sour cream, feta cheese, mustard, basil, paprika, poppy seeds, and salt. Garnish with the capers.

Serve with strips of green pepper, celery chunks, and cauliflower florets.

Sea Clam Dip   *serves 2 to 4*

Easy preparation and delicious! Surround with crisp, fresh
vegetables, such as cauliflower, celery, green peppers, green
beans, and raw mushrooms.

2   cans minced clams
    (6 to 8 ounces each),
    drained (or cooked
    equivalent)
1   cup sour cream (or low-fat
    substitute)
1/4 teaspoon garlic powder

1   tablespoon lemon juice
1/2 teaspoon salt (or salt
    substitute)
    Cayenne pepper, to taste
    Paprika for garnish (optional)
    Chopped parsley for garnish
    (optional)

Blend the drained clams, sour cream, garlic powder, lemon
juice, salt, and cayenne pepper.

Place in a serving bowl and, if desired, garnish with a light
sprinkling of paprika and parsley.

Crab Spread

serves 4

Adds a sparkling new flavor to the start of your meal.

4 ounces cream cheese
(or low-fat substitute)
Dash of ground black
pepper
½ teaspoon garlic powder
1 teaspoon mayonnaise*

2 ounces mild prepared white
horseradish
1 teaspoon fresh lemon juice
1 can (6 to 8 ounces) canned
crab (or cooked equivalent),
minced
chopped parsley
for garnish

Blend together the cream cheese, black pepper, garlic powder, mayonnaise, horseradish, and lemon juice.

Sprinkle the minced crab on top and if desired garnish with chopped parsley.

*Do not use low-fat mayonnaise for Craving-Reducing Meals or Snacks as low-fat varieties of mayonnaise often contain added sugars. For an easy low-fat Craving-Reducing mayonnaise alternative, thin "regular" mayonnaise with a little water at a time and mix well.

Craving-Reducing Breakfast Choices

SPECIAL NOTE:
Due to the special nature of Craving-Reducing foods, that is, that they are low in carbohydrates, many of the Craving-Reducing Breakfast Choices that follow must rely on eggs and/or other higher-fat foods to replace carbohydrate-rich flours. For lower-fat Craving-Reducing breakfast alternatives, see pages 180–81.

Smooth and Cheesy-Good Omelet   *serves 2*

This unusually tasty breakfast treat will quickly disappear from the serving plate. Serve it hot and keep it coming.

Olive oil or low-fat spray to grease pan
4 large mushrooms, sliced
1 tablespoon chopped hot green pepper (optional)

¹/₄ teaspoon dried basil
4 eggs (or low-fat substitute)
¹/₄ cup cottage cheese or cream cheese (or low-fat equivalent)
Ground black pepper, to taste

In oiled pan, sauté the mushrooms and hot peppers. Add the basil.

Beat the eggs and place them in a medium-sized oiled or sprayed skillet set over medium heat. Flip when semisolid.

Pour in the mushroom and pepper mixture. Add the cheese and fold the omelet in half. Cook until firm.

Add black pepper to taste. Serve warm.

Mushroom Crustless
Breakfast Quiche
serves 2

A snappy breakfast dish readily made ahead of time and served hot
or cold as a special treat.

1 teaspoon butter
(or low-fat substitute)
1/4 cup cream (or whole milk)*
4 ounces Monterey Jack
cheese, grated (or low-fat,
low-salt alternative)
2 cups sliced mushrooms
Dash of dried basil, paprika,
and ground black pepper

2 eggs, lightly beaten*
1/2 package frozen whole-leaf
spinach, thawed, liquid
squeezed out (optional)
1/8 cup bacon bits* (optional)

Preheat the oven to 325°F.

Butter the bottom and sides of a 9-inch pie pan (preferably
glass or ceramic) or a glass loaf pan.

In a medium saucepan, heat the cream (or milk alternative)
until scalded. Remove from the heat and quickly stir in the grated
cheese.

When the cheese is melted, add the mushroom slices, basil,
paprika, and pepper.

Cool for 5 minutes. Add one egg at a time and, if desired, the
spinach. Mix well.

Add the bacon bits if desired. Mix well.

Pour the mixture into the pie pan, place it in the oven, and
bake until the custard is set (45 to 50 minutes).

Serve warm or cold.

*In this recipe, low-fat substitutes cannot be used in place of this item. Always
follow your physician's recommendations.

Cottage Cheese Muffins   *serves 1 or 2*

A light and delicate muffin to get you going for the rest of the day.

1 teaspoon sweet butter (or low-fat substitute)	1/4 cup regular cottage cheese (or low-fat substitute)
2 eggs*	1 tablespoon soy flour†
1/4 teaspoon cream of tartar	1/2 packet sugar substitute

Preheat the oven to 300°F.

Coat the muffin cups with room-temperature butter (or substitute).

Separate the egg whites and egg yolks. Beat the egg whites until frothy. Add cream of tartar and continue to beat until stiff peaks form.

In a medium-sized bowl, combine the egg yolks, cottage cheese, soy flour, and sugar substitute. Mix well. Add the mixture to the beaten egg whites and fold in gently.

Fill each muffin cup 2/3 full with batter.

Bake the muffins until they are golden-brown and they spring back when touched with the back of a fork (25 to 30 minutes).

Remove and serve.

---

*In this recipe, low-fat substitutes cannot be used for this item. Always follow your physician's recommendations.
†Available in most health food stores; see page 210 for purchasing details.

Cinnamon "Bread"   *serves 2*

An exquisite and tasty bread that is high in protein, low in carbohy-drates, and low in fat.

½ teaspoon butter (or low-fat substitute)	½ teaspoon ground cinnamon
4 eggs*	2 tablespoons soy flour†
¾ teaspoon cream of tartar	1 packet sugar substitute
¼ cup regular cottage cheese (or low-fat substitute)	

Preheat the oven to 300°F.

Butter the sides and bottom of a 4   7-inch loaf pan.

Separate the egg whites and yolks. Beat the egg whites until frothy. Add the cream of tartar and continue to beat until stiff but moist peaks form.

In a medium-sized bowl, combine the cinnamon and soy flour. Add the beaten egg yolks, cottage cheese, and sugar substitute. Mix well but do not overmix.

Gently fold the egg-yolk mixture into the beaten egg whites.

Pour the mixture into the prepared pan and bake until the loaf is brown and it springs back when touched with the back of a fork (40 to 45 minutes).

*In this recipe, low-fat substitutes cannot be used in place of this item. Always follow your physician's recommendations.
†Available in most health food stores; see page 210 for purchasing details

Cottage Cheese Soufflé   *serve 2 to 3*

This breakfast pleaser is very light, easy, and delicious.

1 teaspoon butter (or low-fat substitute)

4 eggs*

1 teaspoon cream of tartar

2 cups regular cottage cheese (or low-fat substitute)

½ packet sugar substitute

Preheat the oven to 300°F.

Butter a 9-inch round baking pan.

Separate the egg whites and yolks. Beat the egg whites until frothy but not stiff. Add the cream of tartar and continue to beat until you can form high peaks.

In a medium-sized bowl, combine the cottage cheese, egg yolks, and sweetener and mix well. Fold in the egg whites, gently.

Pour the mixture into the baking pan and place it in oven. Bake for 25 to 30 minutes. Turn the heat to broil and broil top for 2 to 3 minutes. Be careful not to burn the soufflé.

*In this recipe, low-fat substitutes cannot be used in place of this item. Always follow your physician's recommendations.

Western Omelet

serves 2 to 3

A Craving-Reducing twist on an old favorite.

4 large mushrooms, sliced	Butter, olive oil, or
1 slice ham, chopped (or	low-fat pan spray
low-fat or low-salt	1/4 teaspoon dried basil
substitutes)	4 eggs (or low-fat substitute)
1 tablespoon chopped	1/4 cup shredded Swiss or
green pepper (optional)	Cheddar cheese (or low-
1/8 fresh small tomato,	fat substitute)
diced *or* 1 teaspoon	Ground black or cayenne
onion	pepper, to taste

Sauté the mushrooms, ham, green pepper, and tomato or onion in a skillet with a little butter, olive oil, or low-fat pan spray. Add the basil.

Beat the eggs. Add the eggs to a separate skillet that contains a little hot butter, olive oil, or low-fat substitute. Cook over medium heat. Flip when semisolid.

Pour in the mushroom and ham mixture. Add the cheese and fold the omelet in half. Cook until the cheese has melted.

Add pepper to taste and serve warm.

Breakfast Pancakes   *serves 2*

An appetizing breakfast change.

2 eggs*
1/2 teaspoon cream of tartar
1 cup regular cottage cheese
   (or low-fat substitute)

1 tablespoon soy flour†
1/2 packet sugar substitute
1 teaspoon butter (or low-fat
   substitute)

Separate the egg whites and yolks. Beat the whites until frothy. Add the cream of tartar and continue to beat until stiff, dry peaks form.

In a medium-sized bowl, combine the egg yolks, cottage cheese, soy flour, and sweetener. Mix well. Gently fold the yolk mixture into the beaten egg whites.

Place a square griddle over moderate heat. Melt the butter, but do not let it burn.

Pour enough batter to form four 3-inch pancakes on the hot griddle. Cook until brown on one side (about 2 minutes), then turn and brown on the other side.

Stack and serve hot.

*In this recipe, low-fat substitutes cannot be used in place of this item. Always follow your physician's recommendations.
†Available in most health food stores; see page 210 for purchasing details.

Craving-Reducing Fish, Seafood, and Poultry

Sole Triumph   *serves 3 to 4*

A quick and tantalizing preparation for one of the finest-tasting fish.

1½	pounds sole fillets	2 tablespoons finely chopped
1	tablespoon lemon juice	broccoli florets
2	teaspoons olive oil	Coarsely ground black
½	teaspoon dried basil	pepper, to taste

Preheat the oven to 425°F.

Arrange the fillets in a single layer in a suitable baking dish.

In a small bowl, combine the lemon juice, olive oil, basil, and broccoli. Mix thoroughly and sprinkle over fillets. Pepper to taste.

Bake, uncovered, for 10 to 12 minutes, or until the flesh flakes easily with a fork.

Broiled Swordfish   *serves 3 to 4*

A wonderful new recipe that transforms a simple fish into a feast that will delight you as well as guests.

1 teaspoon butter or low-fat spray for greasing pan	Ground black pepper, to taste
	1/8 teaspoon paprika
	1/4 cup olive oil
1 1/2 pounds swordfish steaks	2 tablespoons dried basil
	2 tablespoons lemon juice
Salt (or salt substitute), to taste	Watercress for garnish (optional)

Place a greased broiler rack or broiling pan at level about 2 inches below the broiler element.

Preheat the broiler.

Wash the steaks and sprinkle them with the salt, pepper, and paprika.

Place the steaks on the preheated broiler rack.

Coat the top of the steaks with 1/2 of the olive oil and broil for 3 minutes.

Turn the steaks and coat with the remaining olive oil, then sprinkle with sweet basil, and broil for 4 to 5 additional minutes.

Sprinkle with the lemon juice and, if desired, garnish with watercress.

Baked Fish and Sour Cream   *serves 3 to 4*

This mouth-watering selection is a sumptuous choice for a quick lunch or dinner.

1½ pounds white fish or flounder fillets
1 clove garlic
1 tablespoon butter (or low-fat substitute)
½ teaspoon paprika
1 cup sour cream (or low-fat substitute)
½ teaspoon chopped fresh parsley
¼ teaspoon chopped fresh dill

Preheat the oven to 350°F.

Cut the garlic clove lengthwise and rub the exposed surfaces on both sides of each fillet.

Make a butter-paprika paste and rub it on both sides of each fillet.

Place the fillets in an ovenproof dish and cover with the sour cream.

Cover the dish and bake for 40 to 50 minutes (or until fillets flake with fork).

Remove the dish from the oven, uncover, and sprinkle with the parsley and dill. Serve immediately.

Poached Salmon Steak   *serves 3 to 4*

From the Pacific Northwest to your table in a matter of 25 to 30 minutes of cooking time.

2 tablespoons butter (or low-fat substitute)	1/4 cup white or wine vinegar
1/4 cup chopped onion	Salt (or salt substitute), to taste
1/4 cup chopped green pepper	White peppercorns, to taste
1/4 cup chopped celery	1 large salmon steak, about 2 pounds
1 quart water	

In a large skillet, melt the butter, then add the onion, green pepper, and celery.

Sauté the mixture for 5 to 8 minutes. Add the water, vinegar, salt, and peppercorns and simmer for 5 minutes.

Bring the liquid to a boil as you wrap the steak in coarse cheesecloth.

Submerge the steak in the boiling liquid. Immediately lower the heat and allow the steak to simmer for 25 to 30 minutes.

Remove the steak, carefully unwrap it and serve it hot.

At Craving-Reducing Meals, add one of the sauces from this chapter. At Reward Meals, add any sauce of choice.

Baked Bluefish   *serves 3 to 4*

Humble but luscious.

1 tablespoon vegetable oil	2 cloves garlic, finely minced
1 bluefish, 2 to 3 pounds, cleaned and split	1 tablespoon lemon juice
1 teaspoon sesame oil (optional)	Lemon wedges
	Parsley sprigs for garnish (optional)

Preheat the oven to 425°F.

Spread the vegetable oil over the surface of a large, shallow baking pan.

Place the bluefish cut-side up in the baking pan and sprinkle the surface uniformly with the sesame oil, garlic, and lemon juice.

Bake, uncovered, until the flesh flakes with fork (20 to 25 minutes).

Serve with lemon wedges. If desired, garnish with parsley.

Shrimp with an Oriental Twist   *serves 2*

A robust dish to satisfy the finicky fish eaters in the family.

1 pound parboiled shrimp, shelled and deveined
Butter or low-fat spray for greasing baking pan
Salt (or salt substitute), to taste
1/2 cup diced celery
1/2 cup sliced mushrooms

1 tablespoon teriyaki sauce (or low-salt substitute)
2 tablespoons toasted sesame seeds
1/2 teaspoon dried, crumbled thyme leaves
1/4 cup melted butter (or low-fat substitute)

Preheat the oven to 350°F.

Arrange the shrimp in a buttered shallow baking pan.

Salt to taste.

Combine the celery, mushrooms, teriyaki sauce, sesame seeds, thyme, and melted butter, and pour the mixture over the shrimp.

Bake, uncovered, for about 8 minutes.

Serve warm or as a delicious cold leftover.

Herby Crabmeat Salad   *serves 3 to 4*

A luncheon taste treat that requires very little preparation time.

1 pound raw crabmeat
4 tablespoons olive oil
Salt (or salt substitute), to taste
Coarsely ground black pepper, to taste

1 tablespoon lemon juice
$1/2$ tablespoon dried basil
$1/2$ tablespoon chopped scallions
$1/2$ tablespoon dried tarragon
Parsley for garnish (optional)

Remove all bits of nonedible material from the crabmeat.

In a skillet, heat the olive oil until hot and add the crabmeat and stir continually until thoroughly cooked (about 3 minutes).

Remove the skillet from the heat and add the salt, pepper, lemon juice, basil, scallions, and tarragon. Mix thoroughly.

Garnish with parsley, if desired, and serve.

Shrimp with Spices   *serves 2 to 4*

A splendid surprise—yours to enjoy at any lunch, snack, or as the start of a wonderful dinner.

1 pound medium shrimp	1/3 cup olive oil
2 tablespoons celery leaves	1/4 cup white or wine vinegar
1 tablespoon mixed pickling spices	1 tablespoon capers and juice
	2 teaspoons celery seeds
1/2 teaspoon salt (or salt substitute)	1/2 teaspoon salt
	Cayenne pepper, to taste
1 bay leaf	

Place the shrimp in a saucepan filled with boiling water, adding the celery leaves, pickling spices, and salt.

Reduce the heat to a simmer, cover the pan, and cook for 5 minutes, then drain. Peel and devein the shrimp under cold running water.

In a shallow dish, layer the shrimp.

Place the bay leaf, olive oil, vinegar, capers and juice, celery seeds, salt, and cayenne pepper in a small bowl and combine well, add shrimp and mix well, then cover the dish.

Chill for at least 24 hours, occasionally spooning the marinade over the shrimp.

Serve cold over a bed of lettuce, if desired.

Chicken in Olive Sauce   *serves 3 to 4*

A sure taste delight.

1 tablespoon olive oil
4 skinned, boneless
  chicken breasts
2 tablespoons lime juice
1 tablespoon wine vinegar
1 clove garlic, crushed

4 tablespoons sliced pitted
  black olives
4 tablespoons sliced pitted
  green olives
4 tablespoons dried basil
  Ground black pepper, to taste
  Green pepper rings for
  garnish (optional)

In a large skillet, heat the olive oil and brown the chicken over medium-high heat. Lower the heat, cover, and cook until tender (8 to 10 minutes).

Remove the chicken to a serving plate and keep warm.

Combine the lime juice, vinegar, garlic, black and green olives, and basil in the skillet used for the chicken. Gently heat.

Slice the chicken, top with olive sauce, and season with pepper to taste. If desired, arrange on plates with green pepper rings.

Chicken and Broccoli   *serves 3 to 4*

A stir-fry that is easily prepared in advance or served up "on the spot."

2 pounds chicken breasts, boneless and skinned	3/4 cup chicken stock
2 tablespoons olive oil	2 tablespoons teriyaki sauce (or low-salt substitute)
2 tablespoons minced ginger root	2 tablespoons mayonnaise*
6 cups chopped broccoli florets and stems	2 tablespoons water
3/4 pound mushrooms, sliced	4 cups sliced red or green cabbage
2 tablespoons dry sherry (or cooking wine)	Ground black pepper, to taste

Cut the chicken into thin strips (pinky-sized). Set aside.

In a large, heavy skillet, heat the oil until very hot. Carefully add the chicken and 1 tablespoon of ginger root to skillet. If sticking occurs, add a bit more oil. Stir continually and slowly for about 2 minutes. Remove the chicken from the skillet and set it aside.

Reheat the skillet. Combine the broccoli, mushrooms, and remaining ginger root and stir continually for 2 minutes. Add a little water if sticking occurs.

Mix the sherry, chicken stock, and teriyaki sauce, and pour the liquid mixture over the broccoli mixture in the skillet. Cover, and let steam for 2 minutes.

Stir in the chicken mixture, mayonnaise, water, and bring to a boil.

Add the cabbage, stir for 1 minute, or until cabbage is crisp. Season to taste with black pepper. Serve hot.

---

* Do not use low-fat mayonnaise for Craving-Reducing Meals or Snacks as low-fat varieties of mayonnaise often contain added sugars. For an easy low-fat Craving-Reducing mayonnaise alternative, thin "regular" mayonnaise with a little water at a time and mix well.

Sultry Lemon Chicken   *serves 3 to 4*

A wonderful summer delight that is something that can be enjoyed in the winter as well.

4 large chicken breasts, boneless and skinned	1/4 teaspoon dried basil
	1/4 teaspoon cayenne pepper, or to taste
2 tablespoons lemon juice	
2 teaspoons olive oil	1/4 teaspoon teriyaki sauce (or low-salt substitute)
2 cloves garlic, minced	

Rinse the breasts thoroughly and arrange them in a single layer in a shallow baking dish.

In a small bowl, combine the lemon juice, olive oil, garlic, basil, cayenne, and teriyaki sauce and mix well.

Pour the mixture over the chicken and turn to cover both sides of the chicken.

Cover and refrigerate overnight for best results.

Cook the chicken over hot coals on a greased grill or broil in a conventional oven until thoroughly cooked, approximately 6 minutes per side.

CRAVING-REDUCING MEATS:
Beef, Pork, Lamb, and Veal

Saucy Sirloin Steak
serves 3 to 4

A hearty steak with a saucy twist that will delight the palate.

3 tablespoons olive oil
1 tablespoon sesame oil
2 large sirloin steaks (1½ to 2 pounds)
½ cup chopped scallion bulbs
2 tablespoons chopped fresh chives

1 tablespoon red wine vinegar
½ cup dry red wine
Coarsely ground black pepper, to taste
Parsley sprigs for garnish (optional)

In a deep skillet, combine the olive oil and sesame oil and heat over medium heat.

When hot, add the steak and cook for 8 to 10 minutes on each side, depending on the desired degree of doneness (rare, medium, well-done).

When ready, set the steak on a platter and cover. Raise the burner heat to medium-high and add the scallions, chives, and vinegar to the oil at the bottom of the skillet and stir for 20 seconds.

Add the wine and simmer for 1 minute. Raise the burner heat to medium-high and return the steak to the skillet. Cook for 1 minute on each side and remove the skillet from the heat.

Slice the steak crosswise into thin slices and serve topped with the sauce from the bottom of the skillet. Season to taste with black pepper.

Garnish with parsley sprigs, if desired.

Spicy Beef   *serves 4 to 6*

This tasty hot dish is also delicious served for a cold lunch, snack, or dinner the following day.

2-pound chuck roast
White or wine vinegar
Dry red wine
1 cup chopped scallions
1 bay leaf
1 teaspoon ground cinnamon
1 teaspoon ground allspice
1 teaspoon ground cloves

1 teaspoon ground black pepper
1 teaspoon salt
  (or salt substitute)
2 cups sliced mushrooms
2 stalks celery, trimmed and
  minced
1 tablespoon butter
  (or low-fat substitute)

In a medium-sized pot, place the roast and enough vinegar and wine in 1:1 proportions to cover the roast 1 inch above the top.

Add the scallions, bay leaf, cinnamon, allspice, cloves, pepper, and salt. Cover the pot and refrigerate and marinate overnight.

When ready, preheat the oven to 275°F. Remove the meat from the marinade and set the liquid aside.

Place the meat in a roasting pan and pour in ½ of the marinade liquid. Add 2 cups water, cover, and roast for about 3 hours. Baste several times.

Sauté the mushrooms and celery in the butter until golden-brown. Add the mixture to the roasting pan for the last ½ hour of cooking. Baste twice.

When ready, slice the meat and serve hot.

Enjoy with cooked wine-rich marinade at Reward Meals only.

Beef and Celery Ragoût

serves 4 to 6

A simple but elegant dish that will always be a hit.

2 pounds lean boneless beef
1 tablespoon garlic powder
6 stalks celery, cut into strips
3 cups beef bouillon
2 cups sliced mushrooms
2 cups broccoli florets
½ cup chopped fresh parsley

3 cloves, gently crushed
1 teaspoon dried thyme
1 teaspoon salt
(or salt substitute)
Coarsely ground black pepper,
to taste.

Preheat the broiler.

Cut the beef into 1-inch cubes and sprinkle with the garlic powder.

Place the beef on a broiling rack and place it in the oven about 4 inches below the broiling element and brown it on all sides (about 15 minutes).

Transfer the beef to a Dutch oven. Add the celery, beef bouillon, mushrooms, parsley, cloves, thyme, salt, and pepper and cover the pan.

Bring the liquid to a boil, reduce the heat, and simmer until the beef is tender (approximately 1¼ hours). Add broccoli and continue simmering (about 10 minutes).

Serve hot.

Green Pepper Steak   *serves 3 to 4*

This easy-to-make luncheon or dinner choice is a favorite for a wintry day. It keeps well for a delicious leftover the next day.

¼ cup olive oil
1 teaspoon teriyaki sauce (or low-salt substitute)
¼ cup finely chopped celery (½ stalk and ½ leaves)

1 cup sliced green pepper
8 very thinly sliced minute steaks
½ cup sliced mushrooms
1 clove chopped garlic

In a large skillet, thoroughly combine the olive oil and teriyaki sauce. Sauté the celery and green pepper until slightly soft.

Push vegetables to one side in the skillet. Add the steaks to the other side and brown on one side (about 2 minutes), then turn the steaks and brown them on the other side (about 1 minute).

Add the mushrooms and garlic. Stir and continue to sauté until tender.

Serve warm.

Peppered Fillet of Beef
serves 3 to 4

A tantalizing and delightful cut of beef.

1 beef fillet (about 2 pounds), rolled and tied	1 tablespoon paprika
3 large cloves garlic, slivered	1 tablespoon coarsely ground black pepper
2 tablespoons teriyaki sauce	1 teaspoon dried basil

Preheat the oven to 425°F.

Using a sharp-pointed knife, poke 1-inch slits into the surface of the fillet and insert a garlic sliver into each slit, until all slivers are used. Try to distribute them evenly over the surface.

Brush the teriyaki sauce over the surface and sprinkle with the paprika, black pepper, and basil.

Place the fillet on a roasting rack in a shallow roasting pan. Insert a meat thermometer into thick part of roast, and place the roast in the oven.

After 15 minutes, reduce the heat to 350°F. and roast until it reaches the desired doneness (rare, medium, or well-done).

Hamburgers with Dill   *serves 3 to 4*

Another delectable form of ground beef. If you prefer a low-fat
alternative, ground turkey makes a fine substitute.

2	pounds ground round steak (or other suitable lower-fat cut)	2	teaspoons olive oil
			Teriyaki sauce, salt, or salt substitute, to taste
1	teaspoon dried dill		Ground black pepper, to taste

Combine the meat with the dill and divide into six equal
burgers.

Heat the oil in a deep skillet set over medium heat until it
becomes quite hot (about 2-3 minutes).

Sprinkle teriyaki sauce or salt to taste on the bottom of the pan
and add the burgers.

Sear both sides of the burgers, reduce the heat, and continue to
cook until desired doneness (rare, medium, well-done).

Sprinkle each burger with black pepper to taste.

Herby Lamb Loin
serves 3 to 4

This special treat is tasty and easy to prepare in advance.

1 pound boneless lamb loin	1/4 teaspoon dried oregano
1 tablespoon ground black pepper	1 tablespoon dried basil
	1/2 cup chopped fresh parsley
2 cloves garlic, minced	2 tablespoons teriyaki sauce (or low-salt substitute)

Slice the lamb into thin pieces and place them in a medium-sized bowl.

Combine the pepper, garlic, oregano, basil, parsley, and teriyaki sauce in a small bowl, and mix well.

Immediately pour the mixture over the lamb. Cover and refrigerate overnight.

Remove the lamb from the marinade and broil it (or grill it over hot coals) for 2 to 3 minutes per side.

Serve with steamed broccoli or cauliflower.

Peppered Lamb

serves 3 to 4

A spicy special treat.

Coarsely ground black pepper, to taste

2 pounds lamb chops, thin-cut

2 teaspoons salt (or salt substitute)

¼ cup (4 tablespoons) butter (or low-fat substitute)

1 teaspoon teriyaki sauce (or low-salt substitute)

Lemon juice, to taste

Parsley sprigs for garnish (optional)

Sprinkle black pepper on a cutting board and press the lamb chops into the pepper and work it into both sides of the meat using the palms of your hands.

Sprinkle a large heavy skillet with salt and then heat. When the salt begins to brown, place the steaks in the skillet and brown them on both sides over high heat. Reduce the heat and cook the steaks to the desired doneness (rare, medium, well-done).

In a small pan, combine the butter, teriyaki sauce, and lemon juice and heat until warm but not boiling. Pour the mixture over the chops.

Serve immediately and, if desired, garnish with parsley sprigs.

Roast Lamb with Herbs   *serves 9 to 12*

A wonderful recipe that is easy and great for company.

1 lamb roast, about 3 pounds	1/2 teaspoon ground ginger
1 clove garlic, crushed	1 bay leaf
1 teaspoon salt (or salt substitute)	1/2 teaspoon dried thyme
	1/2 teaspoon dried sage
2 tablespoons coarsely ground black pepper (or to taste)	1/2 teaspoon dried marjoram
	1 tablespoon teriyaki sauce (or low-salt substitute)
1 teaspoon dried basil	1 tablespoon olive oil

Preheat the oven to 350°F.

Place the meat on a rack in a roasting pan.

In a small bowl, combine the garlic, salt, pepper, basil, ginger, bay leaf, thyme, sage, marjoram, teriyaki sauce, and olive oil and mix thoroughly.

Make slits in the lamb and rub the mixture into the slits and over the entire surface of the lamb.

Insert a meat thermometer into the thickest part of the roast, and place the pan in the oven. After 10 minutes, reduce the heat to 300°F. and roast to the desired doneness (rare, medium, or well-done).

Pork and Vegetable Bounty   *serves 3 to 4*

A delicious and simple pork recipe.

	pork tenderloin, about 1½ pounds	½	pound mushrooms, sliced
2	tablespoons butter (or low-fat substitute)	½	teaspoon dried rosemary
1	medium green pepper, cut into strips	6	pitted green olives, sliced
½	cup dry white wine	2	tablespoons lemon juice
			Parsley sprigs for garnish (optional)

Cut the pork into 1-inch crosswise slices.

Place the butter in a skillet set over medium heat. When hot, sauté the pork strips until golden-brown. Lower the heat. Add the green pepper strips.

In a small pot, bring the wine to a boil. Carefully pour the heated wine over the meat. Immediately add the mushrooms and the rosemary. Cover the skillet and simmer for ½ hour.

Add the olives and lemon juice.

If desired, serve with a parsley garnish.

Pork Roast

serves 4 to 5

A wonderful taste treat that is not only delightful to the eye but also to the nose, tongue, and stomach.

1	boneless pork roast, almost 2 pounds		Paprika, to taste
1	tablespoon teriyaki sauce (or low-salt substitute)	3	tablespoons olive oil
		2	tablespoons sesame oil
		2	cloves garlic, crushed

Preheat the oven to 350°F.

Place a meat thermometer in the thickest part of the pork roast and place the roast on a rack in a roasting pan with a 1-inch water level on the bottom.

Pour the teriyaki sauce over the top of the roast, then sprinkle with paprika to taste.

Combine the oils, pour the mixture over the top of the roast, and sprinkle on the garlic.

Roast for about 2½ hours (until appropriate temperature is reached on the meat thermometer).

Ham and Cabbage

serves 3 to 4

A new switch on an old favorite.

1	small head red or green cabbage	¹/₄	cup chopped fresh parsley
4	teaspoons butter (or low-fat substitute)		Finely ground black pepper, to taste
1	cup sour cream (or low-fat substitute)	3	four-ounce fully cooked, deboned ham slices
¹/₂	cup grated Swiss cheese (or low-fat substitute)	1	cup chopped green pepper Coarsely ground black pepper, to taste

Preheat the oven to 350°F.

Cut the cabbage into quarters, then split each quarter in half.

Place 1 inch water in a deep skillet, add the cabbage, and turn the burner heat to high. Cover and cook for 3 minutes. Turn off the heat, pour off the water, and keep covered.

In a saucepan, melt the butter, and add the sour cream, Swiss cheese, parsley, and pepper to taste. Stir until the cheese is melted.

Lightly grease a shallow baking pan.

Arrange the ham and cabbage in the pan, sprinkle with the green pepper, and pour the sauce over all. Sprinkle with coarsely ground black pepper to taste.

Bake for 20 minutes.

Serve with spicy or regular mustard.

Asparagus-Ham Delight   *serves 4*

A great use for leftovers that produces a dish good enough for guests.

12 fresh, thick asparagus spears	1 cup grated Cheddar cheese (or low-fat substitute)
4 four-ounce fully cooked, thick deboned ham slices	1/2 teaspoon salt (or salt substitute)
2 tablespoons butter (or low-fat substitute)	2 teaspoons lemon juice
4 tablespoons sour cream (or low-fat substitute)	1 tablespoon Dijon mustard

Preheat oven to 350°F.

Place 1 inch water in a deep skillet, add the asparagus, and turn the burner heat to high. Cover and heat for 2 to 3 minutes. Turn off the heat, pour off the water, and keep the skillet covered.

In a medium casserole dish, arrange the ham slices and place 3 asparagus spears over each.

In a small saucepan, melt the butter, then reduce the heat and add the sour cream, grated Cheddar, salt, lemon juice, and Dijon mustard, stirring until completely mixed.

Pour the sauce over the asparagus and ham.

Place the casserole in the oven and cook until hot (8 to 10 minutes).

Serve warm or cold.

Lemony Veal

serves 3 to 4

A wonderful contrast in flavors.

2	tablespoons olive oil		Lemon peel, to taste
1/2	cup chopped scallions	2	tablespoons olive oil
1 1/2	pounds cubed boneless veal	4	tablespoons sour cream (or low-fat substitute)
1/2	cup chicken broth	2	teaspoons dried tarragon
1/2	cup large green olives, pitted	1	tablespoon lemon juice
2	stalks celery, diced		Ground black pepper, to taste
			Salt (or salt substitute), to taste

In a flameproof casserole dish, heat the oil over low heat. Add the scallions and sauté for 3 minutes.

Add the veal cubes and quickly brown them over medium-high heat. Turn off the heat and set aside.

In a small bowl, combine the broth, olives, celery, lemon peel, olive oil, sour cream, tarragon, and lemon juice.

Add the mixture to the casserole, and simmer until the veal is tender (about 1 hour). Pepper and salt to taste.

Savory Veal Chops

serves 4 to 6

A wonderfully tasty dish with a delicate flavor.

2	large cloves garlic, crushed		Coarsely ground black pepper, to taste
2	tablespoons dried sage	8	thick veal chops
2	tablespoons dried rosemary		Parsley sprigs for garnish
2	tablespoons dried thyme		(optional)

Preheat the broiler.

In a small bowl, combine the garlic, sage, rosemary, thyme, and pepper. Mix well.

Coat both sides of the chops with the mixture and press the mixture into the chops with the palms of the hands. Cover and refrigerate overnight.

Broil the chops for about 4 minutes per side, and serve hot.

If desired, garnish with parsley sprigs.

Craving-Reducing Salads, Dressings, and Vegetables

Caesar Salad
serves 2

An old standby salad with a twist.

Salt (or salt substitute), to taste
1 large clove garlic, peeled
1 teaspoon dry mustard
1 tablespoon lemon juice
Cayenne pepper, to taste
2 tablespoons olive oil

1 bunch lettuce, spinach, or greens
1 tablespoon grated imported Swiss cheese (or cheese of choice or low-fat substitute)
2/3 can anchovies, drained (optional)
1 egg boiled for 60 seconds*†

Sprinkle salt on the bottom of a large wooden bowl and generously rub the bottom and sides with the garlic clove.

Add the mustard, lemon juice, and cayenne pepper to taste.

Stir with a wooden spoon until the salt dissolves.

Rinse the lettuce or other greens well. Dry with paper toweling and tear the lettuce into bite-size pieces and place them in the bowl.

Sprinkle with the grated cheese. Add the anchovies if desired.

Break the egg over the salad.

Thoroughly mix by tossing gently until the ingredients are distributed uniformly.

---

* In this recipe, low-fat substitutes cannot be used in place of this item. Always follow your physician's recommendations.
† Use certified salmonella-free eggs only.

Cucumber Salad with Dressing   *serves 3 to 4*

A wonderful change of pace.

1   cup sour cream
    (or low-fat substitute)
1   teaspoon chopped chives
½ teaspoon salt
    (or salt substitute)

Ground black pepper, to taste
1   tablespoon wine vinegar
2   medium cucumbers,
    peeled and sliced thinly
Paprika for garnish

In a large bowl, combine the sour cream, chives, salt, pepper, and vinegar.

Add cucumbers and toss lightly.

Garnish with paprika and serve on a bed of lettuce.

Oregano Chicken Salad with Dressing

serves 3 to 4

This easy-to-make salad favorite is great for leftover chicken. Add a side vegetable or extra chicken or other protein if you like, or serve the salad all alone; it makes a complete Craving-Reducing lunch or snack in itself.

2 cups cold cooked, cubed chicken
1 cup diced celery
$1/4$ cup chopped chives or scallions

$1/3$ cup plain sour cream or mayonnaise* (or low-fat sour cream substitute)
$1/4$ teaspoon dried oregano
Ground black pepper and salt (or salt substitute), to taste

In a large bowl, combine the chicken, celery, chives or scallions, sour cream (or mayonnaise), and oregano; mix lightly with a fork.

Cover and refrigerate for at least 2 hours.

Just before serving, add pepper and salt to taste.

* Do not use low-fat mayonnaise for Craving-Reducing Meals or Snacks as low-fat varieties of mayonnaise often contain added sugars. For an easy low-fat Craving-Reducing mayonnaise alternative, thin "regular" mayonnaise with a little water at a time and mix well.

Monkfish Salad with Dressing   *serves 3 to 4*

A light and tasty meal that has passed review with flying colors many times.

3 cups diced monkfish or
   fish of choice, poached
   or broiled
3 cups diced celery
1/2 green pepper, chopped
1/4 cup mayonnaise*
1/4 cup dried basil
1/4 cup chopped scallions

1 tablespoon chopped pitted
   green olives
3 or 4 large lettuce leaves,
   for garnish (optional)
   Coarsely ground black pepper,
   to taste
   Radishes and olives for garnish
   Favorite dressing

In a large bowl, combine the fish, celery, green pepper, mayonnaise, basil, scallions, and olives. Toss gently.

Line another large bowl with the lettuce leaves and spoon the contents of the first bowl over them; pepper to taste.

Garnish with radishes and olives and serve with your favorite dressing.

---

* Do not use low-fat mayonnaise for Craving-Reducing Meals or Snacks as low-fat varieties of mayonnaise often contain added sugars. For an easy low-fat Craving-Reducing mayonnaise alternative, thin "regular" mayonnaise with a little water at a time and mix well.

Tossed Green Salad   *serves 3 to 4*

This salad can be varied in many different ways. Use it as a basic
and let your creative mind take over. Make sure that you use only
the Craving-Reducing vegetables listed on page 121.

4   cups torn lettuce leaves   1/2 cup alfalfa or bean sprouts
    (any type)   8   medium radishes
1   cup sliced celery   4   scallions
1   cup sliced cucumber   Favorite dressing
1/2 cup chopped red cabbage   Coarsely ground black pepper,
1/2 cup sliced mushrooms   to taste

In a large bowl, combine the lettuce, celery, cucumber,
cabbage, mushrooms, sprouts, radishes, and scallions. Toss lightly.
   Add your favorite dressing and toss lightly again.
   Pepper to taste and serve.

Egg and Broccoli Salad
with Dressing   *serves 3 to 4*

A subtle and simple delight.

1 small head broccoli, cut into florets (cauliflower or green beans may be substituted)	1/8 teaspoon black pepper 1/8 teaspoon dried basil or parsley
1 tablespoon red wine vinegar	3 tablespoons olive oil 3 eggs, hard-cooked*
1/8 teaspoon salt (or salt substitute)	3/4 cup mayonnaise† Paprika, for garnish (optional)

Add the broccoli to a medium-sized pot containing 1/2 inch of boiling water, then cover and steam (3 to 4 minutes).

Drain the remaining water from the pot and add the vinegar, salt, pepper, basil (or parsley), and oil while still hot. Cool and refrigerate for several hours or overnight.

Separate the yolks from the whites of the cooled hard-cooked eggs. Set the yolks aside and slice the whites, mixing them with the cooled broccoli mixture. Add the mayonnaise and combine.

Carefully spoon the mixture into a shallow serving bowl. Sprinkle with grated egg yolk and paprika, if desired.

* In this recipe, low-fat substitutes cannot be used in place of this item. Always follow your physician's recommendations.
† Do not use low-fat mayonnaise for Craving-Reducing Meals or Snacks as low-fat varieties of mayonnaise often contain added sugars. For an easy low-fat Craving-Reducing mayonnaise alternative, thin "regular" mayonnaise with a little water at a time and mix well.

Shrimp Salad with Dressing   *serves 3 to 4*

The fruits of the sea always provide a satisfying salad for any meal
of the day.

6 tablepoons virgin olive oil	1 teaspoon dried basil Water for boiling shrimp
1 tablespoon lemon juice	16 medium shrimp shelled and deveined
1 teaspoon Dijon mustard	
1/4 teaspoon plus	2 heads romaine lettuce (or other green of choice)
1/8 teaspoon salt (or salt substitute), Ground black pepper to taste	1 bunch watercress, large stems removed

First make the dressing. In a small bowl, combine the olive oil,
lemon juice, mustard, 1/4 teaspoon salt, pepper, and basil. Mix
thoroughly.

In a large pot, heat water and boil the shrimp until red (about 5
minutes at a boil).

In a large bowl combine the cucumber, 1/8 teaspoon salt,
lettuce, and watercress. Gently toss the greens until thoroughly
mixed.

Add the shrimp, top with the dressing, and toss gently.

Chill for 1 hour, then serve.

Chef's Salad   *serves 3 to 4*

A wonderfully satisfying and filling lunch or unusual dinner salad.

3 cups torn lettuce (or greens of choice)	6 to 8 large lettuce leaves
1 cup cooked chicken or turkey,* cut into thin strips	4 hard-cooked eggs, cut in half lengthwise (optional)
1 cup cooked roast beef or ham*	8 radishes, cut in half
1 cup hard cheese, cut into thin strips	8 pitted olives, black or green Coarse black pepper, to taste Favorite salad dressing

In a large bowl, combine the lettuce, poultry, beef or ham, and cheese. Toss gently.

Line another large bowl with the lettuce leaves, add the salad mixture and eggs, cut-side up.

Garnish with radishes and olives, pepper to taste, and serve with your favorite dressing.

* For Craving-Reducing Meals or Snacks, use only meats and poultry that are home-made or that you are certain contain no added sugars or fillers. In addition, note that many delicatessen varieties of these meats and poultry may contain added MSG, so avoid these as well.

Italian Mozzarella Salad
with Dressing

serves 3 to 4

A refreshing salad that is fun to make and eat. You can vary the recipe to taste.

1 cup diced celery	2 tablespoons olive oil
1 cup diced green pepper	2 tablespoons lemon juice
1 cup sliced mushrooms	1 tablespoon mayonnaise*
1 cup small mozzarella cheese slices	1/4 teaspoon dried thyme
	1/4 teaspoon dried basil
3 tablespoons wine or white vinegar	1/4 teaspoon dried oregano
	Ground black pepper, to taste

In a large salad bowl, combine the celery, pepper, mushrooms, and mozzarella. Set aside.

In a small bowl, combine the vinegar, olive oil, lemon juice, mayonnaise, thyme, basil, and oregano; mix thoroughly.

Pour the dressing mixture over the salad and toss until the mixture is uniformly distributed. Pepper to taste.

May be served immediately or chilled for later use.

* Do not use low-fat mayonnaise for Craving-Reducing Meals or Snacks as low-fat varieties of mayonnaise often contain added sugars. For an easy low-fat Craving-Reducing mayonnaise alternative, thin "regular" mayonnaise with a little water at a time and mix well.

Spinach Salad with Dressing   *serves 2*

"Olive oil" not withstanding, even Popeye would find this salad to be a wonderful change at your Craving-Reducing lunch or as the start of your evening Reward Meal. Serve it with your favorite dressing.

1 pound fresh spinach	1/2 cup chopped mushrooms
1 clove garlic	6 tablespoons thin
2 tablespoons olive oil	sliced scallions
3 teaspoons lemon juice	2 hard-cooked eggs, thick-
1/4 cup crumbled crisp	sliced across (optional)
cooked bacon	Favorite salad dressing

Wash the spinach several times thoroughly. Remove the tough stems, pat dry with paper toweling, and wrap in damp paper toweling. Refrigerate for about 1 hour.

Cut the garlic clove in half and rub the cut surface over the inside surface of a large bowl. Coat the inside of the bowl with the olive oil and lemon juice.

Tear the chilled spinach into bite-sized pieces and place in the bowl prepared above.

Add the bacon, mushrooms, and scallions. Toss lightly.

Arrange the egg slices around edge of salad and serve with your favorite dressing.

Fresh Seafood Salad   *serves 3 to 4*

A cold seafood salad that makes a complete and tasty Craving-Reducing lunch or snack or a wonderful starter for your Reward Meal.

2/3 pound medium shrimp, shelled and deveined
1/4 pound sea scallops
1/4 pound fresh codfish, monkfish, or other fish of choice
1/2 cup coarsely chopped cucumber
1/2 cup chopped celery
1/2 cup chopped scallions
Coarsely ground black pepper, to taste
Favorite salad dressing

Boil, broil, or sauté the shrimp, scallops, and fish. Cool.
In a large bowl, combine the cooled shrimp, scallops, and fish. Add the cucumber, celery, scallions, and pepper to taste.
Add your favorite dressing and toss lightly.
Cover and chill for 2 hours.
Serve on a cool bed of large lettuce leaves.

Bean Sprout Salad
with Dressing

serves 3 to 4

Take advantage of this simple but delightful salad.

2   cups fresh sprouts,
    bean or alfalfa (or lettuce,
    arugula, or greens of
    choice)
1/4 cup chopped green pepper
1/4 cup chopped celery
1/2 cup thinly sliced cucumber
1   clove garlic, minced

1/4 cup olive oil
2   tablespoons vinegar
1/2 teaspoon salt
    (or salt substitute)
1/4 teaspoon cayenne pepper
    (optional)
1   tablespoon sesame seeds

In a large bowl, gently combine the sprouts (or greens), green pepper, celery, and cucumber.

In a small bowl, combine the garlic, oil, vinegar, salt, cayenne pepper (if desired), and sesame seeds and mix thoroughly.

Chill both bowls, separately, for at least 1 hour.

Spoon generous portions of the dressing over each serving of salad.

Garlic Dressing

Makes about 1 cup

An aromatic salad dressing that is a tasty complement to any green salad, or served as a wonderful raw vegetable dip.

½ teaspoon mild dry
  mustard
Salt (or salt substitute),
to taste
Coarsely ground black
pepper, to taste

2 cloves garlic, finely minced
1 tablespoon tarragon vinegar
3 tablespoons lemon juice
1 cup olive oil

In a bowl or large jar, combine and mix the mustard, salt, and black pepper.

Add the garlic, vinegar, lemon juice, and oil to the mixture and stir until thoroughly mixed.

Let sit at room temperature for an hour before serving.

Green Garden Mayonnaise   *Makes about 1 cup*

A tempting dressing with a mild and creamy texture.

1 stalk celery with leaves	1 tablespoon dried basil
5 spinach leaves	1/2 teaspoon lemon juice
5 scallions, chopped fine	1/2 cup mayonnaise*

In a blender or food processor, chop the celery and leaves, spinach, and scallions.

Add the basil, lemon juice, and mayonnaise. Blend well.

Use as topping for vegetables, fish, chicken, or fresh green salads.

---

*Do not use low-fat mayonnaise for Craving-Reducing Meals or Snacks as low-fat varieties of mayonnaise often contain added sugars. For an easy low-fat Craving-Reducing mayonnaise alternative, thin "regular" mayonnaise with a little water at a time and mix well.

Creamy Herbal Dressing   *Makes about 1 cup*

This delicate and creamy dressing will brighten any salad.

½ cup cottage cheese
   (or low-fat substitute)
½ cup sour cream
   (or low-fat substitute)
½ teaspoon spicy mustard

¼ teaspoon dried tarragon
½ tablespoon dried basil
Salt (or salt substitute), to taste
Ground black pepper, to taste

In a blender, food processor, or mixing bowl, process cottage cheese until smooth. Add the sour cream, mustard, tarragon, and basil. Salt and pepper to taste.

Refrigerate overnight.

Mustard-Garlic Vinaigrette   *makes about 1 cup*

A tangy but simple dressing that is a great addition to any salad.

2 cloves garlic, minced
2 teaspoons Dijon mustard
2 tablespoons lemon
  juice
1/3 cup water
1/4 cup olive, vegetable
  or walnut oil

1 teaspoon grated imported
  Swiss cheese (or other
  cheese of choice, or low-fat
  substitute)
  Ground black pepper, to taste

In a blender, food processor, or mixing bowl, combine the garlic, mustard, lemon juice, and water until well mixed. Continue mixing while gradually adding oil. Add the cheese and ground pepper to taste.

Let sit for 2 minutes before serving.

Steamed Cauliflower
and Cheese

serves 3 to 4

Simple, quick, but very tasty.

4 cups cauliflower florets (broccoli can be substituted)	1 cup sharp Cheddar cheese (or low-fat substitute), shredded
1/2 cup water	Cayenne or ground black pepper, to taste

Heat the water and cauliflower over high heat in a covered skillet.

Turn off the heat, remove the cover, and sprinkle the cheese over the cauliflower florets.

Return the cover and let stand for 2 minutes only.

Season to taste with cayenne or black pepper.

Serve immediately.

Garlic and Green Beans

serves 3 to 4

Once you get your first taste, this side vegetable dish will disappear in no time.

1/2 cup water
1/8 teaspoon salt (or salt substitute)
1 pound fresh green beans, trimmed

1/4 cup (4 tablespoons) butter (or low-fat substitute)
1 clove garlic, crushed
Ground black pepper, to taste

In a deep skillet set over high heat, add the water, 1/2 of the salt, and the green beans.

Cover and cook over high heat until the beans are barely tender (approximately 3 1/2 minutes).

Place beans in a serving dish and cover to keep warm.

In a small saucepan set over medium heat, combine the butter and garlic. Mix well as butter melts.

Pour the mixture over the beans. Add remaining salt and pepper to taste and serve warm with any entree.

Savory Spinach
serves 3 to 4

Popeye's favorite vegetable served in a wonderful new way to entice family, guests, or Popeye to the lunch table.

2 tablespoons sesame seeds	1 tablespoon teriyaki sauce (or low-salt substitute)
1½ pounds fresh spinach	1 teaspoon Dijon mustard
1 tablespoon sesame oil	
2 tablespoons red wine vinegar	Ground black pepper, to taste

In a dry, clean skillet set over medium heat, add the sesame seeds and gently shake and heat until several seeds take on color or some begin to pop. Remove from the heat and set aside.

Wash the spinach and cut into large pieces.

Add the spinach to a large, deep skillet set over medium heat, cover, and steam in the water clinging to the leaves. Cook the spinach until wilted (about 2 to 3 minutes). Immediately add cold water to the pan to cover the spinach.

Drain and gently squeeze out as much moisture as possible. Place the spinach in a medium-sized bowl and set aside.

In a small bowl combine the sesame oil, vinegar, teriyaki sauce, and mustard. Mix thoroughly.

Add this mixture to the spinach, toss gently, and sprinkle with sesame seeds. Season to taste with black pepper.

Serve hot, warm, or cold.

Tangy Cabbage   *serves 3 to 4*

Everyone will love this spicy dish; it's guaranteed to add a special flavor to your meal.

3 cups water	1/8 teaspoon dried oregano
1/4 teaspoon salt	1/8 teaspoon dried basil
4 cups shredded red or green cabbage	1 bay leaf
2 small hot, green chili peppers	1 large clove garlic, quartered lengthwise
1/8 teaspoon ground cumin	1/2 cup white, wine, or tarragon vinegar

In a large bowl, combine 1 1/2 cups water and the salt. Mix well.

Add the cabbage and soak for 8 to 12 minutes. Drain and discard the liquid.

In a medium-sized saucepan, combine the cabbage, chili peppers, cumin, oregano, basil, bay leaf, garlic, vinegar, and the remaining water.

Cover. Bring to a rapid boil. Remove from heat immediately, uncover, and let cool.

Serve with your favorite entree.

Craving-Reducing Vegetarian (Non-Meat) Choices

Breakfast Tofu Stir-Fry, Western Style
serves 2 to 3

A no-egg omelet treat.

1½ formed tofu squares, ¼ fresh small tomato, diced
    about 4   4 inches   Olive oil or low-fat pan spray
4   large mushrooms, sliced ¼ teaspoon dried basil
1   slice vegetarian "ham,"*   Ground black pepper or
    chopped   cayenne pepper, to taste
2   tablespoons chopped green
    or red pepper

Place the tofu squares on paper toweling and place a heavy plate on top, to release some of the water held by the tofu. Leave for a few minutes.

Sauté the mushrooms, "ham," chopped pepper, and tomato in a little olive oil or a spray-"oiled" pan until the vegetables blend and become semisoft. Add the basil.

Cut the tofu into small squares and add it to the mushroom, "ham," pepper, and tomato mixture. Sauté for 3 to 4 minutes.

Add black or cayenne pepper to taste and serve warm.

*Check nutritional labels. At Craving-Reducing Meals and Snacks, all "vegetarian" meat alternatives should contain 4 grams or less of carbohydrate per average serving.

Breakfast "Salami" and Tofu Stir-Fry

serves 2 to 3

A hearty no-egg breakfast surprise.

1½ formed tofu squares, about 4 4 inches	Olive oil or low-fat pan spray
3 slices vegetarian "salami,"* diced	Ground black pepper or cayenne pepper, to taste

Place the tofu squares on paper toweling and place a heavy plate on top, to release some of the water held by the tofu. Leave for a few minutes.

Sauté the "salami" for 3 minutes in a little olive oil or a spray-"oiled" pan.

Cut the tofu into small squares and add it to the "salami." Sauté for 3 to 4 minutes.

Add black or cayenne pepper to taste and serve warm.

---

*Check nutritional labels. At Craving-Reducing Meals and Snacks, all "vegetarian" meat alternatives should contain 4 grams or less of carbohydrate per average serving.

Tofu Oriental   *serves 2 to 3*

A wonderful, rich change.

2 formed tofu squares, about 4   4 inches
  Olive oil or low-fat pan "spray"
½ cup diced celery
½ cup sliced mushrooms

1 tablespoon teriyaki sauce (or low-salt substitute)
2 tablespoons toasted sesame seeds
½ teaspoon dried, crumbled thyme leaves

Place the tofu squares on paper toweling and place a heavy plate on top, to release some of the water held by the tofu. Leave for a few minutes.

Oil or spray the bottom of a medium-sized frying pan. Add the tofu; warm for 1 minute. Combine the celery, mushrooms, teriyaki sauce, toasted sesame seeds, and thyme and pour the mixture over the tofu. Sauté the tofu for another 3 to 4 minutes.

Serve warm or as a delicious cold leftover.

Spicy Tofu

serves 2 to 3

This tasty hot dish is also delicious served cold for a lunch, snack, or dinner the following day.

2 formed tofu squares, about 4 4 inches	⅛ teaspoon ground cloves
White or wine vinegar	⅛ teaspoon ground black pepper
Dry red wine	⅛ teaspoon salt
2 tablespoons chopped scallions	(or salt substitute)
	1 cup sliced mushrooms
⅛ teaspoon ground cinnamon	1 stalk celery, trimmed and
⅛ teaspoon ground allspice	minced

Place the tofu squares on paper toweling and place a heavy plate on top, to release some of the water held by the tofu. Leave for a few minutes.

Cube the tofu and place in a medium-sized bowl. Add equal amounts of vinegar and wine to cover the tofu. Mix the scallions, cinnamon, allspice, cloves, pepper, and salt in a separate bowl and add to the tofu marinade. Cover and marinate overnight.

Drain off the marinade. Sauté the mushrooms and celery in butter, olive oil, or a spray-"oiled" pan until the celery starts to brown. Add the tofu and sauté for 3 to 4 minutes.

Serve warm or as a delicious cold leftover.

Vegetarian "Burgers" in White Wine

serves 3 to 4

A simple but elegant dish that will wake up your tastebuds.

2 tablespoons olive oil	2 stalks celery, thin sliced
4 vegetarian "burgers"*	Salt (or salt substitute), to taste
1/2 cup chopped cauliflower (or broccoli florets)	Ground black pepper, to taste
1/2 cup sliced mushrooms	1/2 cup water
	1/2 cup dry white wine

Preheat the oven to 375°F.

In a large frying pan, coat the bottom with oil, set the pan over moderate heat, and brown the "burgers" (3 minutes per side).

In an ovenproof casserole dish, combine the cauliflower, mushrooms, and celery. Place the browned "burgers" on top of the vegetables. Sprinkle with salt and pepper to taste. Top with water and white wine.

Bake the casserole until most of the liquid has evaporated (about 50 to 60 minutes). Baste occasionally.

Serve hot, straight from the casserole.

*Check nutritional labels. At Craving-Reducing Meals and Snacks, all "vegetarian" meat alternatives should contain 4 grams or less of carbohydrate per average serving.

Vegetarian Parsley-Butter "Burgers"

serves 3 to 4

A sure-fire taste delight that perks up any Craving-Reducing (or Reward) Meal.

4 teaspoons butter (or low-fat substitute)	4 vegetarian "burgers"*
2 teaspoons chopped fresh parsley	1 clove garlic, crushed

In a large mixing bowl, mix 3 teaspoons of the butter with the parsley. Chill until solid.

Place the remaining butter in a large frying pan and heat until melted. Add the "burgers" and fry on both sides until brown (4 to 5 minutes).

Spread the garlic over both sides of the "burgers" and serve hot, each "burger" topped with a small scoop of the parsley butter.

*Check nutritional labels. At Craving-Reducing Meals and Snacks, all "vegetarian" meat alternatives should contain 4 grams or less of carbohydrate per average serving.

Vegetarian "Burger" Delight   *serves 3 to 4*

This tasty dish will add new spice to your meals; wonderful with a fresh salad.

1 teaspoon olive oil
1 tablespoon butter
  (or low-fat substitute)
1 clove garlic, minced
4 vegetarian "burgers"*
4 sticks celery, chopped
1/2 cup dry red wine
1/2 cup water
2 bay leaves

2 tablespoons chopped fresh
  parsley
  Salt (or salt substitute), to taste
  Ground black pepper, to taste
1 teaspoon dried thyme
1 cup sour cream (or low-fat
  substitute)
1/2 teaspoon paprika
1 tablespoon teriyaki sauce
  (or low-salt substitute)

Preheat oven to 375°F. and oil a deep casserole dish with olive oil.

In a small saucepan, melt the butter and sauté the garlic. Brown "burgers" on both sides (3 minutes per side), then place the "burgers" in casserole dish.

Add the celery to the hot oil from the "burgers" and sauté for 5 minutes. Add the wine, water, bay leaves, parsley, salt, pepper, and thyme, and heat for 5 minutes, stirring continually.

Pour the mixture over the "burgers," cover and bake for 1 hour.

Immediately before serving, remove the "burgers" from the casserole dish. Carefully and quickly stir the sour cream, paprika, and teriyaki sauce into the hot "burger" sauce in the casserole dish. Mix well.

Return the "burgers" to the dish and cover with sauce.

Serve hot.

*Check nutritional labels. At Craving-Reducing Meals and Snacks, all "vegetarian" meat alternatives should contain 4 grams or less of carbohydrate per average serving.

Vegetarian Oriental "Burger" Casserole
serves 3 to 4

A tantalizing and delightful change.

1 tablespoon olive oil	1 teaspoon grated fresh
1 tablespoon butter	ginger root
(or low-fat substitute)	4 vegetarian "burgers"*
1 large green pepper,	1/4 cup water
chopped	1 cup sour cream (or low-fat
4 sticks celery, chopped	substitute)
2 cloves garlic, crushed	1 tablespoon teriyaki sauce
	(or low-salt substitute)

Preheat the oven to 350°F. and add the oil to a deep casserole dish and spread it around the bottom.

Put the butter in a saucepan and melt it over medium heat. Add the pepper, celery, garlic, and ginger and sauté until light brown.

Break the vegetarian "burgers" into small pieces (about 1 inch square) and add them to the saucepan, stirring together for 4 minutes. Pour the mixture into the casserole.

In a small bowl, combine the water, sour cream, and teriyaki sauce and pour this mixture over the casserole mixture. Cover and bake for 30 to 35 minutes.

---

*Check nutritional labels. At Craving-Reducing Meals and Snacks, all "vegetarian" meat alternatives should contain 4 grams or less of carbohydrate per average serving.

Marinated "Burgers," Vegetarian Style
serves 3 to 4

A delectable dish that can be enjoyed time and time again.

¹/₄ cup water	1 teaspoon ground ginger
2 stalks celery with leaves	¹/₄ cup teriyaki sauce
1 cup chopped broccoli florets	(or low-salt substitute)
(or cauliflower florets)	¹/₂ tablespoon lemon juice
¹/₃ cup olive oil	4 vegetarian "burgers"*
1 clove garlic, minced	

Preheat the broiler.

In a blender combine the water and celery. Blend the mixture to a purée.

In a large, deep bowl, combine the celery purée, broccoli, olive oil, garlic, ginger, teriyaki sauce, and lemon juice. This will serve as a marinade for the "burgers."

Break up the "burgers" into bite-sized pieces and place them in the marinade. Mix gently, cover, and refrigerate overnight.

Drain off the marinade and place it in a saucepan. Heat and let simmer. Place the "burger" chunks in a shallow pan and place under the broiler until the burgers are nicely brown (8 to 10 minutes).

Put the "burger" chunks on plates and serve the sauce on the side.

*Check nutritional labels. At Craving-Reducing Meals and Snacks, all "vegetarian" meat alternatives should contain 4 grams or less of carbohydrate per average serving.

Vegetarian "Burgers" Deluxe   *serves 3 to 4*

A specialty that is easy to prepare.

3 tablespoons olive oil	2 tablespoons white wine
1 tablespoon butter (or low-fat substitute)	2 tablespoons dry red wine
	2 tablespoons water
4 vegetarian "burgers"*	2 egg yolks†
1/4 green pepper, chopped	1/4 cup heavy cream (or low-fat substitute)
1 clove garlic, finely minced	
Salt (or salt substitute), to taste	1/4 cup sour cream (or low-fat substitute)
Ground black pepper, to taste	1 tablespoon chopped fresh parsley

Coat the bottom of a large frying pan with 1 tablespoon of the oil. Brown the "burgers" over medium heat (3 minutes per side).

Remove the "burgers" from the pan.

Add the remaining oil to the frying pan. Add the green pepper, garlic, salt, and pepper, and sauté.

Stir in the red and white wine and the water, and simmer for 4 minutes.

In a small bowl, combine the egg yolks, heavy cream, and sour cream. Mix thoroughly.

Reduce the heat. Add the cream mixture to the pan with the wine and pepper mixture and stir well.

Add the parsley and the browned "burgers." Bring to a simmer, turn off the heat.

Serve hot.

---

*Check nutritional labels. At Craving-Reducing Meals and Snacks, all "vegetarian" meat alternatives should contain 4 grams or less of carbohydrate per average serving.

†In this recipe, low-fat substitutes cannot be used in place of this item. Always follow your physician's recommendations.

Sautéed Vegetarian "Burgers"   *serves 3 to 4*

A wonderful contrast in flavors.

1 tablespoon olive oil	1 clove garlic, crushed
4 vegetarian "burgers"*	Ground black pepper, to taste
6 tablespoons dry white wine	Salt (or salt substitute), to taste
1/2 teaspoon dried basil	Parsley sprigs for garnish
1/2 tablespoon lime juice	(optional)

In a large frying pan, place the oil and "burgers." Brown the "burgers" over medium heat (3 minutes per side), then remove the "burgers" from the pan.

To the frying pan add the white wine, basil, lime juice, and garlic and cook for 2 minutes.

Bring to a slow boil for 3 minutes. Return the "burgers" to the pan and heat for an additional 3 minutes.

Pepper and salt to taste.

If desired, garnish with parsley.

*Check nutritional labels. At Craving-Reducing Meals and Snacks, all "vegetarian" meat alternatives should contain 4 grams or less of carbohydrate per average serving.

Vegetarian Pepper "Steaks"   *serves 3 to 4*

A hearty meal with a saucy twist. Great for cold winter days or a refreshing change anytime.

4 vegetarian "steaks"*	1/4 cup dry red wine
1/2 teaspoon sesame oil	Salt (or salt substitute), to taste
2 tablespoons olive oil	Ground black pepper, to taste
1/2 tablespoon butter	1 clove garlic, crushed
(or low-fat substitute)	

Set the "steaks" on a plate, then combine both oils in a small bowl.

Quickly dip the "steak" into the oil mixture (coat both sides) and return them to the plate.

Pour the remaining oil into a large frying pan, place the pan over medium heat, and when oil is hot, brown the "steaks" for 3 minutes per side.

Lower the heat, cover the pan, and cook the "steaks" for 6 minutes.

Remove the "steaks," place them on a platter and keep them warm.

To the pan in which the "steaks" were browned, add the butter, wine, salt and pepper to taste, and garlic. Mix well.

Turn up the heat and bring the ingredients to just under a boil. Lower the heat and cook for 4 minutes.

Immediately pour the sauce over the "steaks" and serve.

*Check nutritional labels. At Craving-Reducing Meals and Snacks, all "vegetarian" meat alternatives should contain 4 grams or less of carbohydrate per average serving.

Vegetarian Gingered "Steak"   *serves 3 to 4*

A spicy, aromatic treat for lunch.

2 tablespoons olive oil
4 vegetarian "steaks"*
1/4 teaspoon ground
   ginger, or to taste
1 tablespoon finely
   chopped celery

1 tablespoon finely
   chopped fresh chives
1 teaspoon coarsely ground
   black pepper, to taste

Preheat the oven to 350°F.

In a large frying pan, coat the bottom with the oil, place the pan over moderate heat, and when the oil is hot brown the "steaks" (3 minutes per side).

Put the "steaks" in an ovenproof dish and place it in the oven.

In the frying pan with the heated oil, combine the ginger, celery, and chives. Mix thoroughly.

Return the "steaks" to the pan and cook with the sauce for 2 minutes.

Serve immediately and sprinkle with pepper to taste.

*Check nutritional labels. At Craving-Reducing Meals and Snacks, all "vegetarian" meat alternatives should contain 4 grams or less of carbohydrate per average serving.

Vegetarian "Steaklets" in Wine   *serves 3 to 4*

A delectable and spicy lunch.

2 tablespoons olive oil	1 tablespoon white horseradish
4 vegetarian "steaklets"*	1 clove garlic, crushed
1/4 cup water	2 tablespoons dry
1/4 cup mayonnaise†	white wine

Preheat the oven to 350°F.

In a large frying pan, place the oil and the "steaklets." Brown the "steaklets" (3 minutes per side), then remove them from the pan and place them on a platter in the warm oven.

To the frying pan, add the water, mayonnaise, horseradish, and garlic, and wine and bring the mixture to a boil.

Pour the hot sauce over the "steaklets" and serve immediately.

*Check nutritional labels. At Craving-Reducing Meals and Snacks, all "vegetarian" meat alternatives should contain 4 grams or less of carbohydrate per average serving.

†Do not use low-fat mayonnaise for Craving-Reducing Meals or Snacks as low-fat varieties of mayonnaise often contain added sugars. For an easy low-fat Craving-Reducing mayonnaise alternative, thin "regular" mayonnaise with a little water at a time and mix well.

Vegetarian "Steaklet" Delight   *serves 3 to 4*

A delicious and simple change of pace that will delight any luncheon guests.

2 tablespoons olive oil	1 cup sliced mushrooms
4 vegetarian "steaklets"*	1/4 pound Cheddar cheese
2 cloves garlic, crushed	(or cheese of choice, or low-fat
6 pitted green olives,	substitute), grated
coarsely chopped	1/4 cup water
1/2 teaspoon spicy mustard	Parsley sprigs for garnish
1 teaspoon chopped scallions	(optional)

Preheat the oven to 350°F.

Spread 1 tablespoon of the oil on the bottom of a deep casserole dish.

In a large frying pan, heat the remaining olive oil and add the "steaklets." Brown them on both sides (about 2 to 3 minutes per side), then set them aside on a plate.

Spread the garlic on both sides of the "steaklets" and place the "steaklets" on the bottom of a prepared casserole dish.

To the frying pan used for the "steaklets," add the olives, mustard, scallions, and mushrooms. Turn the heat to medium and sauté for 3 to 4 minutes.

Pour the sauce over the "steaklets." Add the cheese and the water. Cover and bake for 50 minutes.

If desired, add a garnish of parsley. Serve hot.

*Check nutritional labels. At Craving-Reducing Meals and Snacks, all "vegetarian" meat alternatives should contain 4 grams or less of carbohydrate per average serving.

Eggs, Indian Style
serves 2

A wonderful variation for the versatile egg.

4 eggs*
2 tablespoons olive oil
1 tablespoon sesame oil
1 clove garlic, finely minced
1 tablespoon curry powder
2 tablespoons sour cream
(or low-fat substitute)

$\frac{1}{2}$ cup water
1 tablespoon lemon juice
Salt (or salt substitute), to taste
Coarsely ground black pepper, to taste
2 tablespoons chopped fresh parsley
1 tablespoon slivered lemon rind

In a saucepan of boiling water, place the eggs and hard-cook them (will take about 10 minutes). Set them aside to cool.

In a medium-sized frying pan, combine the olive oil and sesame oil. Place the pan over medium heat and when the oil is hot add the garlic and sauté.

Add the curry powder, sour cream, water, lemon juice, salt and pepper to taste and stir to combine. Reduce the heat and allow the mixture to cook until just about at the boiling point.

Remove the eggs from their shells and slice them lengthwise. Add the egg slices to the mixture in the frying pan. Stir gently.

Turn off the heat, stir in the parsley and lemon rind, and serve immediately.

*In this recipe, low-fat substitutes cannot be used in place of this item. Always follow your physician's recommendations.

Herby Eggs

serves 2

A wonderfully tasty dish with a delicate flavor.

1 tablespoon butter (or low-fat substitute)	1 tablespoon chopped fresh tarragon
1/2 cup heavy cream*	Salt (or salt substitute), to taste
1/2 cup sour cream (or low-fat substitute)	Coarsely ground black pepper, to taste
4 eggs*	Chopped fresh parsley for garnish (optional)
2 tablespoons chopped fresh basil	

Preheat the oven to 350°F.

In a small pan, melt the butter and then brush melted butter on the insides of individual custard cups. Place the cups in a baking tray filled with water.

Break the eggs into a small bowl. Mix until thoroughly beaten.

In a saucepan, combine the cream and sour cream and heat just to boiling.

Lower the heat and add the eggs, stirring constantly. Continue to stir and add the basil, tarragon, and salt and pepper to taste.

Fill the custard cups about 3/4 full with the mixture from the saucepan. Place the baking pan with the cups and water into the oven and bake for 20 minutes. Insert a knife into the contents of one cup. If it comes out clean, then it is ready. If not, cook for an additional 5 minutes.

Serve hot and, if desired, garnish with parsley.

*In this recipe, low-fat substitutes cannot be used in place of this item. Always follow your physician's recommendations.

Curried Eggs
serves 2 to 4

An unusual combination that will quickly become an "old favorite."

4   eggs*
1/4 teaspoon curry powder
1/2 tablespoon chopped
    dill pickle
1/2 teaspoon mild mustard
1   tablespoon sour cream
    (or low-fat substitute)

Finely ground black pepper,
to taste
Salt (or salt substitute), to taste
1   tablespoon capers
2   to 4 large iceberg lettuce leaves
1/2 teaspoon paprika

In a saucepan of boiling water, place the eggs and hard-cook (will take about 10 minutes). Cool the eggs, peel, and slice them in half lengthwise. Remove the yolks and set the white halves aside.

Place the yolks into a mixing bowl with the curry, dill pickle, mustard, sour cream, black pepper and salt to taste, and capers. Mix thoroughly and spoon equal portions of the yolk mixture into the white halves.

Place the lettuce leaves on a platter, arrange the egg-filled halves on the lettuce, sprinkle with paprika, and serve.

*In this recipe, low-fat substitutes cannot be used in place of this item. Always follow your physician's recommendations.

Spicy Omelet   *serves 2*

A quick recipe that will spark the palate and perk up any lunch.

4 eggs (or equivalent
   low-fat egg substitute)
   2-ounce can green
   chilies (chili peppers) in
   brine,drained and
   finely chopped

1 teaspoon butter
   (or low-fat substitute)
   Salt (or salt substitute), to taste
   Ground black pepper, to taste
   Parsley sprigs for garnish
   (optional)

Thoroughly beat the eggs in a mixing bowl and add the chilies.

In a small saucepan, melt the butter, then reduce the heat and add the egg mixture, and season to taste with salt and black pepper.

Turn the heat to medium-high and cook until done to the desired consistency (1 to 3 minutes).

If desired, garnish with parsley before serving.

Asparagus and Egg Casserole   *serves 3 to 4*

This elegant luncheon casserole dish is a delight by itself or with a salad of your choice.

½ tablespoon butter (or low-fat substitute)	1 cup heavy cream*
8 asparagus spears, parboiled	2 hard-cooked eggs, sliced*
	Salt (or salt substitute), to taste
¼ cup grated Cheddar cheese (or low-fat substitute)	½ cup sliced fresh mushrooms
	Ground black pepper, to taste
	⅛ pound imported Swiss cheese sliced

Preheat the oven to 350°F.

Grease the bottom and sides of a medium-sized casserole.

Arrange 4 of the asparagus spears on the bottom of the casserole.

Cover with ½ of the egg slices, salt and pepper to taste, and top with ⅛ cup of the Cheddar cheese and ½ cup of the cream.

Top with the remaining asparagus spears and cover with the remaining egg slices, salt and pepper to taste, and the rest of the Cheddar cheese and cream.

Place the Swiss cheese slices over the top and bake in the preheated oven for 30 minutes.

Remove and serve hot.

---

*In this recipe, low-fat substitutes cannot be used in place of this item. Always follow your physician's recommendations.

Green Bean–Cheese Casserole with Sour Cream
serves 4

A delicious and simple change of pace that will delight you as well as your family or guests.

1 tablespoon olive oil	1 cup sour cream
2 cups green beans,	(or low-fat substitute)
tips removed	1/2 pound Cheddar cheese
1 clove garlic, crushed	(or cheese of choice
Salt (or salt substitute),	or low-fat substitute), grated
to taste	1 tablespoon dried basil
Coarsely ground black	1 teaspoon dried rosemary
pepper, to taste	

Preheat the oven to 375°F. and oil a deep casserole dish.

Cut the green beans into 2-inch sections and place them in a skillet with 1/2 inch water at the bottom.

Cover, turn up the heat, and cook for 4 minutes. Remove from the heat immediately, drain off the water, and arrange the green beans in the bottom of the prepared casserole dish.

Sprinkle the garlic and salt and pepper to taste over the green beans.

In a separate bowl, mix the sour cream and cheese and then pour the mixture over the green beans, spreading the sauce to all sides of the casserole.

Sprinkle the surface with the basil and rosemary. Cover. Bake for 15 to 20 minutes.

Serve warm.

CHAPTER 12

REWARDING RECIPES

CARBOHYDRATE-RICH TEMPTATIONS

*R*emember that your daily Reward Meal is made up of a balance of Craving-Reducing vegetables and proteins along with Carbohydrate-Rich foods such as fruit, fruit juice, bread, pasta, potatoes and other starchy vegetables, rice, desserts, etc. A balanced Reward Meal is essential to craving and weight reduction, and while some of the individual recipes that follow may be carbohydrate-rich, the rest of the meal must include appropriate amounts of salad and Craving-Reducing vegetables and protein (see page 112 for important details on balancing your Reward Meal). Never select only, or mostly, carbohydrate-rich foods as your Reward Meal—always include an appropriate balance of Craving-Reducing foods as well.

The Carbohydrate-Rich Recipes that follow should be included in your Reward Meal only. They are examples of some of the foods that you are free to enjoy, once a day, every day, during these meals.

Reward Meal foods may be baked, boiled, broiled, fried (with breading or batter), poached, roasted, or sautéed. As always, keep in mind your physician's advice regarding fat, salt, and other dietary recommendations. For suggestions on easy ways to include dietary recommendations into this program, see page 214, and for some Reward Meal examples, see page 195.

You are free to include any recipe you like in your balanced daily Reward Meal* but, in addition, we have included some of our favorite Reward Meal Recipes:

As with Craving-Reducing Meal recipes, we have included low-fat alternatives for those people who have concern about fat in their diets.

Remember that you are free to adjust these recipes to account for changes in number of desired servings. Reduce a recipe by $1/2$ or by $3/4$ if you are cooking for only one or two, or enjoy making the full recipe and refrigerating the remainder for the next day. It's always a good idea to freeze appropriate "leftovers" for future meals (place them in serving-size plastic freezer bags or containers for an easy meal that is always ready to go. Remember that if a recipe contains only Craving-Reducing foods, you can have them at any meal, but if they contain any Carbohydrate-Rich foods, be sure to save the dish for your next Reward Meal (see page 121 for food lists).

As always, you are free to go back for "seconds" or even "thirds" at times,* but each time you go back, be certain to balance your Carbohydrate-Rich foods with the right proportion of Craving-Reducing foods as well.

*Always keep your own physician's recommendations in mind.

Reward Meal Appetizers and Dips

Easy Chicken Liver Pâté   *serves 3 to 4*

This exciting appetizer will have everyone asking for your recipe.

½ pound chicken livers
½ (14 ounce) can chicken
  broth
2 hard-cooked eggs*
½ cup chopped onion

2 tablespoons chicken fat or
  butter (or low-fat substitute)
  Salt (or salt substitute), to taste
  Coarsely ground pepper,
  to taste

Place the chicken livers in a large saucepan, add the broth, and simmer until done (8 to 10 minutes).

In a blender, combine the livers and some of the liquid in which the livers were cooked. Purée.

Add the chicken fat or butter or low-fat substitute to a deep frying pan and lightly brown the onion. Blend all ingredients by hand or food processor to make a paste.

Season to taste with salt and pepper. (Other possible flavorings include curry powder or cognac; season to taste.)

Serve the pâté in a bowl surrounded by crisp, fresh vegetables or buttered (or low-fat substitute) toast quarters. Excellent also with Ritz crackers.

*In this recipe, low-fat substitutes cannot be used in place of this item. Always follow your physician's recommendations.

Marinated Strips of Pork   *serves 3 to 4*

This is a finger-lickin' good appetizer served on toothpicks. These
pork strips will disappear from the serving plate faster than you can
bring them out. Serve them hot and be prepared to keep them
coming.

1 large boneless pork tenderloin	1 tablespoon minced onion
1 cup teriyaki sauce (or low-salt substitute)	1 clove garlic, minced
	1/4 cup sesame seeds
1 tablespoon sugar	1 tablespoon olive oil

Trim all the fat from the tenderloin, and if the tenderloin is
thick, split it lengthwise.

In a medium-sized bowl, combine the teriyaki sauce, sugar,
onion, garlic, sesame seeds, and pork. Cover. Marinate in the
refrigerator for 3 to 4 hours, basting and turning frequently.

Preheat the oven to 375°F.

Remove the pork from the refrigerator, drain, and set the
marinade aside.

Oil a medium-sized roasting pan, place the pork in the pan,
and roast it until tender (35 to 40 minutes).

Add the marinade to the pan and simmer for an additional 20
minutes.

Remove the pork, cut it into thin slices, and serve the pieces on
cocktail toothpicks, with the marinade for dipping.

Shrimp Mayonnaise   *serves 3 to 4*

A delectable starter for any meal.

1/2 cup mayonnaise
(or low-fat substitute)
1/8 cup chili or salsa sauce
1 teaspoon finely chopped
onion
1 teaspoon dried basil
Dash cayenne pepper

1 tablespoon white, wine, or
tarragon vinegar
1/2 teaspoon Worcestershire
sauce
1/2 teaspoon prepared white
horseradish
1 pound shrimp
1 cup shredded lettuce

In a medium-sized bowl, combine the mayonnaise, chili or salsa sauce, chopped onion, basil, cayenne, vinegar, Worcestershire sauce, and horseradish. Blend well with a rotary mixer.

Cover and refrigerate until ready to serve.

Cook the shrimp for 5 minutes at a full boil. Peel, devein, and refrigerate them until ready to serve.

When ready to serve, arrange the shrimp on shredded lettuce.

Spoon the mayonnaise mixture over the shrimp. Serve cool.

Swedish Meatballs   *serves 3 to 4*

A true reward.

1 egg*
1/2 cup milk
   (or low-fat substitute)
1/4 cup dry bread crumbs
3 tablespoons butter
   (or low-fat substitute)
1/4 cup chopped onion
1/2 pound ground chuck
1/4 pound ground pork
   Salt (or salt substitute),
   to taste

Ground black pepper, to taste
1/4 teaspoon dried basil
1/8 teaspoon ground allspice
1/8 teaspoon ground cardamom
1/8 teaspoon ground nutmeg
2 tablespoons flour
4 ounces (1/2 cup) condensed
   beef broth
1/2 cup heavy cream
   (or low-fat substitute)

In a large bowl, beat the egg and then combine the milk and bread crumbs.

Melt 2 tablespoons of the butter in a large skillet and sauté the onion until soft (4 to 5 minutes); remove the onion with a slotted spoon and add it to the mixture in the bowl. Add the chuck, pork, salt and pepper to taste, basil, allspice, cardamom, and nutmeg. Mix well until all the ingredients are blended.

Cover and refrigerate for 1 hour. When chilled, shape the mixture into 20 to 25 meatballs and sauté and brown them in the large skillet in which the remaining butter has been melted. Remove the meatballs and place them in a 2-quart casserole.

Pour the drippings from the skillet into a measuring cup and return 1/4 of the drippings to the skillet. Stir in the flour and more salt and pepper to taste.

Heat the mixture in the skillet while gradually adding the beef broth; stir constantly until it boils.

Remove the skillet from the heat and stir in the cream until smooth.

Pour the mixture over the meatballs in the casserole and bake for 30 minutes. Serve hot.

*In this recipe, low-fat substitutes cannot be used in place of this item. Always follow your physician's recommendations.

Egg and Spinach Pie

serves 3 to 4

A satisfying taste-tickler for the wonderful meal to follow.

Pastry for 1 eight-inch
pie crust
½ pound fresh spinach,
washed
2 eggs*
½ cup sour cream
(or low-fat substitute)

¼ cup soft bread crumbs
1 teaspoon butter (or low-fat
substitute)
1 tablespoon grated Swiss
cheese (or low-fat substitute)
Plain or flavored bread crumbs

Preheat the oven to 450°F.

Roll the pastry to ⅛-inch thickness and fit it loosely into an 8-inch pie pan. Using a fork, prick the sides and the bottom of the pastry well and bake it until set but not brown (about 5 minutes).

Remove the pan from the oven and reduce temperature to 350°F.

Coarsely chop the spinach, drain it well, and spread the spinach over the pastry.

Break the eggs over the spinach and cover them with the sour cream.

Combine the bread crumbs, butter, and cheese and sprinkle the mixture over the crust. Return the pan to the oven and bake until the eggs are set (15 to 20 minutes).

Remove the pie from the oven, sprinkle with plain or flavored bread crumbs and serve hot, or chill and serve cold.

---

*In this recipe, low-fat substitutes cannot be used in place of this item. Always follow your physician's recommendations.

Baked Clams   *serves 3 to 4*

A special treat that will beckon you to make it over and over again.

16 cherrystone clams	¹/₄ teaspoon chopped fresh
4 canned water chestnuts,	ginger root
diced	2 teaspoons butter
¹/₄ cup chopped bean	(or low-fat substitute)
sprouts	1 cup milk*
4 scallions, finely chopped	¹/₄ cup grated Parmesan cheese
2 teaspoons teriyaki sauce	(or low-fat substitute)
(or low-salt substitute)	¹/₂ cup sesame seeds

Preheat the oven to 475°F.

Remove the clams from the shells and dice them. Keep the shells.

In a medium-sized bowl, combine the clams, water chestnuts, bean sprouts, scallions, teriyaki sauce, and ginger. Spoon equal quantities into the clam shells.

In a small saucepan set over low heat, melt the butter, add the flour, and stir until blended.

In another saucepan, bring the milk to a boil and add it quickly to the butter-flour mixture. Stir continually until the sauce is smooth and thick. Add the cheese and stir until melted.

Arrange the shells in a baking pan, spoon the sauce over the contents of the shells, and sprinkle with sesame seeds.

Bake for 4 to 5 minutes. Serve hot and enjoy.

*In this recipe, low-fat substitutes cannot be used in place of this item. Always follow your physician's recommendations.

Tuna and Cheese Canapés   *serves 3 to 4*

A basic but luxurious starter for any meal to follow.

½ cup grated imported
   Swiss cheese (or low-fat
   substitute)
¼ cup canned tuna (water-
   or oil-packed), drained

1 tablespoon cooking sherry
   (or other dry wine)
   Ground black pepper, to taste
6 to 8 slices of toast, white or
   whole wheat

Preheat oven to 350°F.

In a medium-sized bowl, combine the cheese, tuna, and wine. Add pepper to taste and blend the mixture well.

Spread the mixture on the toast slices, and bake for 5 minutes in the oven.

Shrimp with Herb Sauce   *serves 3 to 4*

A tasty treat that is always a successful start to any dinner.

20 medium or large shrimp,   1 teaspoon chopped fresh basil
    shelled and deveined   (or 1 teaspoon dried basil)
4   large lettuce leaves   1 teaspoon chopped fresh
¼   cup mayonnaise   chives
    (or low-fat substitute)   1 teaspoon chopped cucumber
                                   Juice of 1 small lemon

Add the shrimp to a large pot of boiling water and cook, stirring occasionally, until the shrimp are red in color and thoroughly cooked (about 5 minutes).

Arrange 5 shrimp on each large lettuce leaf. Cover each with waxed paper or plastic wrap and chill.

Combine the mayonnaise, basil, chives, cucumber, and lemon juice and chill for 1 hour.

Place a toothpick through each shrimp, spoon the mayonnaise sauce over the shrimp, and serve.

Fettuccine with Cream Sauce   *serves 3 to 4*

A dish that has been a tradition since the time that Marco Polo
returned to Italy.

8 cups water
1 teaspoon salt
1/2 pound fettuccine noodles
1/4 cup (4 tablespoons) butter
   (or low-fat substitute),
   softened
1/2 cup heavy cream
   (or low-fat substitute)

1 cup grated Parmesan cheese,
   (or low-fat substitute)
1/2 teaspoon teriyaki sauce
   (or low-salt substitute)
1/2 teaspoon ground black pepper
1/2 cup chopped scallions

Preheat the oven to 300°F.

Place a large casserole dish into the oven to warm.

In a large pot, combine the water and salt and bring to a boil.

Add the fettuccine to the boiling water and gently stir until the
strands are well separated (about 1 minute). Once the water has
returned to a boil, cook until done (7 to 8 minutes).

In a medium-sized bowl, combine the softened butter, cream,
cheese, and teriyaki sauce. Beat until the ingredients are light and
fluffy (well mixed).

Drain the fettuccine well in a colander and transfer it to the
casserole dish that has been warming in the oven.

Pour the butter-cream mixture over the fettuccine, sprinkle the
top with the pepper and chopped scallions, and toss well until
each strand is well coated.

Serve immediately with grated Parmesan cheese and, if you
like, with garlic bread.

Norwegian Fritters   *serves 3 to 4*

An hors d'oeuvre that is sure to surprise and satisfy at the same time.

1 cup olive oil	$1/2$ teaspoon coarsely ground pepper
1 cup grated imported Swiss cheese (or low-fat substitute)	$1/4$ teaspoon dry mustard
2 tablespoons flour	2 egg whites
1 teaspoon dried basil	$1/2$ cup packaged plain dry bread crumbs

Preheat the oven to 375°F.

Pour the oil into a deep skillet and slowly heat to 375°F. (Use a deep-fry thermometer.)

In a medium-sized bowl, combine the cheese, flour, basil, pepper, and mustard.

In a mixer, beat the egg whites until stiff. Add the beaten whites to the bowl containing the other ingredients and mix well.

Make 1-inch fritters (balls) from the mixture and roll each fritter in bread crumbs.

Deep-fry the fritters until golden-brown (1 to 2 minutes). Do not crowd the fritters when frying.

Drain the fritters on paper toweling.

Before serving, heat the fritters in the preheated oven (5 minutes), place on a bed of lettuce, and serve hot with toothpicks and your favorite dipping sauce.

Deluxe Deviled Eggs   *serves 3 to 4*

An old favorite to begin a meal that offers a taste of "wonderful
things to come."

4   hard-cooked eggs,* peeled
4   tablespoons chopped ham,
    chicken, or tuna
2   tablespoons butter
    at room temperature
    (or olive oil)

1   teaspoon teriyaki sauce
    (or low-salt substitute)
    Salt (or salt substitute), to taste
    Ground black pepper, to taste
1   tablespoon mayonnaise (or
    low-fat substitute)

Cut the eggs lengthwise and remove the yolks. Arrange the
whites on a cake rack and add 1/2 tablespoon of the chopped ham,
chicken, or tuna to each half egg-white cavity.

In a mixer, combine the yolks with the butter, teriyaki sauce,
salt and pepper to taste, and mayonnaise. Beat until smooth.
(Optional additions: anchovy paste, dried mustard, paprika, dried
basil, or lemon juice.)

Use a pastry bag with a large star tube and spoon the yolk
mixture into it. Hold the pastry bag close to egg-white cavity and
force the mixture through the tube, moving in a zigzag to form a
pattern.

Place the eggs on a tray lined with large lettuce leaves and
serve chilled.

---

*In this recipe, low-fat substitutes cannot be used in place of this item. Always
follow your physician's recommendations.

California Avocado Halves   *serves 6*

Lots of flavor; a delight that is sure to please the palate.

2	tablespoons chili sauce or salsa	1	teaspoon Worcestershire sauce
2	tablespoons catsup	8	dashes Tabasco sauce
1	tablespoon white vinegar	4	tablespoons lemon juice
2	tablespoons brown sugar	3	large, ripe avocados, chilled

In a medium-sized bowl, combine the chili sauce, catsup, vinegar, brown sugar, Worcestershire sauce, Tabasco, and 2 tablespoons of the lemon juice.

Refrigerate for 3 to 4 hours.

When ready to serve, peel the avocados, cut them in half, and remove the pits. Brush the cut sides with the remaining lemon juice, then fill the cavities with the sauce.

Serve cold.

Spinach Riata and Dip
serves 3 to 4

This little treat is a nice accompaniment to spiced foods or works wonderfully well as a dip.

¼ pound fresh spinach, trimmed and washed (or equivalent frozen)

1 medium cucumber, peeled, seeded, and chopped

2 cups plain yogurt (regular or low-fat)

1 teaspoon ground cumin

¼ teaspoon ground cardamom

Salt (or salt-substitute), to taste

Ground black pepper, to taste

Paprika (mild or hot), to taste

Place the spinach leaves, in a large covered pot with the water clinging to the leaves. Steam over medium heat until the leaves are wilted (3 to 4 minutes).

Remove the pot from the heat, drain the spinach in a colander, and cool to room temperature. (If using frozen spinach, simply defrost and continue as if you had cooked it fresh.) Gently squeeze out the liquid and chop the spinach finely.

Place the cucumber on paper toweling to drain excess liquid.

In a medium-sized mixing bowl, combine the yogurt, cumin, cardamom, and salt and pepper to taste. Add the spinach and cucumber and mix until all ingredients are blended.

Cover and refrigerate for at least 2 hours.

Sprinkle with paprika to taste, and serve with flatbread or vegetables.

Tangy Egg Dip   *serves 4 to 5*

A savory dip that can be readily made ahead of time and served cold.

½ cup mayonnaise
   (or low-fat substitute)
1 tablespoon butter
   (or low-fat substitute)
1 tablespoon lemon juice
1 tablespoon grated onion
1 teaspoon Dijon mustard

1 teaspoon celery seeds
½ teaspoon Worchestershire sauce
Ground black pepper, to taste
4 hard-cooked eggs,* peeled and cut into quarters

In a blender or food processor, combine the mayonnaise, butter, lemon juice, grated onion, mustard, celery seeds, Worchestershire sauce, and pepper to taste.

Add the eggs and blend until smooth.

Chill and serve with fresh vegetables for dipping.

*In this recipe, low-fat substitutes cannot be used in place of this item. Always follow your physician's recommendations.

Curry Dip

serves 5 to 6

A mouth-watering companion for a wide range of garden vegetables.

2 cups mayonnaise (or low-fat substitute)

1/2 cup sour cream (or plain low-fat yogurt combined with 1/2 tablespoon sugar)

1/4 cup minced fresh parsley

2 tablespoons curry powder

4 teaspoons sugar

Salt (or salt substitute), to taste

2 teaspoons lemon juice

2 cloves garlic, crushed (or 1/2 teaspoon garlic powder)

1/4 teaspoon turmeric

Combine the mayonnaise, sour cream, parsley, curry powder, sugar, salt, lemon juice, garlic, and turmeric in a mixing bowl and stir thoroughly.

Refrigerate for 2 hours before serving.

Serve with the fresh vegetables of your choice.

Hot Sausage Dip   *serves 7 to 8*

An exquisite and tasty dip that will complement any dinner party.

1 pound ground pork sausage (or low-fat substitute)

1 medium onion, thinly sliced

1/2 pound mushrooms, thinly sliced

1 cup sour cream (or low-fat plain yogurt plus 1 tablespoon sugar)

1 1/2 tablespoons flour

3/4 cup milk (or 2% low-fat substitute)

1 tablespoon Worcestershire sauce

1 teaspoon teriyaki sauce (or low-salt substitute)

1 teaspoon paprika

In a medium skillet set over medium-high heat, brown the sausage, crumbling it with a fork while cooking. Drain on paper toweling.

Add the onions and mushrooms to the fat in the skillet. Over medium heat, cook until the onions are soft. Drain the fat and return the crumbled sausage to the skillet.

In a small bowl, slowly add the sour cream to the flour and stir. Stir in the milk and seasonings until well blended. Add to the sausage in the skillet and stir until mixed.

Cover the skillet and cook the mixture over moderate heat until thickened.

Serve hot in a chafing dish and enjoy with bowls of crisp chips or vegetables of your choice.

Tangy Salsa Fria   *serves 8 to 10*

This cold salsa is a hot treat for the palate of salsa lovers.

4 cups fresh, peeled tomatoes (or canned Italian plum tomatoes)	4 tablespoons wine vinegar
	2 teaspoons olive oil
	1 teaspoon dried oregano
5 tablespoons chopped green chilies	1 teaspoon dried basil
	1/4 teaspoon dried thyme
2 tablespoons chopped fresh parsley	Ground black pepper, to taste
	Salt (or salt substitute), to taste
2 medium cloves garlic, minced	

In a medium-sized bowl, chop the tomatoes.

Add the chilies, parsley, garlic, vinegar, oil, oregano, basil, thyme, pepper, and salt and mix well.

Chill for 2 hours and serve with crisp chips of your choice.

Savory Salsa Roja

serves 3 to 4

This salsa is always a real pleaser.

3   fresh, ripe tomatoes,   1   large clove garlic, minced
    chopped (or a 16-ounce   1½ teaspoons wine vinegar
    can crushed tomatoes)   1   teaspoon Worcestershire
2   tablespoons diced   sauce
    green chilies   Sugar, to taste
    Salt (or salt substitute),
    to taste

Combine the tomatoes, chilies, salt, garlic, vinegar,
Worcestershire sauce, and sugar to taste in a medium saucepan and
place pan over low-medium heat.

Simmer, uncovered, for 30 to 45 minutes, until thickened.

Cool to room temperature and serve with crisp chips of your
choice.

Reward Meal Desserts

Old-fashioned Rice Custard   *serves 4*

This is a fine finish for any meal. Not too sweet but still a very rich dessert.

4 cups water
1/3 uncooked regular
    white rice
5 cups milk (or low-fat
    substitute)
1 teaspoon salt (or salt
    substitute)

3 eggs*
1/2 cup plus 2 tablespoons sugar
1/4 cup brown sugar
2 teaspoons vanilla extract
1/4 teaspoon cinnamon

Place the water in the bottom of a double boiler. Place the top of the double boiler into place and combine the rice, 4 cups of the milk, and the salt and mix well.

Heat the water to boiling and cook the mixture until the rice is tender (1 hour), stirring occasionally.

Preheat the oven to 350°F.

Grease a 2-quart casserole and place it in a large baking pan.

In a large bowl, combine the eggs, 1/2 cup of the sugar, brown sugar, vanilla, and the remaining 1 cup of milk. Mix well and then stir in the hot rice mixture. Pour the mixture into the prepared casserole, pour hot water into the baking pan to form a 2-inch-deep layer around the casserole.

Mix the cinnamon and the remaining 2 tablespoons sugar together, sprinkle it over the top of the mixture in the casserole, and bake uncovered (about 1 hour) until the blade of a kitchen knife inserted 1 inch from any edge of the casserole comes out clean.

Remove the casserole from the water and cool, then refrigerate for at least 3 hours.

Serve plain or topped with whipped cream (or low-fat substitute).

*In this recipe, low-fat substitutes cannot be used in place of this item. Always follow your physician's recommendations.

Jellied Almond Cream   *serves 5 to 6*

Wonderful at any time of the year.

1	envelope unflavored gelatin	3	eggs, separated*

1   envelope unflavored   3   eggs, separated*
    gelatin   1   teaspoon vanilla extract
¹/₄ cup cold water   1   cup heavy cream, whipped
1¹/₂ cups milk   (or low-fat substitute)
    (or 2% low-fat substitute) ¹/₂ cup sugar
³/₄ cup almond paste

Soften the gelatin in the cold water.

In a double boiler, scald the milk, add the almond paste, and stir until thoroughly mixed.

In a medium-sized bowl, beat the egg yolks, gradually adding the almond mixture.

Return the mixture to the double boiler and cook over hot water, stirring constantly, until the mixture begins to thicken. Continue stirring and add softened gelatin and vanilla. Refrigerate until the mixture starts to set.

Remove the bowl from the refrigerator and fold in the whipped cream. Beat the egg whites and sugar until semistiff, and fold it into the mixture.

Spoon equal portions of mixture into glass serving dishes and refrigerate until firm.

*In this recipe, low-fat substitutes cannot be used in place of this item. Always follow your physician's recommendations.

Iced Lemon Soufflé   *serves 3 to 4*

A simple but elegant chilled dessert that cleanses the palate. It's a marvelous summer treat that works any time of the year.

1 tablespoon unflavored gelatin	1 cup sugar (or sugar substitute equivalent)
½ cup lemon juice	1 cup heavy cream (or low-fat substitute)
1 cup egg whites	

In a mixing bowl, dissolve the gelatin as directed on the package. Add the lemon juice to the gelatin mixture. Set aside.

In a medium-sized bowl, beat the egg whites until foamy only. Add the sugar to the whites and continue to beat until the sugar is dissolved and the whites are glossy. Set aside.

In a clean chilled bowl, whip the cream until stiff. Gently fold the whites and whipped cream into the gelatin mixture. Divide the mixture into 6 individual soufflé dishes and freeze until solid.

Serve plain or with your favorite topping.

Quick and Easy Mocha Pie

serves 5 to 6

A breeze to prepare for the busy person who wants a quick and easy dessert with which to make friends and influence people.

1 commercially prepared chocolate cookie crust	2 small Heath English Toffee bars
1 quart softened coffee ice cream (or low-fat substitute)	2 cups whipped cream (or low-fat substitute)
	1 tablespoon coffee liqueur

Place the softened ice cream into the crust and spread it out evenly.

Place the Heath Bars into a sturdy plastic bag and close securely. With a hammer or some hard instrument, break the Heath Bars into small pieces. In a small bowl, mix the whipped cream and liqueur and then spoon the mixture into the crust.

Sprinkle the broken Heath Bar pieces over the whipped cream, then freeze for 2 or more hours.

Let sit at room temperature for $1/2$ hour before serving.

Creamy Fudge Cake   *serves 5 to 6*

A favorite dessert that is always right and seem to disappear almost as fast as you set it out. It freezes well, so you can put separate portions away for future Reward Meal treats.

1 teaspoon butter (or low-fat substitute)	1/2 cup sour cream (or low-fat substitute)
1 cup sifted all-purpose flour	2 ounces unsweetened chocolate, melted
3/4 cup sugar	
1/2 teaspoon baking soda	1 egg
1/4 teaspoon salt (or salt substitute)	1/2 teaspoon vanilla extract
	1/4 cup hot water
1/4 cup shortening	

Preheat the oven to 350°F.

Grease the bottom and sides of an 8   8-inch cake pan.

In a medium-sized bowl, sift together the flour, sugar, baking soda, and salt. Add shortening and sour cream and blend for 2 minutes.

Add the chocolate, egg, vanilla, and hot water, and blend again for another two minutes.

Empty the contents of the bowl into a greased pan and place the pan in the oven, baking until the center of the cake rebounds to a slight touch (about 30 to 35 minutes).

Remove the pan from the oven and cool for 5 minutes. Remove the cake from the pan and cool it on a rack.

Enjoy it plain or with the frosting of your choice.

Rice Grete

serves 3 to 4

A creamy delight for you alone, a special friend, the family, or a notable "bring along" to a party.

2 cups milk (or low-fat substitute)

1/3 cup uncooked white rice

1/4 teaspoon salt (or salt substitute)

1 tablespoon sugar

1 teaspoon vanilla extract

1/4 cup chopped blanched almonds

1 cup heavy cream, whipped (or low-fat substitute)

1 cup pitted Bing cherries in heavy syrup

2 teaspoons cornstarch

In a large saucepan set over high heat, bring the milk to a boil and quickly stir in the rice. Lower the heat immediately, cover, and cook until tender (40 to 45 minutes), stirring occasionally.

Remove the saucepan from the heat and add the salt, sugar, vanilla, and almonds. Mix well. Chill in the refrigerator.

Fold in 1/3 of the whipped cream until thoroughly combined with the chilled mixture. Repeat twice more with the remaining thirds.

Drain the cherries and reserve 3/4 cup of the juice, adding water if there is not enough juice.

Mix 1 tablespoon juice with the cornstarch to make a smooth paste. Place the remaining juice in a small saucepan, stir in the cornstarch paste, and heat until thickened, stirring constantly.

Remove from the heat and add the cherries. Serve lukewarm over the rice mixture.

Crème Brûlée   *serves 5 to 6*

This wonderful long-time French favorite will always be the height
of elegance at any special dinner.

2	cups heavy cream*	5	tablespoons sugar
1	tablespoon vanilla extract	4	egg yolks*
			Brown sugar, to taste

In a medium saucepan, combine the cream and vanilla and
heat until warm.

In a medium-sized bowl, combine the sugar and egg yolks and
mix well.

Pour the mixture into the saucepan and mix the contents
thoroughly. Divide the mixture into 6 individual ovenproof dishes.
Place the dishes in a shallow pan filled with 1 inch of water. Place
the pan in the oven and cook until set (40 to 50 minutes).

Remove the pan from the oven, sprinkle the top with brown
sugar, place under the broiler element, and broil until the sugar is
melted.

Serve plain or with any topping that you think might add an
interesting twist.

*In this recipe, low-fat substitutes cannot be used in place of this item. Always
follow your physician's recommendations.

Walnut Crumb Cake Smoothie   *serves 6 to 8*

A delectable classic old-fashioned cake that will satisfy the sweet tooth and the tummy.

1 cup shortening	3 cups fine graham cracker
1 cup sugar	crumbs
4 eggs*	1 cup finely chopped walnuts
2 teaspoons vanilla	3 teaspoons baking powder
extract	1 cup milk (or low-fat substitute)

Preheat the oven to 350°F.

In a medium bowl, combine the shortening, sugar, eggs, and vanilla.

In a separate bowl, combine the cracker crumbs, walnuts, and baking powder, adding the result to the shortening mixture.

Add the milk and mix thoroughly.

Pour mixture into a greased 8-inch cake pan (4 inches deep).

Place the pan in the oven and bake until done (30 to 35 minutes). Remove the pan from the oven and remove the cake and cool on a wire rack.

This cake is great without frosting, but feel free to add a topping of your choice.

*In this recipe, low-fat substitutes cannot be used in place of this item. Always follow your physician's recommendations.

Key Lime Pie
serves 6 to 8

This remarkable recipe is sure to make family and guests sit up and take notice.

1 cup sugar
1/4 cup flour
3 teaspoons cornstarch
1/4 teaspoon salt
(or salt substitute)
2 cups water
3 egg yolks* (whites will be used for meringue)
1 tablespoon butter (or low-fat substitute)

1/4 cup lime juice,
Grated rind of 1 lime (or lemon)
Baked 9-inch pastry shell

Standard meringue pie topping:
3 egg whites
1/4 teaspoon cream of tartar
6 tablespoons sugar

In a medium-sized saucepan, combine the sugar, flour, cornstarch, and salt. Add the water gradually, stirring continually.

Cook over medium-low heat, stirring constantly, until thickened.

Beat the egg yolks and gradually add them to the saucepan, stirring continually for 2 minutes.

Remove from the heat and stir in the butter, lime juice, and rind. Allow to cool for 5 minutes, then pour into the pastry shell and cool for 30 minutes.

Preheat the oven to 425°F.

Beat the egg whites until frothy and light. Add cream of tartar and beat until the whites hold a peak. Gradually add the sugar and beat until the meringue is glossy and stiff.

Pile this meringue on top of the pie and spread it to the edge to prevent shrinking when browning. Place the pie in the oven and bake until the meringue is brown on top, about 5 to 7 minutes.

Cool and serve.

*In this recipe, low-fat substitutes cannot be used in place of this item. Always follow your physician's recommendations.

Fresh Pears in Wine   *serves 3 to 4*

A light and rewarding finish for the simplest to the most elegant
meal.

$1/3$ cup water

4 large pears, peeled
   and cored

$2/3$ cup sugar

$1/2$ cup dry red wine

$1/3$ cup orange juice

Grated peel of orange

Whipped cream (or low-fat
substitute) (optional)

Add the water, pears, sugar, wine, juice, and orange peel to a
large saucepan set over medium heat. Cover and simmer until the
pears are soft (about 30 minutes).

Remove the saucepan from the heat and serve hot, if desired,
or chill and serve. A dash of whipped cream (or low-fat substitute)
is optional.

Simply Gingerbread   *serves 6 to 8*

This excellent standard is a nice way to end any menu.

1	teaspoon butter (or low-fat substitute)	1½	teaspoons ground ginger
1	tablespoon vinegar	1	teaspoon ground cinnamon
¾	cup milk (or low-fat substitute)	⅓	cup shortening
2	cups sifted flour	½	cup sugar
2	teaspoons baking powder	1	egg (or low-fat substitute)
¼	teaspoon baking soda	¾	cup molasses
½	teaspoon salt (or salt substitute)		

Preheat the oven to 350°F.

Butter an 8   8-inch deep cake pan.

In a medium-sized bowl, add the vinegar to the milk and set aside.

Sift together the flour, baking powder, baking soda, salt, ginger, and cinnamon. Sift a second time.

In a small bowl, cream the shortening, add the sugar gradually, and combine well. Add the egg and whip until fluffy. Add the molasses and blend well.

To the bowl with milk and vinegar (curdled by this time), add, ¼ at a time, the dry ingredients. Stir until mixed before adding the next ¼.

Empty the contents into the greased cake pan and place it in the oven for 45 to 50 minutes, or until the surface at the center of the cake rebounds with the light touch of a finger. Remove from the oven and then from the pan and cool before serving. Frosting is optional.

Pecan Pie   *serves 6 to 8*

A southern specialty that is easy to prepare and even easier to enjoy at the end of the meal.

8 ounces cream cheese (or low-fat substitute)	1½ teaspoons vanilla extract
½ cup sugar	1 unbaked standard 9-inch pie shell in pie pan
4 eggs*	1 cup pecan halves
¼ teaspoon salt (or salt substitute)	1 cup corn syrup

Preheat the oven to 375°F.

In a medium-sized bowl, combine the cream cheese, ¼ cup of the sugar, 1 of eggs, the salt, and ½ teaspoon of the vanilla. Mix thoroughly until thick and smooth. Pour the mixture into the pie shell and cover with the pecans.

In a small bowl, combine the remaining 3 eggs, the remaining sugar, the corn syrup, and the remaining vanilla. Mix thoroughly and pour it over the mixture in the pie shell.

Place in the oven and bake until set (35 to 40 minutes).

*In this recipe, low-fat substitutes cannot be used in place of this item. Always follow your physician's recommendations.

Banana Fritters   *serves 3 to 4*

This wonderful dessert tops off any meal.

2/3 cup flour

1/2 tablespoon sugar

1/2 teaspoon baking powder

1/2 teaspoon salt
  (or salt substitute)

1 egg (or low-fat substitute)

1/3 cup milk (or low-fat
  substitute)

1/2 teaspoon corn oil

1/2 teaspoon vanilla extract

1 teaspoon grated lemon peel

2 large, semiripe bananas, peeled

1/2 tablespoon lemon juice

2 cups salad oil (or vegetable
  shortening)

Flour, as needed

Confectioners' sugar,
  as needed

In a small mixing bowl, combine the flour, sugar, baking powder, and salt, mixing thoroughly.

In a medium-sized mixing bowl, combine the milk, corn oil, vanilla, and lemon peel and mix thoroughly.

Mixing continually, slowly add the contents of the small bowl and stir until the mixture is smooth.

Slice the bananas diagonally into 1/2-inch sections and sprinkle each chunk with lemon juice. Heat oil or shortening in a deep skillet (heated contents should be at least 2 inches deep) until a temperature of 375°F. is reached (use a deep-fry thermometer).

Coat the banana chunks with flour, shake off excess. Use a fork to dip each coated chunk into the mixture in the bowl and then hold it 1/2 inch above hot oil. Using a knife, gently dislodge the chunk so that it falls gently into the oil. Continue with all pieces.

Deep-fry until golden-brown, remove with a slotted spoon, and drain on paper toweling.

Sprinkle with confectioners' sugar and serve hot.

Sponge Heaven
serves 6 to 8

A nice and light dessert that can be served plain or with your
favorite fillings or toppings.

³/₄ cup sifted cake flour	³/₄ cup sugar
1 teaspoon baking powder	¹/₂ teaspoon almond extract
¹/₄ teaspoon salt	2 tablespoons water
4 eggs,* separated	

Preheat the oven to 375°F.

In a medium-sized bowl, sift together the flour, baking powder,
and salt.

Beat the egg whites until stiff, gradually adding half of the sugar
(6 tablespoons).

Beat the egg yolks until thick and gradually add the remaining
sugar. Continue beating until very thick and then blend in the
almond extract. Gradually add the water while beating the mixture.
Then fold in the egg-white mixture.

About one-third at a time, sift in the flour mixture, folding it
into the egg-white mixture, before sifting in the next third.

Pour the mixture into a jellyroll pan or shallow cookie pan that
has been lined with baking parchment. Place it in the oven and
bake it until done (15 to 18 minutes).

Remove the pan from the oven and carefully turn the cake onto
a cooling rack. Cut the cake in half and enjoy it plain or fill it with
any desired frosting or filling mixture.

*In this recipe, low-fat substitutes cannot be used in place of this item. Always
follow your physician's recommendations.

Grandma's Pound Cake   *serves 6 to 8*

A wonderful dessert on its own, but with a little imagination it can be served with toppings of many kinds.

3/4 cup butter (or low-fat substitute)	2 cups flour
2 cups confectioners' sugar	2 tablespoons brown sugar
3 large eggs*	1 teaspoon vanilla extract
	1 teaspoon lemon juice

Preheat the oven to 325°F.

In a medium-sized bowl, combine the butter and confectioners' sugar and beat until fluffy. One at a time, add the eggs and beat thoroughly. Add the vanilla and lemon juice and mix again. Finally, slowly add the flour and mix thoroughly.

Grease a 9x5-inch loaf pan and pour in the mixture. Place the pan in the oven and bake until the cake is golden (1 hour).

Cool and serve plain or with your favorite topping, or top with your favorite glaze and serve. Set your imagination free.

---

*In this recipe, low-fat substitutes cannot be used in place of this item. Always follow your physician's recommendations.

Scottish Pecan Shortbread   *serves 5 to 6*

This wonderful dessert will put a lilt in your smile and a sparkle in
your eye.

1 cup (2 sticks) butter*	½ cup finely chopped pecans
½ cup sugar	1 cup flour

Preheat the oven to 300°F.

In a medium-sized bowl, combine the butter and sugar, mixing
thoroughly. Add the pecans and flour and mix again.

With your hands, knead the dough until it appears blended.
Divide the dough into four equal parts.

Take ¼ of dough and, on a floured board, roll it into a 9-inch
circle about ¼ inch thick. Cut the circle into 4 wedges immediately
and transfer them to a large greased cookie sheet. Using a fork,
prick each wedge several times.

Repeat the process for each remaining quarter. Use a second
greased cookie sheet if necessary.

Place the sheets in the oven and bake until the wedge edges
barely turn brown. Don't overbake.

Cool on cookie sheets until solid, then transfer to cooling racks.

*In this recipe, low-fat substitutes cannot be used in place of this item. Always
follow your physician's recommendations.

Apple Cream Pie   *serves 5 to 6*

Always a favorite, apple pie comes in many variations. This one is a variation with a wonderful hint of cream that will make you happy you waited for this reward.

1 teaspoon sugar	4 Granny Smith apples, peeled and cored
1¼ cups flour	½ cup sugar
6 tablespoons butter (or low-fat substitute)	½ cup heavy cream*
2 tablespoons vegetable shortening	1 egg*
3 tablespoons cold water	1 teaspoon fruit liqueur
	Ground cinnamon, to taste

Preheat the oven to 375°F.

In a medium-sized bowl combine the sugar, flour, butter, and shortening. Mix until crumbly. Add the water and mix until the ingredients appear to hold together.

Using the back of a spoon, press the ingredients into the sides and bottom of a 9-inch pie pan. Place the pan into the oven and bake until the crust is light brown (15 to 20 minutes). Remove the pan from the oven.

Cut the apples into thin slices, arrange them neatly in the pan, and put the pie back in the oven for 15 minutes, then remove it from the oven and set it aside.

In a medium-sized bowl, combine the sugar, cream, egg, and fruit liqueur. Mix thoroughly and pour over the apples.

Return the pan to the oven and cook until the custard sets (20 minutes).

Cool on a rack and sprinkle with cinnamon.

Serve either at room temperature or chilled. Top with a fruit sherbet if you wish.

*In this recipe, low-fat substitutes cannot be used in place of this item. Always follow your physician's recommendations.

Reward Meal Fish, Seafood, and Poultry

Baked Fish with Wine   *serves 3 to 4*

A light and tasty entree to satisfy the fussiest fish eater.

1½ pounds fillets of mild fish
4 tablespoons butter (or low-fat substitute)
1 cup dry white wine
1 clove garlic, minced
Ground black pepper, to taste
1 teaspoon teriyaki sauce (or low-salt substitute)
12 medium mushroom caps
Parsley sprigs
4 lemon wedges

Preheat the oven to 350°F.

Rinse the fillets and set aside.

Grease a large baking dish using 1 tablespoon of the butter.

Pour the wine all over the fillets, sprinkle with the garlic and pepper to taste, and dot each fillet with butter (2 tablespoons in total). Place the tip of an oven thermometer into the deepest part of the thickest fillet and place the dish in the oven. Bake until done (thermometer reads 140°F.).

Add the remaining tablespoon of butter to a medium-sized skillet and melt over medium heat.

Cut the mushroom caps in half and add to the hot skillet along with the teriyaki sauce. Sauté until the mushrooms are soft (3 to 4 minutes).

Remove the dish from the oven, transfer the fillets to serving plates, and pour the liquid from the skillet over the fillets.

Garnish with mushrooms and parsley, and serve with lemon wedges.

Fillet of Sole with Herbs   *serves 3 to 4*

This flatfish has a sweet and delicate meat that makes a wonderful entree that is quick and easy to prepare.

2   medium sole fillets
1/2 cup plus 1 teaspoon butter (or low-fat substitute)
2   tablespoons lime juice
1   tablespoon dried tarragon

1/2 teaspoon minced garlic
2   tablespoons chopped fresh chives
Salt (or salt substitute), to taste
Paprika, to taste
Parsley sprigs for garnish (optional)

Preheat the oven to 350°F.

In a small skillet, melt the butter and use half to brush on the fillets. Sprinkle with the lime juice.

Grease a large baking dish and arrange the fillets in the dish. Cover the dish, place it in the oven, and cook until fish is fork-tender (18 to 20 minutes).

To the remaining melted butter in the skillet, add the tarragon, garlic, chives, and salt and paprika to taste.

Remove the fillets from the oven.

Slightly heat the contents of the skillet and pour the mixture over the fish.

If desired, garnish with parsley sprigs.

Breaded Fish Fillets

serves 3 to 4

A main course that is good for you and tastes great.

2 pounds fish fillets
(your choice of fish)
½ cup seasoned packaged
bread crumbs
1 egg

¼ cup olive oil for frying
6 lemon wedges
Parsley sprigs for garnish
(optional)

Rinse the fillets, pat them dry on paper toweling, and cut into serving-size pieces.

Spread the bread crumbs on a large dish or platter.

In a small dish, beat the egg with a fork. Dip the fish in the beaten egg, moistening both sides, and then dip the fish into the crumbs, coating both sides well.

In a large skillet, carefully heat the oil until hot. Add enough fish pieces to cover the bottom of the skillet. Reduce the heat to medium and sauté until golden-brown (4 to 5 minutes). Turn the pieces over and sauté the other side (4 to 5 minutes).

Remove the fish to a serving platter, garnish with lemon wedges, and, if desired, parsley sprigs.

If you like, serve with your favorite relish or sauce.

Black Peppercorn Tuna   *serves 3 to 4*

This fantastic peppery dish will wake up your tastebuds.

1 tablespoon fresh-crushed black pepper	4 teaspoons olive oil
	4 medium tuna steaks
2 tablespoons teriyaki sauce (or low-salt substitute)	1/4 cup chicken broth
	1/4 cup dry white wine
2 tablespoons lemon or lime juice	4 thin lemon slices

Preheat the oven broiler.

In a small bowl, combine the pepper, teriyaki sauce, and juice. Mix and set aside.

Coat both sides of each tuna steak thinly with olive oil, place the tuna steaks on a broiling tray, and broil each side for 5 to 6 minutes. Turn off the heat but leave the tuna in the oven.

In a large skillet set over medium-high heat, combine the peppercorn mixture, broth, and wine.

Stirring continually, cook over high heat until the sauce is light brown. Reduce the heat to low, remove the tuna from the oven, and lay the steaks in the skillet. Sauté each side for 1 minute.

Place the tuna steaks on a serving dish, pour the remaining sauce over the steaks, and garnish with lemon slices.

Broiled Lobster Tails   *serves 2 to 3*

The best part of the lobster is the tail, and here is one simple way
to enjoy this seafood delicacy.

4   medium-large lobster tails
1/4 cup lime juice
1/4 cup olive oil
1   teaspoon mild paprika
1   teaspoon salt (or salt
    substitute), to taste
1   clove garlic, minced

1   teaspoon dried tarragon
1   teaspoon dried basil
1   tablespoon butter (or low-fat
    substitute)
    Melted butter (or low-fat
    substitute)

Preheat the broiler.

Using a strong scissors, carefully cut along both sides of the
under-cover of the tail. Slightly crack the upper shell with a cleaver
and bend the sides up so that the tails lie flat.

In a large shallow dish, combine the lime juice, olive oil,
paprika, salt, garlic, tarragon, and basil. Mix well and marinate the
lobster tails for 3 hours.

Remove the tails from the marinade. Lightly coat the exposed
meat with butter. Broil for 5 minutes per side.

Place the lobster tails on plates and serve with melted butter or
low-fat substitute as well as any desired side dishes.

Shrimp in Wine Sauce   *serves 3 to 4*

A special and sumptuous seafood treat.

2 teaspoons olive oil	1/2 cup chicken broth
1 medium onion, chopped	1 pound medium shrimp,
3 cloves garlic, cut in	shelled and deveined
quarters	Salt (or low-salt substitute),
1 cup dry white wine	to taste
1/4 cup lemon juice	Coarsely ground black pepper,
	to taste

To a large skillet set over low heat, add the oil, onion, and garlic, stir well, and cook over medium heat until the onions begin to turn golden.

Mix in the wine and broth, turn up the heat to high, and cook until the liquid starts to boil. Reduce the heat and simmer for 2 minutes.

Add the shrimp and quickly mix, coating all the shrimp. Cover and cook until all the shrimp turn pink (4 to 5 minutes).

With a slotted spoon, transfer the shrimp to a serving dish, add the salt, pepper, and lemon juice to taste, and pour the contents of the skillet over the shrimp.

Serve plain or over rice.

Batter-Fried Shrimp   *serves 3 to 4*

A restaurant favorite that can be prepared and served at home with little muss or fuss.

1 teaspoon salt	1 cup flat beer
1/3 teaspoon coarsely ground black pepper	1 pound medium shrimp, shelled and deveined
1 clove garlic, minced	1/4 cup olive oil for frying
2 eggs,* separated	
1 tablespoon melted butter (or low-fat substitute)	

In a medium-sized bowl, combine the salt, pepper, garlic, egg yolks, and melted butter. Mix thoroughly, cover, and refrigerate (4 hours or more).

Just prior to use, beat the egg whites and fold them into the batter.

Heat the oil in a deep-fat fryer to 370°F. or heat the oil in a large skillet.

Coat the shrimp with batter and deep-fry until golden-brown. Drain on paper toweling, set on a platter, and serve.

If desired, serve with lemon wedges, tartar sauce, or any relish that pleases you.

Fried Clams

serves 5 to 6

Clams have always been one of man's favorite bounties from the sea, and here is one more wonderful way to serve them.

2 cups sour cream (or plain low-fat yogurt combined with 2 tablespoons sugar)
4 tablespoons sweet-pickle relish
1 teaspoon salt (or salt substitute)
½ teaspoon Tabasco sauce
2 teaspoons minced garlic

1 quart clams
1 egg (or low-fat substitute)
¼ teaspoon paprika
1 cup packaged flavored bread crumbs
¼ cup olive oil for frying

In a small bowl, combine the sour cream, relish, salt, tabasco sauce, and garlic, Mix thoroughly. Refrigerate the sauce for 2 hours or more.

Shuck the clams, drain, and set aside, reserving 2 tablespoons of the clam liquid.

In a small bowl, combine the liquid, egg, and paprika. Mix thoroughly.

In another small bowl, place the bread crumbs.

Dip the clams first in the liquid, then in the bread crumbs, and set aside.

In a large skillet, heat the oil over medium heat. When the oil is hot, sauté the clams until done (3 to 4 minutes per side).

Drain the clams on paper toweling and serve with the sour cream sauce.

Chicken Kiev   *serves 4*

A delight to the eyes and the palate as well.

2 large whole chicken breasts, skinless and boneless
$1/2$ cup chilled butter (or low-fat substitute)
Salt (or salt substitute), to taste
Ground black pepper, to taste

2 tablespoons chopped fresh chives
Flour for dredging
2 eggs, lightly beaten*
$2/3$ cup fresh bread crumbs
$1/4$ cup olive oil for deep-frying

Place the chicken breasts between sheets of waxed paper and pound with a mallet until thin. Avoid splitting the flesh. Remove the waxed paper.

Cut the butter into four finger-shaped pieces. Place one piece of butter in the center of each breast, salt and pepper to taste, add $1/2$ tablespoon chives to each breast, and roll up like an envelope, letting sides overlap (no fasteners necessary, as flesh will adhere).

Lightly dredge each roll in flour, dip into beaten eggs, and roll in bread crumbs. Refrigerate for 1 hour.

Fill a deep-fat fryer or deep pan with enough olive oil to cover the breasts. Heat oil to 360°F. Add each breast gradually and cook until brown on all sides.

Drain on absorbent paper toweling and serve hot.

---

*In this recipe, low-fat substitutes cannot be used in place of this item. Always follow your physician's recommendations.

Golden Roast Chicken
with Stuffing
serves 5 to 6

A holiday favorite, but it can be served all year long.

4　cups white bread cubes
4　tablespoon dried basil
2　tablespoons chopped
　　fresh parsley
1/4　teaspoon salt
　　(or salt substitute)
2　tablespoons butter
　　(or low-fat substitute)
1　cup chopped celery

1/4　cup chopped onion
　　4-to 5-pound chicken,
　　ready for cooking
1　tablespoon melted butter
　　(or low-fat substitute)
　　Garlic powder, to taste
　　Paprika, to taste
　　Coarsely ground black pepper,
　　to taste

Preheat the oven to 350°F.

In a large bowl, combine the bread cubes, basil, parsley, salt, and pepper. Mix well.

In a medium skillet, melt the butter. When butter is hot, add the celery and onion, reduce heat, sauté until golden (8 to 10 minutes).

Add the contents of the skillet to the bread mixture and blend well. Set the dressing aside.

Remove all excess parts and wash the chicken inside and out. Spoon the dressing into the body cavity and fold over the skin flap. Insert a meat thermometer into the thickest part of the inner thigh.

Place the chicken on a roasting rack set into a roasting pan. Brush the outside of the chicken with melted butter and sprinkle on garlic powder, paprika, pepper, and salt to taste.

Place the open pan into the oven and roast the chicken until the thermometer reaches the desired temperature (about 1 1/2 to 2 hours). A loose tent of foil placed over for the first 3/4 hour of the roasting process will reduce excess browning.

Remove the bird from the oven and place it on a large serving platter. Remove all the stuffing, place it in a large bowl, then remove to a warm oven that has been turned off.

Let the chicken stand for 10 minutes, then carve and serve with the dressing.

Chicken Breasts Napoleon   *serves 5 to 6*

Exotic, but simple and quick to prepare.

3 large chicken breasts,
   boned and skinned
3 tablespoons butter
   (or low-fat substitute)
6 thin slices Virginia ham
6 small, thin slices
   imported Swiss cheese
   (or low-fat substitute)

½ cup minced shallots
12 medium mushroom caps
1 cup dry wine
1 cup chopped tomatoes
⅓ cup heavy cream*
⅓ cup chopped fresh parsley

Rinse the chicken breasts and flatten between sheets of waxed paper with a mallet or cleaver until very thin.

In a large skillet, heat the butter until hot but not brown. Take one piece of chicken, move it around in the hot butter, on both sides, until it is no longer pink (2 to 3 minutes). Immediately place the chicken breast in a large, flat dish. On one half of the top of the breast, place a piece of ham and a piece of cheese. Fold the other half over the first half.

Repeat the process for each thin breast.

To the drippings in the skillet, add the shallots and mushrooms and sauté for about 3 minutes.

Add the wine and tomatoes and simmer for 3 minutes more, then add the cream.

Without boiling, add the stuffed chicken breasts to the sauce and simmer for 3 minutes, turning the pieces once or twice.

Sprinkle with parsley and serve over wild rice.

---

*In this recipe, low-fat substitutes cannot be used in place of this item. Always follow your physician's recommendations.

Chicken Cacciatore   *serves 4*

An outstanding dish with a tomato sauce and mushroom base that delights the nose and pleases the palate.

2-pound chicken broiler-fryer, cut into pieces

3 tablespoons olive oil

2 tablespoons butter (or low-fat substitute)

1 large can (32 ounces) whole tomatoes, diced

Salt (or salt substitute), to taste

Ground black pepper, to taste

$3/4$ cup dry red wine

1 teaspoon dried oregano

1 teaspoon dried basil

2 tablespoons chopped fresh parsley

1 cup diced green pepper

$1/2$ teaspoon minced garlic

4 tablespoons flour

3 tablespoons water

12 medium mushrooms

Wash and pat dry all the chicken parts.

In a 6-quart pan, combine the oil and butter, and heat.

Place 4 pieces of chicken on the bottom of the pan, brown well on both sides, and remove from the pan. Repeat for the remaining pieces of chicken.

Return all browned chicken parts to the pan and add the canned tomato pieces, salt and pepper to taste, wine, oregano, basil, parsley, green pepper, and garlic. Cover and simmer until the chicken is tender (45 to 50 minutes).

In a small bowl, combine the flour and water and stir until smooth. Pour the mixture into the pan and stir to combine.

Add the mushrooms and cook over low heat until the sauce is thickened (10 to 15 minutes).

Serve warm with pasta (traditional) or rice or noodles (new and terrific).

Yogurt Chicken Breasts   *serves 5 to 6*

A tradition among Mideastern, Russian, and Indian cultures, yogurt is used to give chicken a succulent flavor that allows blended spices to penetrate the meat, making the eating a joy.

3	whole chicken breasts, with bone but skinned		Salt (or salt substitute), to taste
1½	cup plain yogurt (or low-fat yogurt)		Ground black pepper, to taste
3	cloves garlic, minced	3	teaspoons olive oil
3	teaspoons dried tarragon	1	medium onion, thinly sliced
		1½	cups thinly sliced mushrooms
		3	teaspoons cornstarch
		½	cup water

Preheat the oven to 350°F.

Rinse the chicken, pat dry with paper toweling, and set aside in a large shallow pan.

In a medium bowl, combine the yogurt, garlic, tarragon, and salt and pepper to taste.

Spoon the contents of the bowl over the chicken. Let stand (7 to 8 minutes), then turn over and let stand again (7 to 8 minutes).

While the chicken marinates, place the oil in a large skillet and heat. Add the onion and mushrooms and sauté (2 minutes).

In a small dish, combine the cornstarch and water. Mix well. Pour the mixture into the skillet with the onions and mushrooms and stir until thickened.

Remove the chicken from the shallow pan and place in a casserole or baking dish.

Add the skillet contents to the marinade and mix thoroughly. Pour it over the chicken, cover, and bake for 25 minutes. Uncover, and bake until the chicken is tender when pierced with the tines of a fork (10 to 15 minutes).

Serve over rice or noodles.

Golden-Fried Chicken *serves 3 to 4*

This all-time southern favorite and delight is right at any time of the year.

3½-pound broiler-fryer, cut into sections
¼ cup flour
¼ cup flavored packaged bread crumbs

Salt (or salt substitute), to taste
Ground black pepper, to taste
¼ cup olive oil for frying
Sprigs of parsley for garnish (optional)

Wash the chicken pieces and damp-dry with paper toweling.

In a 1-gallon plastic bag combine the flour, bread crumbs, and salt and pepper to taste. Add 2 pieces of chicken at a time, shake to coat evenly with the mixture, and remove to a plate. Repeat the process until all the pieces of chicken have been coated.

To an electric skillet, add the oil and heat to 375°F., or heat the oil, carefully, in a large skillet set on a standard range.

Add the chicken, a few pieces at a time, and brown on all sides. Remove to a clean plate lined with paper toweling. Repeat the process until all pieces have been browned but not fully cooked.

Carefully drain all the fat from the skillet and then return 2 tablespoons fat to the skillet. Reduce the heat to 300°F. (or lower range heat) and add all the chicken pieces, skin-side down.

Cover and cook for 30 minutes. Uncover, turn all pieces over, and cook uncovered for 15 minutes.

Remove the chicken and place on a serving platter. If desired, garnish with parsley and serve hot.

Chicken Paprikash   *serves 4 to 6*

A simple but remarkable recipe credited to the Hungarians but now enjoyed by people around the world.

	4-pound oven-stuffer roaster (or boneless, skinless breast equivalent)	2	cloves garlic, minced
		3	tablespoons mild paprika
		2	teaspoons salt (or salt substitute)
3	tablespoons butter (or low-fat substitute)	2	cups chicken broth
3	tablespoons olive oil	2	teaspoons flour
2	cups chopped onion	2	cups sour cream (or plain, low-fat yogurt plus 2 tablespoons sugar)
1	cup diced green pepper		

Cut the chicken into sections and wash all the parts. Set aside.

To a large, heavy pot, add the butter and olive oil, and heat until the butter is melted.

Add the onion, green pepper, garlic, and paprika. Simmer until the onion is golden-brown.

Add the salt and broth and bring the contents of the pot to a boil. Reduce the heat to a simmer, add the chicken, and cover and cook until the chicken is tender (about 1 hour). Remove the chicken pieces to a plate.

In a small bowl, combine the flour and sour cream.

Reduce the heat to just below boiling and slowly stir the flour–sour cream mixture into the pot containing the chicken sauce. Heat and stir but do not boil, and cook for 5 additional minutes.

Served traditionally over wide noodles, but tastes just as wonderful all alone or on a bed of rice.

Reward Meal Meats:
Beef, Pork, Lamb, and Veal

Ragoût of Beef
serves 5 to 6

This good old standard stays surprisingly delicious.

1½ tablespoons butter	Ground black pepper,
1 large onion, chopped	to taste
2 cloves garlic, whole	2 large tomatoes, chopped
2 pounds bottom round,	1 cup diced celery
cut into 1-inch cubes	½ ounce dried black
1 teaspoon paprika	mushrooms
Salt (or salt substitute),	Water, as needed
to taste	2 tablespoons flour

Place a skillet over medium heat and melt the butter. Add the onion and garlic and sauté until the onion is transparent.

Discard the garlic and add the meat, paprika, and salt and pepper to taste. Stir until browned.

Add the chopped tomatoes and lower the heat. Cover and simmer. After 1 hour, add the diced celery.

As meat simmers, wash the mushrooms and place them in a medium saucepan to soak in 1 cup water for 15 to 20 minutes.

Boil the mushrooms in their soaking liquid for 3 to 4 minutes.

Add them to the meat mixture 15 minutes after adding the celery. Continue to simmer for 30 to 45 additional minutes.

When the meat is tender, reduce the heat. In a separate bowl, blend the flour and ¼ cup water and add, stirring, to the meat mixture. Cook, stirring, until the liquid is thickened.

Serve all alone or over noodles or rice.

Jamaican Pot Roast   *serves 5 to 6*

A special new pot roast that provides a welcome change and is a taste delight.

Flour, for dredging	3 tablespoons olive oil
Salt (or salt substitute), to taste	1/2 cup chopped onion
	1 clove garlic, finely chopped
Ground black pepper, to taste	1/2 teaspoon dried basil
3 pounds rump roast of beef	2 cups canned tomatoes with liquid
	1/2 teaspoon ground ginger

Combine the flour, salt, and pepper. Dredge the meat in the mixture.

In a Dutch oven, heat the oil, add the meat, and keep turning until browned well on all sides.

Add the onion, garlic, and basil. Stir until the onions start to brown. Add the tomatoes and ginger. Cover tightly and simmer until tender (2 to 2 1/2 hours). (Alternately, you may brown the meat, then simmer with the remaining ingredients in a slow cooker until fully done.)

Remove and place the roast on a heated platter.

Beef Stew with Wine and Herbs   *serves 3 to 4*

A rich, hearty main course that will warm you all winter.

1½ pounds stewing beef, cubed

⅔ cup dry red wine

1 large bay leaf

1 clove garlic, sliced

Salt (or salt substitute), to taste

½ teaspoon black pepper, to taste

2 tablespoons olive oil

1½ cups beef stock

1 stalk celery with leaves, diced

1 medium onion, sliced

Few sprigs parsley

¼ teaspoon dried thyme

4 cloves garlic

1 piece ginger root

Cornstarch

To a large bowl, add the meat, wine, bay leaf, garlic, and salt and pepper to taste. Refrigerate and marinate for 3 to 4 hours, turning frequently.

Remove the meat and set on a plate. Set the marinade aside.

Place the olive oil in a Dutch oven and heat. Add the meat and brown on all sides.

In a medium saucepan set over low-medium heat, add the marinade, beef stock, celery, onion, and herbs and spices tied in a piece of cheesecloth.

Add the contents of the saucepan to the meat, cover, and simmer until the meat is tender (2½ to 3 hours). Add water if necessary. (Alternately, you may brown the meat, then cook with the remaining ingredients in a slow cooker until fully done.)

Other vegetables may be added if desired. Cook until the added vegetables are tender.

Discard the bag of herbs and set the meat on a hot platter.

Use cornstarch in a little cold water to thicken the gravy (½ teaspoon cornstarch for each cup of broth). Add the mixture to the liquid in the Dutch oven and stir for 2 minutes over medium heat.

Pour the sauce over the meat and serve immediately.

Classic New England Beef Dinner *serves 3 to 4*

A enjoyable dinner to prepare and a joy to eat.

1 2-pound corned beef brisket	3 large potatoes, peeled
1 clove garlic	6 small onions, peeled
1 whole clove	1 small head cabbage
6 whole black peppercorns	2 tablespoons butter (or low-fat substitute)
1 bay leaf	1/2 cup chopped fresh parsley
4 medium carrots, peeled	

Rinse the corned beef and place it in a kettle and add just enough cold water to cover the meat.

Add the garlic, clove, peppercorns, and bay leaf.

Bring to a boil, reduce the heat, and simmer (5 to 6 minutes). Skim off the surface, cover, and continue to simmer (3 to 3 1/2 hours).

Add the carrots, potatoes, and onions. Cut the cabbage into 8 wedges and add them to the pot and simmer for an additional 1/2 hour.

Remove the meat from the pot, then slice the meat thinly across the grain. Remove the vegetables and serve along with the meat.

Add a spicy mustard sauce as a fine accompaniment.

Beef Goulash

serves 3 to 4

A mainstay from Hungary and Rumania alike, this seldom-made delight is both easy to prepare and makes a memorable meal.

1/4 cup olive oil	1 1/2 teaspoons salt
4 cups chopped onions	(or salt substitute)
1 1/2 pounds beef chuck,	1 tablespoon sweet paprika
cubed	1 small can tomato paste

Set a heavy 2-quart saucepan over medium heat and add the oil and onions. Sauté until the onions are brown.

Add the beef, stirring until the beef has lost all of its redness. Add the salt, paprika, and tomato paste.

Lower the heat, cover, and simmer very slowly until the beef is tender (1 to 2 hours). Check often, adding a little water if the meat begins to stick.

Dish it out, alone or on noodles, and wait for the raves.

Steak Supreme   *serves 3 to 4*

This uncommon dish can be thrown together from commonly stocked ingredients.

2-pound thick sirloin steak	Ground black pepper, to taste
1 clove garlic, cut in half	Dried basil, to taste
1/4 cup olive oil	1/4 cup dry red wine
Salt (or salt substitute), to taste	1 tablespoon butter (or low-fat substitute)

Preheat the oven to 350°F.

Dry the steak with paper toweling. Rub each side with the garlic and set the remaining garlic aside.

Place the oil in a large skillet and set it over high heat until very hot. Brown the steak very well on both sides, 3 to 5 minutes per side.

Remove it from the heat and place the steak in a shallow roasting pan, and add the salt, pepper, and basil to taste. Add the garlic.

Using the top part of the oven, bake for 25 minutes. Remove the steak from the pan and keep it warm in the oven.

Pour off the excess fat from the pan and remove the garlic. Place the pan over direct heat on the range. Add the wine and bring the mixture to a brief boil, stirring to loosen brown bits.

Remove from the heat, stir in the butter, and use as a sauce.

Thin-slice the steak on the diagonal and serve with the sauce on the side.

Beef and Rice Casserole

serves 3 to 4

A hearty dish that satisfies the fussiest meat eaters.

1 pound lean ground beef	Salt (or salt substitute), to taste
1 tablespoon olive oil	
1/2 cup chopped onion	2 teaspoons chili powder
1 cup sliced celery	Ground black pepper, to taste
1/4 cup chopped green pepper	1 teaspoon teriyaki sauce (or low-salt substitute)
1/2 cup uncooked rice	1/2 cup pitted ripe olives (either green or black), cut into large pieces
1 1/2 cups canned tomatoes	
1/2 cup water	

Preheat the oven to 325°F.

In a large skillet set on medium-low heat, heat the oil and brown the beef.

Remove the meat from the pan and add the onion, celery, green pepper, and rice. Cook, stirring, until the contents are browned.

Add the tomatoes, water, salt, chili powder, pepper, teriyaki sauce, meat, and olives and bring to a boil. Pour the mixture into a 2-quart casserole and cover.

Bake until done (45 to 60 minutes).

Serve hot.

Broiled Lamb Chops   *serves 3 to 4*

This simple recipe highlights the delightful taste of lamb.

4   double-thick lamb chops
3   tablespoons olive oil
1   clove garlic, sliced
    Salt (or salt substitute),
    to taste

Ground black pepper, to taste
Butter (or low-fat substitute),
to taste
Herbs of choice—parsley,
rosemary, and/or basil
Lemon juice (optional)

Preheat the oven to broil.

In a large bowl, combine the lamb, olive oil, and garlic, and marinate, covered, in the refrigerator for 1 to 2 hours.

Place the lamb on the broiling rack and place it in the oven about 2 inches from the heat. Brown on both sides, rare (5 minutes per side), medium (6 to 7 minutes per side), or well-done (10 minutes per side).

Transfer the lamb to a warm platter, salt and pepper to taste, and place a pat of butter on each chop.

Sprinkle on the herb of your choice. A sprinkling of lemon juice is optional.

Moroccan Lamb Chops   *serves 3 to 4*

A Middle Eastern delight that will soon become a family classic.

4	double-thick lamb chops		Ground black pepper, to taste
3	tablespoons olive oil	1	teaspoon paprika
1	clove garlic, sliced	4	pats butter (or low-fat
1	teaspoon dried basil		substitute)
1/2	teaspoon dried thyme	1	tablespoon lemon juice
	Salt (or salt substitute),		Parsley sprigs for garnish
	to taste		(optional)

Rinse the chops and set them aside.

In a large bowl, combine the oil, garlic, and herbs and mix well. Add the chops and marinate in the refrigerator, covered, for 2 hours.

Preheat the oven to broil.

Remove the chops and place them on a broiling rack. Place the rack about 2 inches from the heat source. Brown each side for 5 minutes (10 minutes total).

Transfer the chops to a heated serving dish, salt, pepper, and paprika to taste, and put 1 pat of butter in the center of each chop, then sprinkle with lemon juice. If desired, garnish with a sprig of parsley on top of each pat of butter.

Serve with your favorite vegetables and potatoes, noodles, or rice.

Hearty Rack of Lamb

serves 5 to 6

A satisfying Reward Meal dish. Save any leftovers for tomorrow night's Reward Meal appetizer.

3-pound rack of lamb	1/2 cup apricot preserves
1 teaspoon salt	1/4 cup lemon juice
(or salt substitute)	Ground black pepper,
1 clove garlic,	to taste
sliced in half	

Preheat the oven to 300°F.

Cover the end of each rib with aluminum foil to avoid burning. Rub the lamb with the salt and garlic. Avoiding the bone and the fat, insert a meat thermometer into the appropriate center of the rack.

Place the roast on a rack in a shallow roasting pan, fat-side up. Do not cover.

Place the pan in the oven and roast for 30 minutes.

In a medium-sized bowl, combine the apricot preserves, lemon juice, and pepper to taste to make a glaze.

Remove the pan from the oven and spoon half of the glaze on the lamb. Without covering, return the pan to the oven and continue to roast the lamb for 30 additional minutes.

Remove the pan from the oven and repeat the process with the remainder of the glaze. Return the pan to the oven and roast until the desired temperature is reached (175°F. for medium and 185°F. for well-done).

Serve with your favorite vegetables, rice or noodles, and mint jelly.

Lamb Curry   *serves 3 to 4*

An exotic delight that can be made mild or strong, according to
your taste.

1/4 cup butter (4 tablespoons) (or low-fat substitute)	1 teaspoon grated ginger root
1 teaspoon sesame oil	1 tablespoon dried basil
4 medium scallions, chopped	2 teaspoons ground coriander
1 clove garlic, chopped	1/4 teaspoon ground cinnamon
1 pound cubed boneless lamb shoulder	1/2 teaspoon ground cardamom
1 cup plain yogurt (regular or low-fat)	1/4 teaspoon ground cloves
	1/2 teaspoon curry powder, or more to taste

Place the butter and oil in a medium-sized pot and melt the
butter over moderate heat.

Add the scallions and garlic and sauté until the scallions are
soft. Remove the scallions and garlic and set them aside.

Add the lamb to the heated pot and brown on all sides.

Return the scallions and garlic and add the yogurt, ginger, basil,
coriander, cinnamon, cardamom, cloves, and curry. Mix thoroughly
and coat all sides of the lamb with the mixture. Cover and continue
to simmer for 30 minutes.

Serve with rice or couscous.

Stuffed Shoulder of Lamb   *serves 5 to 6*

A delicious main course that will go well with many of your
favorite side dishes.

3 tablespoons butter (or low-fat substitute)	1 grated peel of lemon
1 cup dried mushrooms	Salt (or salt substitute), to taste
1 clove garlic, diced	Ground black pepper, to taste
1/2 pound ham, finely chopped	1/4 cup soft bread crumbs
1 tablespoon finely chopped fresh parsley	2 eggs (or low-fat substitute), lightly beaten
1/4 cup finely chopped onion	1 2-pound boned shoulder of lamb, prepared for stuffing

Preheat the oven to 300°F.

Place a rack in a shallow roasting pan.

In a large skillet set over medium-low heat, melt the butter and
add the mushrooms and sauté until browned. Add the garlic, ham,
parsley, onion, grated lemon peel, salt, pepper, bread crumbs, and
eggs, mixing thoroughly.

Stuff the shoulder with the contents of the skillet and tie
securely with string.

Place the stuffed shoulder on the rack in the roasting pan.
Roast, uncovered, until done (40 minutes per pound).

Skewered Spicy Lamb

serves 3 to 4

A wonderful kebab that can be done in almost no time at all but will receive rave reviews.

1 pound boneless lamb

1 small onion, finely chopped

3 cloves garlic, finely chopped

1 teaspoon grated ginger root

1 teaspoon finely chopped fresh parsley

2 cups of your favorite vegetables—green or red peppers, cauliflower, onion slices, mushrooms, etc.

2 tablespoons red wine vinegar

1 tablespoon hot paprika

1/2 teaspoon ground cinnamon

1/4 cup beef broth

Salt (or salt substitute), to taste

Ground black pepper, to taste

2 tablespoons sesame oil

Cut the lamb into 11/2-inch cubes and place them in a medium-sized mixing bowl.

In another medium-sized mixing bowl, combine the onion, garlic, ginger root, parsley, vegetables, vinegar, paprika, cinnamon, beef broth, salt and pepper to taste, and sesame oil and mix thoroughly.

Transfer the lamb to the bowl containing the mixture. Make sure all of the meat is covered with the marinade. Cover and refrigerate overnight. Turn the meat from time to time while marinating in the refrigerator.

Heat the broiler or grill. Remove the bowl from the refrigerator. Thread the meat and vegetables on metal skewers and place them 4 to 5 inches away from the source of heat and cook for 10 minutes. Turn the skewers. Baste several times with the dripping liquid.

Serve hot on a bed of lettuce or with noodles or rice.

Roast Leg of Lamb   *serves 6 to 8*

A delectable and tender dish that you will enjoy at tonight's Reward
Meal and tomorrow's Craving-Reducing Meals as well.

	5-pound leg of lamb, trimmed	Lemon juice, to taste
1	clove garlic, slivered	Sesame oil, to taste
1	teaspoon dried rosemary	Salt (or salt substitute), to taste
		Ground black pepper, to taste

Preheat the oven to 300°F.

Cut small slits in the surface of the lamb and insert slivers of
garlic. Rub the surface of the meat with the rosemary, lemon juice,
and oil. Salt and pepper to taste.

Insert a meat thermometer in the center of the roast. Place a
rack in a roasting pan and set the meat on the rack and roast until
desired temperature is reached for rare (140°F.—about 1 hour),
medium (160°F.—about 1$1/4$ hours), or well-done (175°F.—about
1$1/2$ hours).

Remove the meat and set on a warming tray for 20 minutes.

Carve and serve with pan gravy (remove fat if appropriate).

Sweet-and-Pungent Apricot Pork

serves 5 to 6

Oriental cuisine is always a favorite, and this wonderful recipe is a contrast in flavors.

2 pounds boneless lean pork, cut into 1-inch cubes

2 cups water

Salt (or salt substitute), to taste

1/4 cup teriyaki sauce (or low-salt substitute)

1 clove garlic, quartered

1/3 cup sugar

1/4 cup cornstarch

1 cup white, wine, or tarragon vinegar

1/2 cup apricot heavy syrup

Coarsely ground black pepper, to taste

2/3 cup canned apricot halves in heavy syrup, drained

In a large saucepan, combine the pork, water, salt to taste, teriyaki sauce, and garlic. Bring to a boil, reduce the heat, cover, and simmer gently (50 to 60 minutes). Remove the garlic and discard. Remove the meat and set the pan with the sauce aside.

In a clean saucepan, combine the sugar, cornstarch, vinegar, syrup, and black pepper to taste until well mixed.

Add the broth from the original saucepan, and cook and stir over medium heat until the sauce becomes semiclear and thick.

Add the pork cubes and apricots and mix thoroughly.

Serve plain or over noodles or brown, wild, or white rice.

Stuffed Pork Chops   *serves 4*

A pork dish with an imaginative twist that will delight your family
or guests. Enjoy the leftovers cold as tomorrow's Reward Meal
appetizer.

4   double-rib pork chops
2   tablespoons olive oil
1   teaspoon sesame oil
1   medium onion, chopped
2   cups chopped
    mushrooms
1/4 cup water
1   cup flavored packaged
    bread crumbs

Salt (or salt substitute),
to taste
Ground black pepper, to taste
1/4 teaspoon dried sage
2   tablespoons sour cream (or
    low-fat plain yogurt and
    dash of sugar)

Preheat the oven to 350°F.

Cut pockets in between the ribs of the pork chops.

Put the olive oil and sesame oil in a deep skillet and heat. Add
the onion and sauté until soft.

Stir in the mushrooms and cook for 2 minutes. Add the bread
crumbs, salt and pepper to taste, and sage. Mix thoroughly. Add the
sour cream to moisten the mixture.

With a spoon, fill the pocket in each chop with stuffing
mixture. Seal each opening with a wooden toothpick. Add the
water to a baking pan and arrange the chops in the pan.

Bake, covered, for 30 minutes.

Remove the cover and continue baking for an additional 30 to
45 minutes.

Serve with your favorite sauce or the natural gravy.

Pork Chinese Style   *serves 3 to 4*

An engaging pork dish that will be the highlight of your most sumptuous meal.

3 tablespoons olive oil	2 tablespoons cornstarch
1/2 chopped onion	1/4 teaspoon sugar
1 1/2 cups roast pork,	Salt (or salt substitute),
cut into small, thin strips	to taste
1 1/2 cups chicken broth	Ground black pepper, to taste
1/2 cup thin sliced celery	2 tablespoons teriyaki sauce
1 cup sliced mushrooms	(or low-salt substitute)
1 cup fresh bean sprouts	2 tablespoons water

Add the oil to a skillet and heat. Add the onion and sauté until transparent.

Add the pork, broth, celery, and mushrooms. Simmer for 5 minutes. Turn the heat to low and add the sprouts.

In a small bowl, combine the cornstarch, sugar, salt and pepper to taste, teriyaki sauce, and water. Add the mixture to the skillet, and stir over medium heat until thickened.

Serve over a bed of Chinese noodles or rice, if desired.

Sliced Ham Surprise   *serves 3 to 4*

Bet you never tasted a ham dish like this!

5 tablespoons butter (or low-fat substitute)	¼ cup grated Parmesan cheese (or low-fat substitute)
4 tablespoons flour	2 hard-cooked eggs, sliced*
2 cups whole milk or half-and-half*	4 slices lean and thick baked ham
Salt (or salt substitute), to taste	8 triangles toast
Ground black pepper, to taste	12 asparagus spears, trimmed and steamed lightly

In a saucepan set over medium heat, melt 4 tablespoons of the butter. Add the flour and stir with a wire whisk until blended.

In another pan, bring the milk to a boil and add immediately to the flour-butter mixture, stirring vigorously.

When thickened, reduce the heat and simmer for 1 minute.

Add the salt and pepper, remove from the heat, and add the cheese, stirring until smooth.

Carefully stir in the egg slices to conclude the sauce preparation.

In a large skillet, sauté the ham slices in the remaining butter, until heated through. Place the toast triangles on a large serving dish, cover with the ham slices, and top each slice with three cooked, drained asparagus spears.

Spoon the egg sauce over the asparagus spears. Serve immediately.

*In this recipe, low-fat substitutes cannot be used in place of this item. Always follow your physician's recommendations.

Hungarian-Style Pork Chops   *serves 3 to 4*

A favorite that will brighten the spirits and satisfy the tummy.

4 loin pork chops	Salt (or low-salt substitute),
1 clove garlic, finely chopped	to taste
1 teaspoon caraway seeds	Ground black pepper, to taste
1 teaspoon paprika	²/₃ cup dry red wine

Place the chops in a large, shallow, heatproof casserole, keeping the chops from touching.

In a medium bowl, combine the garlic, caraway seeds, paprika, salt, and pepper and mix well.

Sprinkle the mixture over the chops. Add the wine and cover. Refrigerate for 2 to 3 hours.

Preheat the oven to 300°F.

Remove the cover, place the casserole in the oven, and bake until tender (50 to 60 minutes). Add more wine if necessary.

Serve with the casserole sauce and buttered noodles, if you like.

Veal with Peppers   *serves 4 to 6*

The delicate flavor of veal with peppers will offer a welcome change.

4 large green peppers,   1 cup chicken broth
   cut in thick slices   1 teaspoon cornstarch
1 tablespoon olive oil   1 teaspoon teriyaki sauce
2 pounds veal,   (or low-salt substitute)
   cut in thin slivers   1 teaspoon dried basil
2 teaspoons sugar   2 tablespoons water
   Salt (or salt substitute),
   to taste

Place the peppers in a saucepan of boiling water, cover, and parboil (3 minutes). Drain immediately and set aside.

In a large skillet, heat the oil. Add the veal, stirring often, and sauté for 2 minutes. Add the peppers, sugar, salt to taste, and broth. Cover and simmer for 10 minutes.

In a small mixing bowl, combine the cornstarch, teriyaki sauce, basil, and water. Add to the veal and stir until thickened (2 to 3 minutes).

Serve alone or over rice or pasta.

Veal Chops Mediterranean   *serves 4*

An easy dish to prepare that has a delicate texture and taste, assuring that it will be long remembered.

4 tablespoons butter (or low-fat substitute)	1 clove garlic, chopped
4 thick loin veal chops	½ cup finely diced ham
1 tablespoon chopped onion	2 cup green olives, pitted and chopped

In a large skillet, heat the butter, then add the chops and brown on both sides over medium heat.

Add the onion, garlic, and ham and stir over medium heat until the onion is transparent.

Turn the chops, cover, and cook over low heat for 20 minutes. Remove the chops to a platter and keep warm.

Add the olives to the skillet and heat for 1 minute.

Pour the skillet ingredients over the chops and serve.

Reward Meal Salads, Dressings, and Vegetables

Green Goddess Cucumber Salad with Dressing
serves 3 to 4

A tantalizing and unusual salad that will spark the most insensitive palate.

Green Goddess dressing:
6   sprigs fresh watercress
6   spinach leaves, washed well
6   stalks fresh tarragon or chervil
$^2/_3$ cup mayonnaise (or low-fat substitute)
1   teaspoon lemon juice

Cucumber salad:
2   medium cucumbers
$^1/_2$ cup cooked green beans, diced
Fresh chives, finely minced

In a medium-sized pot filled with water, simmer the watercress, spinach, and tarragon. Drain and rinse in cold water.

Put the greens on a large plate and use a fork to press out the water until the greens form a pulp.

Place the mayonnaise in a medium-sized bowl, add the lemon juice and greens, and blend well. Refrigerate until needed.

Cut the unpeeled cucumbers in half lengthwise. Place the slices in a large saucepan and cover with water. Simmer for 2 minutes, then remove from the heat. Place in ice water for 5 minutes. Drain and dry thoroughly.

When cold, hollow out the centers of the cucumbers, leaving a shell about $^1/_4$ inch thick.

Fill the hollows with beans and cover with Green Goddess dressing, topping everything with chopped chives.

Hungarian Beet Salad

serves 3 to 4

This delightfully refreshing salad is a wonderful part of any meal.

1 pound red beets	1/2 tablespoon sugar
1 tablespoon white, wine, or tarragon vinegar	1/4 teaspoon caraway seeds
1 tablespoon water	1/2 teaspoon prepared red horseradish
Salt (or salt substitute), to taste	2 eggs (optional) (or low-fat substitute)

In a medium-sized pot of water, cook the beets until tender. Pour off the water, peel and slice, and set aside.

In a small bowl, combine the vinegar, water, sugar, caraway seeds, and horseradish.

Pour the mixture over the beets and refrigerate overnight.

Before serving, if desired, hard-cook the eggs, peel, and serve as garnish to salad.

Spicy Garden Salad with Dressing

serves 3 to 4

A fresh garden salad that is simple and quick to prepare.

1	small head Boston lettuce	1/4	cup lemon juice
1/4	pound fresh spinach, medium leaves	1/3	cup olive oil
			Salt (or salt substitute), to taste
1	dozen large sorrel leaves		Coarsely ground black pepper, to taste
1	small cucumber		
2	medium radishes, cleaned and trimmed	1/2	teaspoon sugar
		1	clove garlic, cut in eighths

Wash all the leafy vegetables well and drain. Break up the lettuce leaves into bite-sized pieces and place in a large salad bowl. After removing the midribs from the spinach and sorrel leaves, repeat the process for them.

Peel the cucumber and thin-slice the cucumber and radishes, adding the slices to the bowl. Cover and refrigerate until ready to use.

In a medium jar with a tight lid, combine the lemon juice, olive oil, salt, pepper, sugar, and garlic, shake well, and refrigerate until ready to use.

When ready, remove the salad bowl and jar from the refrigerator, shake the jar well, remove the cover, and pour the dressing over the salad. Toss the salad until all the pieces are well coated.

Italian Salad with Dressing

serves 3 to 4

Fast and easy to prepare and a pleasure to serve to family and guests alike.

1 medium cucumber	1 tablespoon red wine vinegar
1 bunch radishes, cleaned	1 teaspoon chopped fresh chives
2 oranges, peeled	1 clove garlic, minced
2 tablespoons olive oil	

Peel the cucumber and thinly slice, trim the radishes and thinly slice, and halve and slice the peeled oranges.

In a bowl, combine the cucumber, radishes, and oranges. Mix gently.

In another bowl, combine the oil, vinegar, chives, and garlic. Mix thoroughly and pour over the salad. Toss and serve.

Popeye's Delight Spinach Salad
with Dressing   *serves 3 to 4*

A marvelous use of a wonderful and often unappreciated green vegetable.

½ pound fresh spinach
   leaves, well washed
   Coarse salt (or salt
   substitute), to taste
1 clove garlic, peeled
1 tablespoon lemon juice
3 tablespoons olive oil

Ground black pepper, to taste
1 hard-cooked egg, cut into
   wedges (or low-fat substitute)
1 medium ripe tomato, cut into
   wedges
½ medium red onion,
   sliced into thin rings

Pat the wet spinach leaves between two pieces of paper toweling. Tear the spinach into bite-sized pieces, removing any tough main veins and stems.

In a large wooden bowl, sprinkle salt and rub the inside of the bowl with the garlic clove.

Add the lemon juice and olive oil and refrigerate the bowl for 1 hour. When ready to serve, add the spinach and sprinkle with pepper.

Garnish with egg, tomato wedges, and onion rings.

Toss lightly and serve.

Caesar Salad Roman-Style   *serves 5 to 6*

An old standard that is a complement to any Reward Meal.

Coarse salt (or salt substitute), to taste
1 clove garlic, peeled
1 teaspoon dry mustard
1 tablespoon lemon juice
Teriyaki sauce to taste
3 tablespoons olive oil
3 bunches romaine lettuce leaves, washed
1 tablespoon grated Parmesan cheese (or low-fat substitute)
1 can anchovies, drained
1 egg, boiled 1 minute*
1/2 cup croutons

In a large wooden bowl, sprinkle salt and rub the inside of the bowl with the garlic clove. Add the mustard, lemon juice, and teriyaki sauce and stir until the salt dissolves. Add the olive oil and stir rapidly until everything is blended.

Blot the romaine leaves on paper toweling and tear into bite-sized pieces. Place the pieces in the bowl.

Sprinkle with the Parmesan cheese, add the anchovies and the contents of the egg.

Sprinkle with croutons and mix gently.

Serve immediately or chill for 1/2 hour.

*Use certified salmonella-free eggs only.

Mustard Vinaigrette   *makes about 1 cup*

Spruce up any salad with this tangy vinaigrette.

1/4 cup wine vinegar	1/2 tablespoon dried basil
1 teaspoon dry red wine	Salt (or salt substitute), to taste
2 tablespoons water	Ground black pepper, to taste
1/2 cup chicken broth	1 clove garlic, minced
1 tablespoon Dijon mustard	1 1/2 tablespoons olive oil

In a medium bowl, combine the vinegar, wine, water, broth, mustard, basil, salt and pepper to taste, and garlic.

Add the oil slowly and whisk continually. Just before serving, whisk thoroughly.

Herb Dressing   *serves 3 to 4*

Take advantage of this simple, cool, and satisfying dressing.

1/4 cup olive oil	1/2 tablespoon water
2 teaspoons wine vinegar	Salt (or salt substitute),
1/8 teaspoon dried thyme	to taste
1/8 teaspoon dried marjoram	Ground black pepper,
1/4 teaspoon dried basil	to taste
1/2 tablespoon finely	1/2 tablespoon finely
chopped onion	chopped fresh parsley

In a medium jar, combine the oil, vinegar, thyme, marjoram, basil, onion, water, salt and pepper to taste, and parsley for 1 minute and then let stand.

Makes a great topping for any mixed green salad.

Cucumber-Tomato Triumph Salad with Dressing

serves 3 to 4

This plain dish, with its uncompromising nutrition, taste, and texture, is a wonderful addition to any Reward Meal.

4 tomatoes	¼ cup wine vinegar
2 tablespoons finely chopped fresh basil	½ cup olive oil
2 tablespoons finely chopped fresh parsley	Salt (or salt substitute), to taste
4 tablespoons finely chopped onion	½ teaspoon sugar
4 cucumbers	2 tablespoons capers
	Fresh dill

Peel the tomatoes and cut into halves.

Combine the basil, parsley, and onion. Sprinkle over the tomato halves. Refrigerate for 1 hour.

Peel the cucumbers and slice crosswise. Combine the vinegar, olive oil, salt, and sugar and marinate the cucumbers in the mixture in the refrigerator for 1 hour.

When ready to serve, drain the cucumber slices, retaining the marinade as dressing. Arrange the cucumbers in the center of a large serving platter, sprinkle with the capers and fresh dill. Arrange the tomato halves around the edge.

Serve immediately with the dressing on the side.

Lemon Mayonnaise Dressing   *serves 3 to 4*

A uncomplicated dressing that turns any green salad into a wonderful dish. If you use "regular" mayonnaise (not a low-fat variety that is often sugar-rich), you can save any leftovers for your Craving-Reducing Meals.

1/3 cup mayonnaise (or low-fat substitute)	1 tablespoon dried basil
1 tablespoon heavy cream (or low-fat substitute)	2 teaspoons lemon juice

In a small bowl, combine the mayonnaise, cream, basil, and lemon juice. Mix thoroughly, cover, and refrigerate until ready to use.

Thousand Island Dressing   *serves 3 to 4*

A dressing that is very popular, and for good reason.

1 tablespoon prepared pickle relish

1 tablespoon chopped green pepper

1 tablespoon chopped red pepper

1 tablespoon chopped yellow pepper

1 tablespoon chopped onion

1/2 cup mayonnaise (or low-fat substitute)

1 tablespoon chili sauce

1 tablespoon heavy cream (or low-fat substitute)

In a small bowl, combine the relish, peppers, onion, mayonnaise, chili sauce, and heavy cream, mix thoroughly, and cover and refrigerate until ready to use.

Use on any Reward Meal mixed green salad.

Herby Green Beans   *serves 4 to 6*

Take advantage of this simple but tasty vegetable dish.

2 tablespoons butter
   (or low-fat substitute)
½ cup chopped scallions,
   bulbs and tops
1 pound green beans,
   cleaned and trimmed

1 (28-ounce) can tomato purée
¼ teaspoon dried basil
¼ teaspoon dried rosemary
   Salt (or salt substitute),
   to taste
   Ground black pepper, to taste

In a large skillet set over medium heat, melt the butter and
sauté the scallions for 3 minutes.

Add the green beans and sauté for 2 additional minutes.

Add the tomato purée, basil, rosemary, and salt and pepper to
taste. Cover, reduce the heat, and simmer until the beans are tender
(5 to 6 minutes).

Serve hot or cold.

Sour Cream and Potato Salad   *serves 3 to 4*

This tangy, wonderful combination is a memorable addition to any meal prepared for a gathering of family or friends.

¼ cup sour cream
(or low-fat substitute)

¼ cup mayonnaise
(or low-fat substitute)

3 cups cooked potatoes,
peeled and diced

1 teaspoon chopped onion
or chives

Salt (or salt substitute),
to taste

Ground black pepper,
to taste

Celery seeds, light sprinkle

4 large lettuce leaves

4 spinach leaves

In a medium bowl, combine the sour cream and mayonnaise. Add the potatoes, onion or chives, salt and pepper to taste, and celery seeds. Mix the contents of the bowl lightly but well.

Line a serving platter with a bed of lettuce and spinach leaves and heap the salad on top of the greens.

Serve immediately or after being well chilled.

Orange-Pecan Squash   *serves 3 to 4*

A wonderful dish for the fall, or any other time of the year.

2 small acorn squash,
   halved and seeded
³/₄ tablespoon brown sugar
1 tablespoon butter (or
   low-fat substitute)

1 teaspoon grated orange peel
2 tablespoons fresh
   orange juice
   Salt (or salt substitute),
   to taste
2 tablespoons chopped pecans

Preheat the oven to 350°F.

On a greased baking sheet, place the squash halves cut-side down and bake until tender (30 to 35 minutes).

Scoop out the pulp into a medium-sized bowl until only a thin shell is left. Combine the pulp, brown sugar, butter, orange peel, orange juice, and salt. Stir until the mixture is fluffy.

Spoon the mixture into all four shell halves and sprinkle with the pecans. Place in the oven and bake until the tops just begin to brown (10 to 12 minutes).

Serve warm.

Broccoli-Cauliflower
Sweet Delight
serves 3 to 4

Take advantage of the wonderful combination of cancer-fighting
cruciferous vegetables exploding with fiber and vitamins A and C in
this savory and flavorful dish.

½ pound broccoli florets
½ pound cauliflower florets
1 tablespoon olive oil
2 tablespoons pine nuts
2 cloves garlic, peeled
and flattened.

2 tablespoons seedless raisins
Salt (or salt substitute),
to taste
Ground black pepper,
to taste

Steam the broccoli and cauliflower florets in 1 inch of water in
a covered pan over high heat until tender (4 minutes). Drain.

Add the oil to a large skillet and heat over medium heat. Add
the broccoli and cauliflower to the hot oil and cook until the
vegetables just begin to brown (5 to 6 minutes).

Add the nuts, garlic, and raisins and cook until the garlic and
nuts are lightly golden and the raisins are wilted. Salt and pepper
to taste.

Serve hot, room temperature, or cold.

Reward Meal Soups

Scallop Soup   *serves 4*

A tempting and uncommon soup that is a treat on a cold or rainy day.

2	tablespoons olive oil	1½ pounds sea scallops
1	cup sliced mushrooms	4½ cups chicken broth
¼	teaspoon dried thyme	½ cup dry white wine
1	bay leaf	Coarsely ground black pepper, to taste
1	tablespoon chopped fresh parsley	Salt (or salt substitute), to taste
1	tablespoon chopped scallion	3 tablespoons butter (or low-fat substitute)
1	tablespoon chopped fresh spinach	

In a large saucepan, combine the olive oil, mushrooms, thyme, bay leaf, parsley, scallion, and spinach. Heat until lightly browned. Set the vegetables aside.

In a saucepan, combine the scallops, 1 cup of the broth, and the wine. Cover and cook until the scallops are done (5 to 6 minutes). Strain and remove the scallops. Chop the scallops into medium-sized pieces.

Combine the remaining broth with the sautéed vegetables and bring the broth to a boil. Remove the bay leaf, and purée the vegetables. Add the chopped scallops to the soup.

Bring the soup to a boil, turn off the heat immediately, and add pepper and salt to taste, and the butter.

Cream of Sorrel Soup   *serves 3 to 4*

A remarkable change-of-pace soup that can be served either hot or cold.

½ pound sorrel (sour grass),   2 cups heavy cream
  finely chopped   (or low-fat plain yogurt and
1 teaspoon butter   2 tablespoons of sugar)
  (or low-fat substitute)   Coarsely ground black pepper,
5 cups chicken broth   to taste
4 egg yolks*

In a saucepan, melt the butter, add the sorrel, and sauté until wilted. Set the pan aside.

In a small pot, add the broth and heat to boiling, then keep on low heat.

In a small bowl, combine the egg yolks and cream and mix with a whisk. Add the cream mixture to the broth while constantly stirring. Do not allow the mixture to boil. Remove from the heat, add the sorrel and mix.

Serve hot topped with black pepper to taste, or cool and refrigerate to be served cold.

*In this recipe, low-fat substitutes cannot be used in place of this item. Always follow your physician's recommendations.

Chicken and Mushroom Soup   *serves 3 to 4*

An all time favorite soup with a twist that will leave your family happy and satisfied.

2 stalks celery, chopped	1 large bay leaf
1/2 head lettuce, washed	1 whole clove
1 tablespoon olive oil	Salt (or salt substitute)
2 cups chicken broth	Ground black pepper
1 cup chopped mushrooms	1/4 cup heavy cream, whipped
1/2 cup chopped green or red pepper	2 tablespoons chopped chives

Place the celery and lettuce leaves into the food processor and grind with the finest blade.

In a large saucepan, heat the olive oil, add the celery and lettuce purée, and sauté until soft but not browned. Add the broth, mushrooms, green or red pepper, bay leaf, clove, and salt and black pepper to taste.

Strain the broth and purée the vegetables in the blender. Return the purée to the broth and serve either cool or cold, topped with whipped cream and garnished with chives.

Beef Consommé   *serves 4*

A quick, simple preparation that is welcome on a cold winter's evening.

2 14-ounce cans beef broth	4 tablespoons grated Swiss cheese (or low-fat substitute)
1 soup can water	1 tablespoon lemon juice
2 eggs*	$1/4$ cup finely chopped fresh parsley
Ground black pepper, to taste	
Salt (or salt substitute), to taste	4 thin lemon slices
	2 additional tablespoons chopped fresh parsley

In a medium-sized pot combine the broth and water and bring to a boil over medium heat.

In a bowl, beat the eggs thoroughly. Add pepper and salt to taste.

Combine the egg mixture, the grated cheese, and lemon juice. Add to the boiling broth and whisk until smooth.

Garnish each bowl of soup with a lemon slice and parsley.

*In this recipe, low-fat substitutes cannot be used for this item. Always follow your physician's recommendations.

Cold Cucumber Soup   *serves 3 to 4*

This easy-to-make soup is a favorite for a summertime treat.

2 cups peeled, diced cucumbers	1 clove garlic, minced
Salt (or salt substitute), to taste	2 tablespoons chopped fresh dill
Ground black pepper, to taste	1 cup sour cream (or low-fat substitute or plain low-fat yogurt with 1 tablespoon of sugar)
2 tablespoons olive oil	Ice cubes

Place the diced cucumbers into a medium-sized bowl.

In another medium-sized bowl, combine the salt, pepper, olive oil, garlic, and dill.

Pour the mixture over the diced cucumbers and marinate in the refrigerator for 4 to 6 hours prior to serving.

When ready to serve, add the sour cream and blend well.

In each serving bowl, place 1 or 2 ice cubes and pour in an appropriate quantity of the mixture. If the mixture is too thick, it can be thinned with a small amount of light stock.

Serve immediately.

Cream of Cauliflower Soup   *serves 3 to 4*

This charming and refreshing soup can be served hot or cold. Use
your imagination to vary the recipe.

2 celery stalks with leaves	Dash cayenne pepper
1 cup cauliflower florets	2/3 cup chicken broth
1 clove garlic	1/3 cup heavy cream (or low-fat
1/2 cup water	substitute)
Salt (or salt substitute),	Coarsely ground black pepper,
to taste	to taste

Cut the celery stalks crosswise into 3 parts.

In a medium pot, combine the celery, cauliflower, garlic, and
water. Simmer for 15 minutes.

Transfer the contents of the pot to a blender container and add
salt and cayenne pepper. Cover and blend at high speed.

Uncover while running and slowly add the broth and heavy
cream.

Serve warm or chilled. Season with black pepper to taste.

Romaine Lettuce Soup   *serves 3 to 4*

An uncommon Reward Meal treat that is a delight to make and
wonderful to eat.

1 tablespoon butter (or low-fat substitute)	Salt (or salt substitute), to taste
1 medium stalk celery, diced	Ground black pepper, to taste
2⅔ cups chicken broth	
1 quart chopped romaine lettuce	2 egg yolks*
	⅔ cup heavy cream*

In a large saucepan, melt the butter, add the celery, and cook
until tender (10 minutes).

Add the broth and bring to a boil.

Add the lettuce, salt and pepper, and cook over low heat until
the lettuce is wilted (about 10 minutes).

In a small bowl, combine the egg yolks and heavy cream and
mix thoroughly.

Stir the mixture into the soup and cook, stirring, until the soup
thickens (before boiling).

Season to taste before serving.

---

*In this recipe, low-fat substitutes cannot be used in place of this item. Always
follow your physician's recommendations.

Clam Soup
serves 3 to 4

This makes a nice transition to the cooler weather and change of season.

25 littleneck clams
1/4 cup olive oil
1 clove garlic, minced
2 anchovy fillets, chopped
1 tablespoon dried basil
1/4 cup cooking sherry

1 1/4 cups water
1 teaspoon salt (or salt substitute), or to taste
1 teaspoon ground black pepper, or to taste
1/4 teaspoon dried oregano

Wash and scrub the clams.

In a large saucepan, combine the oil and garlic, and brown over medium heat.

Add the anchovies, basil, and sherry, and cook for 5 minutes.

Add the water, salt, and pepper and cook for 3 to 4 minutes.

Add the clams, cover the pan, and cook until all shells open (or no more than 5 minutes). Add the oregano and cook for 2 additional minutes.

Serve immediately with the garnish of your choice.

Shrimp-Cheese Soup   *serves 4*

Well worth the effort that will produce a delightful bowl of soup.

2 cups sliced mushrooms	Ground black pepper
1 can (16 ounces) chicken	1 teaspoon hot sauce
broth	1 pound shrimp, shelled and
4 ounces Cheddar cheese (or	deveined
low-fat sustitute), grated	Parsley sprigs for garnish
1/2 cup heavy cream*	(optional)

In a large pot, combine the mushrooms and broth. Bring to a boil and cook for 5 minutes.

Reduce the heat to medium-low and add the cheese and cream. Stir and heat until the cheese is melted and blended with the broth. Simmer while preparing the shrimp.

In a large pot of boiling water, add the shrimp and cook until all shrimp are red (5 minutes).

Add the shrimp to the broth and bring to a boil while stirring.

Remove from the heat and, if desired, serve with a garnish of parsley.

---

*In this recipe, low-fat substitutes cannot be used in place of this item. Always follow your physician's recommendations.

Old-fashioned Split Pea Soup   *serves 4*

A wonderful Reward Meal treat that is high in carbohydrates,
so remember to balance with protein and Craving-Reducing
vegetables.

1¹/₂ cups quick-cooking split green peas	¹/₂ teaspoon sugar
	¹/₈ teaspoon dried thyme
2¹/₂-pound cooked ham shank	2 cloves garlic, split
	1 bay leaf
4 cups chicken broth	Salt (or salt substitute), to taste
1 cup chopped onion	Coarsely ground black pepper, to taste
¹/₂ cup chopped celery	
¹/₂ cup sliced carrot	Croutons for garnish (optional)

Fill a large pot or kettle with 1 quart of water, add the peas,
and bring to a boil. Reduce the heat, cover, and simmer for 45
minutes.

Add the ham shank, broth, onion, celery, carrot, sugar, thyme,
garlic, bay leaf, and salt and pepper to taste, cover, and simmer for
1¹/₂ hours.

Remove the pot from the heat, take out the ham shank and
cool, then cut the meat from the bone. Dice the meat and set aside.

Remove the vegetables and liquid from the pot, press through a
coarse sieve, and return to the pot.

Add the diced ham to the pot and slowly reheat, uncovered,
until the soup is hot (15 to 20 minutes).

Serve plain or with a garnish of croutons.

Pumpkin Soup   *serves 3 to 4*

This delightful soup is best served on a cold winter's night, but it can also be enjoyed at any time of the year. Remember that tomatoes are really fruits and that most of the other ingredients are also high-carbo, so balance it appropriately and save it for your Reward Meals only.

3 cups milk (or low-fat substitute)	Salt (or salt substitute), to taste
2 cups canned pumpkin	Coarsely ground black pepper, to taste
2 tablespoons butter (or low-fat substitute)	Pinch nutmeg
2 tablespoons brown sugar	1 cup diced cooked ham

In a medium-sized pot, heat the milk until scalded. Add the pumpkin, butter, sugar, salt and pepper to taste, nutmeg, and ham. Mix thoroughly and heat for 3 minutes, but do not boil. Serve immediately.

Cream of Avocado Soup   *serves 3 to 4*

A wonderful carbohydrate-rich treat.

2   avocados, peeled and   1 tablespoon lemon juice
     seeded   Salt (or salt substitute), to taste
1½ cups heavy cream   Coarsely ground black pepper,
     (or low-fat substitute)   to taste
1½ cups chicken broth   Dill for garnish (optional)

In a blender jar, put the avocados, cream, broth, lemon juice, and salt and pepper to taste. Blend until smooth.

Cover and refrigerate for at least 3 hours.

Serve hot or cold with dill for garnish, if you like.

Cheesy Mushroom Soup

serves 3 to 4

An unusual soup that is tasty and a nice way to introduce a Reward Meal menu.

¼ cup (4 tablespoons) butter (or low-fat substitute)
½ cup diced onion
½ pound mushrooms, sliced
3 tablespoons flour
½ tablespoon dry mustard
1½ cups beef broth

1 cup cream (or milk)
½ pound Cheddar cheese (or low-fat substitute), grated
1 large carrot, peeled and finely shredded
2 tablespoons chopped fresh parsley
Salt (or salt substitute), to taste
Freshly ground black pepper, to taste

In a medium-sized pot set over low heat, melt the butter.

Add the onion and mushrooms and cook, stirring, until the onion is limp and the mushroom liquid nearly disappears.

In a small bowl, mix the flour and mustard. Stir the mixture into the pot. Add the broth, bring to a boil, and stir until thickened.

Remove the pot from the heat and stir in the cream, cheese, carrot, and parsley. Add salt and pepper to taste.

French Onion Soup   *serves 3 to 4*

This restaurant classic is much simpler to prepare than you might think.

¹/₄ cup (4 tablespoons) butter   2   tablespoons grated Parmesan
    (or low-fat substitute)   cheese (or low-fat substitute)
3   cups thinly sliced onions   3   slices imported Swiss cheese
3   cups beef broth   (or low-fat substitute)
3   thick slices French bread

In a large pot or kettle, melt the butter over medium heat. Add the onions and sauté until golden (6 to 8 minutes).

Add the broth and raise the heat to bring the mixture to a boil. Reduce the heat, cover the pot, and simmer for 30 minutes.

Preheat the oven to broil.

Toast the bread on both sides.

Pour the soup into individual ovenproof bowls. Float 1 piece of toast in each bowl, sprinkle Parmesan on top of each piece, and cover with a slice of Swiss cheese. Place the bowls in the broiler and heat until the cheese is bubbly (3 to 5 minutes).

Handle the bowls with pot holders and place each on its own plate to serve. Be careful—remember that the bowls just came out of a hot oven.

Potato and Garlic Soup   *serves 3 to 4*

A simple combination that is tasty and filling without jading your appetite for the rest of your Reward Meal. Remember to balance with protein and Craving-Reducing vegetables for the starchy, carbohydrate-rich potatoes.

2 tablespoons butter*
1 leek, white portion only, cleaned and sliced
8 cloves garlic, peeled
1 pound potatoes, peeled and cubed

3 cups chicken broth
½ teaspoon salt (or salt substitute)
½ cup cream (or milk)*

Put 1 tablespoon of the butter in a medium-sized, heavy-bottomed pot and melt the butter over low heat.

Add the leek and garlic and sauté for several minutes.

Add the potatoes, broth, and salt and allow the mixture to come to a boil. Cover the pot and simmer for 45 to 60 minutes.

Remove the potatoes and garlic cloves from the pot, setting the broth aside.

Together, in a blender, purée small amounts of potatoes and garlic at a time. When smooth, return the purée to the broth. Water may be added if the mixture is too thick.

Add the cream and heat. Add the remaining tablespoon of butter and mix it into the soup.

Serve hot.

*In this recipe, low-fat substitutes cannot be used in place of this item. Always follow your physician's recommendations.

Mexican Soup   *serves 3 to 4*

A wonderful change-of-pace soup that stands out at any meal, but save this treat for Reward Meals only.

2 tablespoons butter (or low-fat substitute)	1 can (16 ounces) whole tomatoes
2 medium potatoes, diced	1 egg*
½ cup chopped onion	½ pound Longhorn cheese, (or low-fat substitute) cut into strips
½ cup green chilies, cut into strips	Salt (or salt substitute), to taste
2 cups water	Ground black pepper, to taste

In a large saucepan set over low-medium heat, melt the butter. Add the potatoes, onion, and green chilies. Turn the heat up to medium and sauté for 5 minutes.

Add the water, cover, reduce the heat, and simmer until the potatoes are nearly done (10 to 15 minutes).

Add the tomatoes, along with their juice, and gently crush them with a fork.

In a small bowl, beat the egg and then add it to the saucepan, allowing the mixture to simmer for 2 to 3 minutes.

Add the cheese strips and stir until the cheese melts (2 to 3 minutes).

Add salt and pepper to taste.

**In this recipe, low-fat substitutes cannot be used in place of this item. Always follow your physician's recommendations.

Minestrone

serves 3 to 4

An opulent and robust Italian soup that warms you all the way through.

6	cups water	1	stalk celery, diced
1/2	cup dried large white beans	1/2	small zucchini, sliced
		1	bay leaf
1/4	pound salt pork, chopped	1/2	cup peeled and diced potatoes
1/4	cup lentils		Salt (or salt substitute), to taste
3	cups beef broth		
1	small onion, chopped		Ground black pepper, to taste
1/2	cup canned tomato purée	1/2	cup peas, fresh or frozen
1/4	cup canned garbanzo beans, drained	1/4	cup elbow pasta
1/2	cup diced carrots		Grated Parmesan cheese, (or low-fat substitute) to taste

In a small bowl with enough water to cover (2 cups), add the beans and soak overnight.

In a large pot or kettle, add the remaining 4 cups water and the pork, and heat to boiling. Reduce the heat immediately and simmer for 10 to 15 minutes.

Drain the beans and add with the lentils to the pot. Simmer until the beans are fork-tender (about 1 hour).

Add the broth, onion, tomato purée, garbanzos, carrots, celery, zucchini, and bay leaf. Simmer for 20 minutes.

Add the potatoes and salt and pepper to taste. Simmer until the potatoes are beginning to get tender when pierced with a fork.

Add the peas and pasta and cook until the pasta is tender (10 to 12 minutes). Add water if the soup is too thick.

Serve hot or cold. Sprinkle each portion with Parmesan cheese when serving.

Sausage Soup Supreme   *serves 3 to 4*

An especially good recipe to serve family and friends.

1 pound hot or mild Italian sausage
1 large head endive, broken into pieces
4 cloves garlic, finely chopped
Salt (or salt substitute), to taste

Ground black pepper, to taste
dried oregano, to taste
chopped fresh parsley, to taste
4 eggs*
Grated Parmesan cheese

Cut the sausage into bite-sized pieces, place in a medium-sized pot, and cover with water. Bring to a boil over low-medium heat and cook for 30 minutes.

Remove from the heat and add the endive, garlic, salt, pepper, oregano, and parsley. Return to the heat and cook for an additional 30 minutes.

In a medium-sized bowl, combine the eggs and Parmesan cheese, and beat until the consistency of heavy cream.

Add to the soup mixture and heat. The soup's "curdled" appearance is normal and desired, so not to worry.

*In this recipe, low-fat substitutes cannot be used in place of this item. Always follow your physician's recommendations.

Reward Meal Vegetarian (Non-Meat) Choices

Vegetarian "Burger" Goulash   *serves 3 to 4*

A tempting entrée for any festive occasion or just a treat for the family.

2 tablespoons olive oil	²/₃ cup dry red wine
1 medium onion, chopped	6 small new potatoes or
1 clove garlic, crushed	2 large baking potatoes, cubed
6 vegetarian "burgers," cubed	Salt (or salt substitute), to taste
¼ cup flour	Ground black pepper,
Paprika	to taste
12 ounces tomatoes, fresh or canned, chopped	½ cup sour cream (or low-fat substitute)

In a large frying pan, heat the olive oil over low-medium heat. Add the onions and garlic and sauté for 4 to 5 minutes.

Coat the "burger" cubes with flour and place in the pan and brown gently (2 to 3 minutes).

Add the paprika, tomatoes, wine, and potatoes. Add salt and pepper to taste. Cover pan and simmer for 25 minutes.

Immediately prior to serving, with pan removed from heat, stir in the sour cream and if desired garnish with additional paprika.

Serve over rice or noodles as a special treat.

Vegetarian "Burgers" with Parsley Butter

serves 3 to 4

A wonderful pan-fried dish with a delicate flavor that is easy to prepare.

4 tablespoons butter (or low-fat substitute)	6 vegetarian "burgers"
2 tablespoons chopped fresh parsley	1 clove garlic, crushed
2 tablespoons olive oil	Ground black pepper, to taste

In a small mixing bowl, combine the butter and parsley. Chill the mixture until firm (about 1 hour).

Put the olive oil in a large frying pan set over low-medium heat. Add the "burgers" and fry until brown on the first side (2 to 3 minutes), then turn and brown on the second side (about 2 minutes).

Place the "burgers" on a large dish and rub the garlic on both sides of the "burgers."

Position the "burgers" on a serving dish and put a small ball of parsley butter on the center of each burger. Pepper to taste.

Serve immediately with a fine accompaniment of rice or pasta and vegetables.

Consummate Vegetarian "Burger"

serves 3 to 4

An aromatic treat that makes fine use of many wonderful ingredients.

1 tablespoon olive oil	4 tablespoons cooking sherry
6 vegetarian "burgers"	
2 tablespoons butter (or low-fat substitute)	4 tablespoons vegetable stock or water
1 medium onion, chopped	2 egg yolks*
2 cloves garlic, crushed Salt (or salt substitute), to taste Pepper, to taste	2 tablespoons heavy cream (or plain low-fat yogurt with dash of sugar)
4 tablespoons dry white wine	2 tablespoons chopped fresh parsley

Put the olive oil in a large frying pan set over medium heat. Add the "burgers" to the pan and brown for 5 minutes, turning often. Remove the pan from the heat and set aside.

Melt the butter in a medium-sized frying pan set over medium heat. Add the onion and garlic, and brown lightly. Add salt and pepper to taste.

Add the wine, sherry, and stock (or water), and stir well. Allow to simmer for 2 to 4 minutes.

In a small bowl, whisk the egg yolks and heavy cream.

Pour the cream mixture into the wine mixture and stir well.

Add the parsley and the browned "burgers," bringing everything to a simmer.

Serve hot.

*In this recipe, low-fat and non-egg substitutes cannot be used in place of this item. Always follow your physician's recommendations.

Vegetarian "Beef" Stroganoff   *serves 3 to 4*

This graceful dish will satisfy the tastebuds of family and guests alike.

3 tablespoons olive oil
1 medium onion, finely chopped
4 cups sliced fresh mushrooms
1 teaspoon paprika
1/4 cup flour

6 vegetarian "steaklets"
2/3 cup dry white wine
3 tablespoons water
4 tablespoons sour cream (or low-fat substitute)
1/2 teaspoon mild prepared mustard

In a medium-sized pan set over low-medium heat, warm the olive oil.

Add the onion, mushrooms, and paprika, and sauté until the onions are translucent (about 10 minutes).

Add the flour and "steaklets," stir well and brown (about 2 minutes).

Add the wine and simmer over low heat until the mixture is thoroughly cooked (12 to 15 minutes), stirring often and adding water if it appears dry.

Add the sour cream and mustard, keeping the mixture warm for 2 additional minutes, without boiling or simmering.

Serve immediately. Add salad, rice, Craving-Reducing vegetables, and top off with some fruit or another tasty dessert.

Vegetarian "Sausage" with Avocados and Fettuccine

serves 3 to 4

A new recipe that will soon become an oft-enjoyed favorite.

1 teaspoon olive oil	1/2 cup heavy cream (or low-fat
6 vegetarian "sausage	plain yogurt with
links," chopped	1/2 tablespoon of sugar)
1/4 teaspoon salt	2 avocados, chopped
(or salt substitute)	1 avocado, sliced
4 cups water	Grated Parmesan cheese
4 ounces fettuccine,	(or low-fat substitute) to taste
packaged or fresh	Ground black pepper,
1/4 cup butter*	to taste
1 teaspoon flour	

To a medium-sized skillet set over medium heat, add the oil and heat. Add the chopped "sausage" and cook until golden (4 to 5 minutes). Set aside.

In a medium-sized pot, add the salt and water. Heat to a boil, add the pasta, and cook until *al dente*. Drain the water and cover the pot to keep the pasta hot.

In a small saucepan set over medium heat, melt the butter. Add the flour and stir. Add the cream and stir constantly while cooking for 5 minutes. Briefly heat the chopped "sausage" in the skillet.

Remove the pasta and place it on a serving platter. Pour the cream sauce over the pasta, add the chopped avocado, 3/4 of the "sausage," 3/4 of the Parmesan cheese, and pepper to taste.

Garnish with the sliced avocado and the remaining "sausage" and serve with the remaining grated cheese.

---

*In this recipe, low-fat and nondairy substitutes cannot be used in place of this item. Always follow your physician's recommendations.

Vegetarian "Sausage" Loaf   *serves 3 to 4*

An unusual "meat loaf" for the vegetarian. It's rich in fiber, and low in calories and fat.

1½ teaspoons olive oil	½ teaspoon hot sauce
2 cloves garlic, chopped	½ pound vegetarian "sausage,"
2 large scallions, chopped	broken into chunks
1 medium tomato,	¼ cup rolled oats
chopped with juice	3 tablespoons oat bran
⅓ cup chopped fresh basil	2 large egg whites, beaten
½ teaspoon dried oregano	Salt (or salt substitute), to taste
4 tablespoons dry red wine	Coarsely ground black pepper,
1 small zucchini, chopped	to taste
1 medium green pepper,	
chopped	

Preheat the oven to 350°F.

Coat the loaf pan with ½ teaspoon of the olive oil. Set aside.

In a saucepan set over medium-low heat, combine the remaining olive oil, garlic, and scallions and cook for 3 minutes. Stir several times during cooking.

Add the tomatoes with their juice, 2 tablespoons of the basil, the oregano, and wine. Simmer for 10 minutes, stirring occasionally.

In a large bowl, combine the contents of the saucepan with the zucchini, green pepper, hot sauce, "sausage," rolled oats, oat bran, egg whites, and salt and pepper to taste. Mix thoroughly.

Transfer the mixture to a loaf pan and spread uniformly.

Place the pan in the oven and bake until golden-brown on top (about 1 hour).

Serve hot or cold.

Vegetarian Pacific Island "Chicken"

serves 3 to 4

A Polynesian pleasure to add to any vegetarian menu.

1 pound vegetarian "chicken steaks"	2 tablespoons lemon juice
	1 tablespoon cornstarch
1/2 cup flour	1/2 cup brown sugar
3 tablespoons teriyaki sauce	1 cup cubed papaya
Salt (or salt substitute), to taste	1 cup diced pineapple
	2 cups sliced banana
1/2 cup olive oil	1 cup sliced water chestnuts
1 cup orange juice	

Preheat the oven to 350°F.

In a large plastic bag, combine serving-size pieces of "chicken," the flour, and 1 teaspoon of the teriyaki sauce. Shake until the "chicken" is thoroughly coated.

Grease a shallow baking pan with a small amount of oil, and at the bottom of the pan form a single layer of coated "chicken" pieces.

Sprinkle the remaining oil over the top of the "chicken."

Place the pan in the oven and bake for 45 to 50 minutes.

In the meantime, in a large saucepan combine the orange juice, lemon juice, cornstarch, sugar, and the remaining teriyaki sauce. Cook over medium heat, continually stirring until the sauce becomes thick and clear.

Add the papaya, pineapple, banana, and water chestnuts and mix thoroughly.

Remove the "chicken" pan from the oven, pour the fruit sauce over the "chicken" in the pan, and heat for 10 more minutes.

Serve plain or over a bed of rice.

Vegetarian Lemon "Chicken" *serves 3 to 4*

Juicy and tender inside, with a golden-crisp outside. You'll love it.

2 eggs*	1/2 teaspoon dried parsley
4 teaspoons lemon juice	1 cup packaged flavored
1/4 teaspoon hot paprika	bread crumbs
4 vegetarian "chicken	Salt (or salt substitute), to taste
steaks," about 3 ounces	Ground black pepper, to taste
each	Lemon slices for garnish
1/2 teaspoon dried basil	(optional)

In a medium-sized bowl, combine the eggs, 3 teaspoons of the lemon juice, and the paprika. Mix thoroughly.

Add the "chicken steaks" and coat both sides, leaving the "steaks" in the bowl.

In a large shallow dish, combine the basil, parsley, bread crumbs, and salt and pepper to taste. Mix well.

Take the "chicken" pieces from the egg mixture and dip into the bread crumb mixture, coating both sides well. Place the coated pieces on a platter and set aside.

Preheat the oven to 400°F.

Grease a large baking pan with oil or an appropriate low-fat spray and make a single layer of coated "chicken" pieces in the pan. Place the pan in the oven and bake until the top is golden-brown (15 minutes). Turn the "chicken" and bake until golden-brown (10 minutes).

Place the "chicken" on a serving platter, and sprinkle with the remaining lemon juice. If desired, garnish with lemon slices and parsley and serve.

*In this recipe, low-fat or non-egg substitutes cannot be used in place of this item. Always follow your physician's recommendations.

Vegetarian "Chicken" and Beans *serves 3 to 4*

A great dish to serve to your "meat-eating" guests.

6	cups water	Salt (or salt substitute),
1	cup dried small white	to taste
	beans	Ground black pepper, to taste
1	medium onion, sliced	Paprika, to taste
2	cloves garlic, minced	Grated cheese (or nondairy
6	vegetarian "chicken" slices	substitute), to taste

In a large saucepan, combine 2 cups of the water and the beans. Soak overnight.

Drain the water and add 4 cups fresh water to just cover the beans. Add the onion and garlic, and cook over medium heat (1^1/$_2$ hours, or until the beans are tender).

Sauté or bake the "chicken" slices as per the package directions. Add salt, pepper, and paprika to taste.

Place the "chicken" on a serving plate, and top with the beans and grated cheese.

Vegetarian "Flounder" Surprise

serves 3 to 4

This tasty dish is worth the effort and goes well with steamed vegetables such as asparagus, broccoli, or Brussels sprouts.

1 cup wild rice
3 cups water
1/4 cup teriyaki sauce (or low-salt substitute)
2 tablespoons butter (or low-fat or nondairy substitute)
1 medium onion, diced
1 stalk celery, diced

1 cup sliced mushrooms
1 cup sliced water chestnuts
1/4 cup slivered almonds
Salt (or salt substitute), to taste
Ground black pepper, to taste
1 1/2 pounds "flounder" fillets (a non-seafood substitute)
1 teaspoon lemon juice
1/4 cup chopped fresh parsley

In a medium-sized pot combine the rice, 3 cups water, and teriyaki sauce. Cook the mixture until the wild rice is tender (40 to 50 minutes).

Preheat the oven to 350° F.

Coat a large baking dish with 1 tablespoon of the butter and set aside.

Transfer the rice and excess liquid to a large mixing bowl.

In a large skillet set over medium heat, melt the remaining butter and add the onion, celery, and mushrooms. Heat and sauté until the onions are light brown (3 to 4 minutes).

Add the contents of the skillet to the bowl with the rice. Add the water chestnuts, almonds, and salt and pepper to taste. Toss lightly.

Spoon the mixture into a greased baking dish, top with the "fish" fillets, and sprinkle with lemon juice. Place the dish in the oven and bake until the "fish" flakes when pierced by fork tines (12 to 15 minutes).

Remove from the oven, garnish with parsley, and serve immediately.

"Seafood" Vegetable Triumph   *serves 3 to 4*

A truly delicious combination dish of tomato stew containing "shell-fish" and "fish." Watch for the signs of delight as your family or guests take their first taste.

1 tablespoon olive oil	2 small zucchini, sliced
1 large carrot, chopped	1 bay leaf
1 large stalk celery, diced	1 teaspoon prepared hot sauce
1 large green pepper, chopped	1 teaspoon dried oregano
1 large red pepper, chopped	1 pound mock "fish" and/or "crab"
1 large onion, chopped	8 green olives
2 large cloves garlic, chopped	8 black olives
2 cups canned whole tomatoes, chopped	1/4 cup chopped fresh parsley
1/2 cup dry red wine	Ground black pepper, to taste

In a large, deep skillet set over medium-low heat, add the oil and coat. Combine the carrot, celery, green pepper, red pepper, and onion. Sauté until the onion is soft (4 to 5 minutes).

Add the tomatoes, wine, zucchini, bay leaf, hot sauce, and oregano. Mix well, raise the heat, and cook until small bubbles appear. Reduce the heat and simmer for 15 minutes.

Add the "fish" and/or "crab," green olives, and black olives. Cover and warm for a minute or two.

Stir in the parsley and pepper to taste.

Serve immediately.

Vegetarian "Scallop" Newburg   *serves 3 to 4*

An appetizing dish that lets you enjoy a delicious taste of the "fruits of the sea."

1/4 cup (4 tablespoons) butter (or low-fat substitute)

2 cups vegetarian "scallops" or "crabmeat"

1/3 teaspoon ground nutmeg

1/2 teaspoon paprika

3 egg yolks,* beaten

1 cup heavy cream (or low-fat plain yogurt and 1 tablespoon sugar)*

1/4 cup cooking sherry

Salt (or low-salt substitute), to taste

Ground black pepper, to taste

In a double boiler, melt the butter, mix in the "scallops," and cook for 3 to 4 minutes.

Add the nutmeg and paprika, and cook for 1 to 2 minutes.

Add the egg yolks and heavy cream. Stir and cook (do not boil) until the liquid is thick.

Add the sherry and salt and pepper to taste.

Serve over buttered and toasted bread of your choice.

*In this recipe, low-fat, non-egg, and nondairy substitutes cannot be used in place of these items. Always follow your physician's recommendations.

Creamy Eggs and Pasta

serves 3 to 4

A wonderfully tasty dish with a hearty flavor.

4   cups water

4   cups uncooked pasta

4   eggs (or egg substitute)
    Salt (or salt substitute), to taste
    Ground black pepper, to taste

2   tablespoons butter (or low-fat or nondairy substitute)

1   cup grated Cheddar cheese (or low fat or nondairy substitute)

In a large, uncovered saucepan, bring the water to a boil and add the pasta. Leave the pan uncovered and boil the pasta until *al dente* (10 to 12 minutes).

While the pasta is cooking, whisk the eggs in a mixing bowl.

Drain the pasta and add to the whisked eggs. Season to taste with salt and pepper and blend well.

In a small frying pan, melt the butter over medium-low heat. Add the egg-pasta mixture to the pan. Raise the heat to medium and let the omelet cook for 1 minute. Sprinkle the grated cheese over the omelet and let cook for 1 to 2 additional minutes.

With a spatula, fold the omelet over and serve immediately. Add lots of crisp raw vegetables and a warm fruit dessert for a great Reward Meal.

Vegetable Delight

serves 3 to 4

This elegant dinner casserole is truly a vegetarian's joy to see, smell, and feast upon. Add some protein, grains, and a salad, then top it off with some fruit or other dessert.

½ teaspoon sesame oil
½ tablespoon olive oil
½ cup green beans, french-cut
½ small-medium zucchini
½ medium yellow squash
½ green pepper, cubed
1 small can whole tomatoes
¼ teaspoon dried basil

Ground black pepper, to taste
¼ teaspoon dried marjoram
¼ teaspoon dried sage
¼ teaspoon dried savory
¼ teaspoon dried thyme
Salt (or salt substitute), to taste
3 slices imported Swiss cheese (or low-fat substitute), grated

Preheat the oven to 375°F.

In a large, deep skillet set over medium heat, combine the sesame oil and olive oil. Add the beans, zucchini, squash, and peppers. Sauté until soft, but do not overcook.

Add the tomatoes with their juice and cut the tomatoes into pieces in the pan. Add the basil, black pepper, marjoram, sage, savory, thyme, and salt. Mix well, cover, and cook for 5 minutes.

Pour the contents of the skillet into an uncovered large casserole, then top with the cheese slices and place in the oven to bake until brown (10 to 15 minutes).

Serve immediately.

Baked Macaroni and Tomato   *serves 3 to 4*

A specialty that is not only a pleasure to prepare but also a delight
to eat.

1 medium can whole tomatoes	1/8 teaspoon dried marjoram 1/8 teaspoon dried oregano
1 small can tomato paste	3 teaspoons olive oil
1/2 tablespoon sugar	1 large onion, sliced thin
Salt (or salt substitute),	1 large green pepper, sliced thin
to taste	1 pound elbow macaroni
Ground black pepper,	6 to 8 thin slices imported
to taste	Swiss cheese (or meltable
1 clove garlic, minced	low-fat or nondairy substitute),
1/8 teaspoon dried basil	to taste
1/8 teaspoon dried chervil	

In a large frying pan set over low heat, combine the tomatoes,
tomato paste, sugar, salt and pepper to taste, garlic, basil, chervil,
marjoram, and oregano. Cook, uncovered, for 1 hour.

Preheat the oven to 350°F.

In a small frying pan set over medium heat, combine 2
teaspoons of the olive oil and the onion and green pepper. Sauté
for 3 minutes.

Boil the elbow macaroni according to the package directions.
Rinse in cold water.

Use the remaining olive oil to coat the inside of the large
casserole. Add in layers the macaroni, sauce, and cheese slices until
the casserole is full. End with sauce and cheese on top.

Place in the oven and bake, uncovered, until the cheese melts
(20 to 30 minutes).

Serve piping hot.

APPENDIX

SELECTED BIBLIOGRAPHY

Abraham AS, Sonnenblick M, Eini M, Shemesh O, and Batt AP. The effect of chromium on established atherosclerotic plaques in rabbits. Am J Clin Nutr, 33: 2294–2298, 1980.

Alemany M. The etiological basis for the classification of obesity. Prog Food Nutr Sci. 13 (1): 46–66, 1989.

Altomare E, Vendemiale G, Chicco D, Procacci V, and Cirelli F. Increased lipid peroxidation in type 2 poorly controlled diabetic patients. Diabetes Metab, 18 (4): 264–271, 1992.

American Psychiatric Association. Diagnostic and statistical manual of mental disorders, 3rd ed. Washington, DC: Am Psychiatric Press, 1987.

Anderson JW. Nutrition management of diabetes mellitus. IN: Modern Nutrition in Health and Disease, 7th ed., ed. by ME Shils and VR Young, Lea & Febiger, Philadelphia: 1204–1229,1988.

Anderson RA. Nutritional role of chromium. The Sci of the Tot Environ, 17: 130–29, 1981.

Anderson RA, Polansky MM, Bryden NA, Roginsk E, Patterson KY, and Reamer DC. Effect of exercise (running) on serum glucose, insulin, glucagon, and chromium excretion. Diabetes, 31: 212–216, 1982.

Anderson RA. Chromium metabolism and its role in disease processes in man. Clin Physiol Biochem, 4: 31–41, 1986.

Anderson RA, Polansky MM, Bryden NA, and Guttman HN. Strenuous exercise may increase dietary needs for chromium and zinc. Sports, Health and Nutrition. Ed. FI Katch, vol 2: 83–88, 1986.

Anderson RA, Polansky MM, Bryden NA, Bhathena SJ, and Canary JJ. Effects of supplemental chromium on patients with symptoms of reactive hypoglycemia. Metab, 36 (4): 351–355, 1987.

Anderson RA. Selenium, chromium, and manganese: (b) chromium IN: Modern Nutrition in Health and Disease, 7th ed., ed by ME Shils and VR Young, Lea & Febiger, Philadelphia: 268–273, 1988.

Anderson RA. Essentiality of chromium in humans. The Sci of the Tot Environ, 86 (1–2): 75–81, 1989.

Anderson RA, Bryden NA, Polansky MM, Reisner S. Urinary chromium excretion and insulinogenic properties of carbohydrates. Am J Clin Nutr, 51 (5): 864–868, 1990.

Anke M. Role of trace elements in the dynamics of atherosclerosis. Z Gesamte Inn Med, 41 (4): 105–111, 1986.

Anselmo J, Vaz F, Correia LG, Pereira E, Lima de Silva F, Pires MT, and Nunes-Correa JC. Influence of body fat topography on glucose homeostasis and serum lipid levels. Acta Med Port, 3 (6): 341–346, 1990.

Aparicio M, Gin H, Potaux L, Bouchet JL, Morel D, and Aubertin J. Effect of a ketoacid diet on glucose tolerance and tissue insulin sensitivity. Kidney Int Suppl, 27: S231–S235, 1989.

Aronow WS, Ahn C, Kronzon I, and Koenigsberg M. Congestive heart failure, coronary events and atherothrombic brain infarction in elderly blacks and whites with systemic hypertension and with and without echocardiographic and electrocardiographic evidence of left ventricular hypertrophy. FASEB J, 67: 295–299, 1991.

Assimacopoulos F and Jeanrenaud JB. The hormonal and metabolic basis of experimental obesity. Clin Endocrinol Metab, 5 (2): 337–365, 1976.

Atrens DM. The questionable wisdom of a low-fat diet and cholesterol reduction. Social Science Medicine, 39 (3): 433–447.

Bagdade JD and Dunn FL. Effects of insulin treatment on lipoprotein composition and function in patients with IDDM. Diabetes, 41 Suppl 2: 107–110, 1992.

Barrett-Connor L. Obesity, atherosclerosis, and coronary heart disease. Annals Intern Med, 103 (6 pt 2): 1010-1019, 1985.

Beck-Nielsen H, Nielsen OH, Damsbo P, Vaag A, Handberg A, and Henriksen JE. Impairment of glucose tolerance: mechanism of action and impact on the cardiovascular system. Am J Obstet Gynecol, 163 (1 Pt2): 292–295, 1990.

Berne C. Insulin in hypertension—a relationship with consequences? J Intern Med Suppl, 735: 65–73, 1991.

Beverly C. Sugary foods may be hazard for those who have breast
cancer. Natural Healing Newsletter, 3 (1G): 5, 1991.

Bhathena SJ, Aparicio P, Revett K, Voyles N, and Recant L. Effect of
dietary carbohydrates on glucagon and insulin receptors in
genetically obese female Zucker rats. J Nutr, 117 (7): 1291–1297,
1987.

Bhathena SJ, Berlin E, Judd JT, Jones J, Kennedy BW, Smith PM,
Jones DY, Taylor PR, and Campbell WS. Dietary fat and men-
strual-cycle effects on the erythrocyte ghost insulin receptor in
premenopausal women. Am J Clin Nutr, 50: 460-464, 1989.

Bierman EL and Chait A. Nutrition and diet in relation to hyperlipi-
demia and atherosclerosis. IN: Modern Nutrition in Health and
Disease, 7th ed., ed. by ME Shils and VR Young, Lea & Febiger,
Philadelphia: 1283–1297, 1988.

Bjorntorp P. Obesity and adipose tissue distribution as a risk factor
for the development of disease. A review. Infusionstherapie, 17
(1): 24–27, 1990.

Black HR. The coronary artery disease paradox: the role of hyperinsulinemia and insulin resistance and its implications for therapy.
J Cardiovasc Pharmacol, 15 Suppl 5: S26–S38, 1990.

Blackburn GL. Medical treatment of obesity. IN: Treatment of Obe-
sity: A Multidisciplinary Approach, presented through the
Department of Education at Harvard Medical School, Nov 7–9.
Ed. by Blackburn GL, Benotti PN, and Mascioli EA, 1991.

Bland J. Nutraerobics. Harper & Row, San Francisco: 1983.

Blendis LM and Jenkins DJA. Nutrition and diet in management of
diseases of the gastrointestinal tract. IN: Modern Nutrition in
Health and Disease, 7th ed., ed by ME Shils and VR Young, Lea
& Febiger, Philadelphia: 1182–1200, 1988.

Block G, Dresser C, Hartman H, and Carol MD. Nutrient sources in
the American diet: Quantitative data from the HANES II survey. I
Vitamins and minerals. AM J Epidemiol, 122: 13–40, 1985.

Boden G, Jadali F, White J, Liang Y, Mozzoli M, Chen X, Coleman E,
and Smith C. Effects of fat on insulin-stimulated carbohydrate
metabolism in normal men. J Clin Invest, 88 (3): 960-966, 1991.

Bogardus C, Lillioja S, Foley J, Christin L, Freymond D, Nyomba B,
Bennett PH, Reaven GM, and Salans L, 1987. Insulin resistance

predicts the development of non-insulin dependent diabetes mellitus in Pima Indians. Diabetes 36 (suppl #1): 47A (abstract).

Bottermann P and Classen M. Diabetes mellitus and arterial hypertension. In search of the connecting link. Z Gesamte Inn Med, 46 (15): 558–562, 1991.

Brands MW and Hall JE. Insulin resistance, hyperinsulinemia, and obesity-associated hypertension. J Am Soc Nephrol, 3 (5): 1064–1077, 1992.

Bray GA. Obesity: historical development of scientific and cultural ideas. Int J Obes, 14 (11): 909–926, 1990.

Bray GA. Obesity, a disorder of nutrient partitioning: The MONA LISA hypothesis. J Nutr, 121: 1146–1162, 1991.

Brindley DN and Rolland Y. Possible connections between stress, diabetes, obesity, hypertension and altered lipoprotein metabolism that may result in atherosclerosis. Clin Sci, 77 (5): 453–461, 1989.

Brindley DN. Mode of action of benfluorex. Recent data. Presse Med, 21 (28): 1330-1335, 1992.

Brought DL and Taylor R. Review: deterioration of glucose tolerance with age: the role of insulin resistance. Age Aging, 20 (3): 221–225, 1991.

Bruning PF, Bonfrer JM, van Noord PA, Hart AA, de Jong-Bakker M, and Nooijen WJ. Insulin resistance and breast cancer risk. Int J Cancer, 52 (4): 511–516, 1992.

Buchanan, TA. Glucose metabolism during pregnancy: normal physiology and implications for diabetes mellitus. Isr J Med Sci, 27 (8–9): 432–441, 1991.

Buhler FR. Cardiovascular risk factors—an integrated sympathetic viewpoint. Schweiz Med Wochenschr, 121 (49): 1793–1802, 1991.

Bunker VW, Lawson MS, Delves HT, and Clayton BE. The uptake and excretion of chromium by the elderly. Am J Clin Nutr, 39: 797–802, 1984.

Butler P, Kryshak E, and Rizza R. Mechanism of growth hormone-induced postprandial carbohydrate intolerance in humans. Am J Physiol 260 (4 Pt 1): E513–E520, 1991. [pub erratum appears in Am J Physiol: 261 (6 Pt 1): E677.]

Cabrijan T, Levanat S, Pekic P, Pavelic J, Spaventi R, Frahm H, Zjacic-Rotkvic V, Goldoni V, Vrbanec D, Misjak M, et al. The role of insulin-related substance in Hodgkin's disease. J Cancer Res Clin Oncol, 117 (6): 615–619, 1991.

Campbell WW and Anderson RA. Effects of aerobic exercise and training on the trace minerals chromium, zinc and copper. Sports Med, 4 (1): 9 –18, 1987.

Ceriello A, Quatraro A, Caretta F, Varano R, and Giugliano D. Evidence for the possible role of oxygen free radicals in the abnormal function of arterial vasomotor in insulin dependent diabetes. Diabetes Meta, 16 (4): 318–322, 1990.

Chandrasekhar Y, Heiner J, Osuamkpe, and Nagamani M. Insulin-like growth factor I and II binding in human myometrium and leiomyomas. Am J Obstet Gynecol, 166 (1 Pt1): 64–69, 1992.

Chaouloff F, Laude D, Merino D, Serrurier B, and Elghozi JL. Peripheral and central consequences of immobilization stress in genetically obese Zucker rats. Am J Physiol, 256 (2 Pt 2): R435–R442, 1989.

Clark MG, Rattigan S, and Clark, DG. Obesity with insulin resistance: experiential insights. Lancet, Nov 26: 1236–1240, 1983.

Contreras RJ and Williams VL. Dietary obesity and weight cycling: effects on blood pressure and heart rate in rats. Am J Physiol, 256 (6 Pt 2): R1209–1219, 1989.

Conway GS, Agrawal R, Betteridge DJ, and Jacobs HS. Risk factors for coronary artery disease in lean and obese women with the polycystic ovary syndrome. Clin Endocrinol (Oxf), 37 (2): 119–125, 1992.

Conway GS, Clark PM, and Wong D. Hyperinsulinemia in the polycystic ovary syndrome confirmed with a specific immunoradiometric assay for insulin. Clin Endocrinol (Oxf), 38 (2): 219–222, 1993.

Creutzfeldt W, Ebert R, Willms B, Frefichs H and Brown JC, Gastric inhibitory polypeptide (GIP) and insulin in obesity: Increased response to stimulation and defective feedback control of serum levels. Diabetologia, 14: 15–24, 1978.

Coulston AM, Liu GC, and Reaven GM. Plasma glucose, insulin and lipid responses to high-carbohydrate low-fat diets in normal humans. Metab, 32 (1): 52–56, 1983.

Coulston AM, Hollenbeck CB, Swislocki ALM, Chen Y-DI and Reaven GM. Deleterious metabolic effects of high-carbohydrate, sucrose-containing diets in patients with non-insulin-dependent diabetes mellitus. Am J Med, 82: 213–220 (Feb), 1987.

Daly PA and Landsberg L. Hypertension in obesity and NIDDM. Role of insulin and sympathetic nervous system. Diabetes Care, 14 (3): 240-248, 1991.

DeFronzo RA and Ferrannini E. Insulin resistance. A multifaceted syndrome responsible for NIDDM, obesity, hypertension, dyslipidemia, and atherosclerotic cardiovascular disease. Diabetes Care, 14 (3): 173–194, 1991.

Del Prato S. Hyperinsulinemia. Causes and mechanisms. Presse Med, 21 (28): 1312–1317, 1992.

Devlin JT and Horton ES. Hormone and nutrient interactions. IN: Modern Nutrition in Health and Disease, 7th ed., ed. by ME Shils and VR Young, Lea & Febiger, Philadelphia: 570-584, 1988.

Dietz WH. Obesity. J Am Coll Nutr, 8 Suppl: 13S-21S, 1989.

Di Pietro S and Suraci C. Metabolic abnormalities in first-degree relatives of type 2 diabetics. Boll Soc Ital Biol Sper, 66 (7): 631–638, 1990.

Doeden B and Rizza R. Use of a variable insulin infusion to assess insulin action in obesity: defects in both kinetics and amplitude of response. J Clin Endocrinol Metab, 64 (5): 902–908, 1987.

Dorner G, Plagemann A, Ruckert J, Gotz F, Rohde W, Stahl F, Kurschner U, Gottschalk J, Mohnike A, and Steindel E. Teratogenic maternofoetal transmission and prevention of diabetes susceptibility. Exp Clin Endocrinol, 91 (3): 247–258, 1988.

Drash A. Relationship between diabetes mellitus and obesity in the child. Metab, 22 (2): 337–34, 1973.

Du Cailar G, Ribstein J, Pasquie JL, Simandoux V, and Mimran A. Left systolic ventricular function and metabolic disorders in untreated hypertensive patients. Arch Mal Coeur Vaiss, 85 (8): 1071–1073, 1992.

Dustan H. Obesity and hypertension. Ann Int Med, 103 (6 Pt 2): 1047–1049, 1985.

Dyer KR and Messing A. Peripheral neuropathy associated with functional islet cell adenoma in SV40 transgenic mice. J Neuropathol Exp Neurol, 48 (4): 399–412, 1989.

Dzurik R, Malkova J, and Spustova V. Essential hypertension and insulin resistance. Cor Vasa, 33 (4): 294–300.

Eaton SB and Konner MJ. Stone age nutrition: implications for today. ASDC J Dent Child, 53 (4): 300-303, 1986.

Eaton SB, Konner M, and Shostak M. Stone agers in the fast lane: chronic degenerative diseases in evolutionary perspective. Am J Med, 84 (4): 739–749, 1988.

Einhorn D and Landsberg L. Nutrition and diet in hypertension. IN: Modern Nutrition in Health and Disease, 7th ed., ed. by ME Shils and VR Young, Lea & Febiger, Philadelphia: 1277, 1988.

Ellis EN, Kemp SK, Frindik JP, and Elders MJ. Glomerulopathy in patients with Donohue syndrome (leprechaunism). Diabetes Care, 14 (5): 413–414, 1991.

Ellison RC, Newburger JW, and Gross DM. Pediatric aspects of essential hypertension. J Am Diet Assoc 80: 21–25, 1982.

Epstein M and Sowers JR. Diabetes mellitus and hypertension. Hypertension, 19 (5): 403–418, 1992.

Eriksson LS, Thorne A, and Wahren J. Diet-induced thermogenesis in patients with liver cirrhosis. Clin Physiol, 9 (2): 131–141, 1989.

Facchini F, Chen YD, Hollenbeck CB, and Reaven GM. Relationship between resistance to insulin-mediated glucose uptake, urinary uric acid clearance, and plasma uric acid concentration. JAMA, 266 (21): 3008–3011, 1991.

Farquhar JW, Frank A, Gross RC, and Reaven GM. Glucose, insulin, and triglyceride responses to high and low carbohydrate diets in man. J Clin Invest, 45 (10): 1648–1656, 1966.

Feraille E, Krempf M, Chabonnel B, Bouhour JB, and Nicolas G. Arterial hypertension in patients with obesity. Role of hyperinsulinism and insulin resistance. Rev Med Interne, 11 (4): 293–296, 1990.

Ferrari P, Weidmann P, Shaw S, Giachino D, Riesen W, Allemann Y, and Heynen G. Altered insulin sensitivity, hyperinsulinemia, and dyslipidemia in individuals with a hypertensive parent. Am J Med, 91 (6): 589–596, 1991.

Fisher JA. The Chromium Program. Harper & Row, N.Y.: 311pp, 1990.

Flack JM and Sowers JR. Epidemiologic and clinical aspects of insulin resistance and hyperinsulinemia. Am J Med, 91 (1A): 11S-21S.

Flodin NW. Atherosclerosis: An insulin-dependent disease? J Amer Coll Nutr 5: 417–427, 1986.

Fontbonne A and Eschwege E. Diabetes, hyperglycemia, hyperinsulinemia and atherosclerosis: epidemiological data. Diabetes-Metab, 13 (3 Pt 2): 350-353, 1987.

Fontbonne A, Charles MA, Thibult N, Richard JL, Claude JR, Warnet JM, Rosselin GE, and Eschwege E. Hyperinsulinemia as a predictor of coronary heart disease mortality in a healthy population: the Paris Prospective Study, 15-year follow-up. Diabetologia, 34 (5): 356–361, 1991.

Fontbonne A and Eschwege E. Insulin and cardiovascular disease. Paris Prospective Study. Diabetes Care, 14 (6): 461–469, 1991.

Foreyt JP and Goodrick GK. Factors common to successful therapy for the obese patient. IN: Treatment of Obesity: A Multidisciplinary Approach, presented through the Department of Education at Harvard Medical School, Nov 7–9, Ed. by Blackburn GL, Benotti PN, and Mascioli EA, 1991.

Foster DW. Insulin resistance—a secret killer? N Eng J Med, 320 (11): 733–734, 1989.

Friedman JM and Leibel RL. Tackling a weighty problem. Cell, 69: 217–220, 1992.

Fuh M M-T, Shieh S-M, Wu D-A, Chen Y-D I, and Reaven GM, 1987. Abnormalities of carbohydrate and lipid metabolism in patients with hypertension. Arch Intern Med, 147: 1035–1038 (Jun).

Fujimoto S. Studies on the relationships between blood trace metal concentrations and the clinical status of patients with cerebrovascular disease, gastric cancer, and diabetes mellitus. Hokkaido Igaku Zasshi, 62 (6): 913–932, 1987.

Garg A, Helderman JH, Koffler M, Ayuso R, Rosenstock J, and Raskin P. Relationship between lipoprotein levels in vivo insulin action in normal young white men. Metabolism, 37 (10): 982–987, 1988a.

Garg A, Bonanome A, Grundy SM, Zhang Z and RH Unger. Comparison of a high-carbohydrate diet with a high-monounsaturated-fat diet in patients with non-insulin-dependent diabetes. New Engl J Med, 319: 829–34, 1988b.

Garg A, Grundy SM, and Unger RH. Comparison of effects of high and low carbohydrate diets on plasma lipoproteins and insulin sensitivity in patients with mild NIDDM. Diabetes, 41 (10): 1278–1285, 1992.

Geiselman PJ. Sugar-induced hyperphagia: is hyperinsulinemia, hypoglycemia, or any other factor a "necessary" condition? Appetite, 11 Suppl 1: 26–34, 1988.

Geiselman PJ and D Novin. The role of carbohydrates in appetite, hunger and obesity. Appetite: J Intake Res, 3: 203–223, 1982.

Ginsberg H, Olefsky JM, Kimmerling G, Crapo P, and Reaven GM. Induction of hypertriglyceridemia by a low-fat diet. J Clin Endocrinol Metab, 42: 729–735, 1976.

Gong EJ and Heald FP. Diet, nutrition, and adolescence. IN: Modern Nutrition in Health and Disease, 7th ed., ed. by ME Shils and VR Young, Lea & Febiger, Philadelphia: 969–981, 1988.

Grimaldi A, Sachon C, Bosquet F, and Doumith R. Intolerance to carbohydrates: the seven questions. Rev Med Interne, 11 (4): 297–307 1990.

Groop LC and Eriksson JG. The etiology and pathogenesis of non-insulin-dependent diabetes. Ann Med, 24 (6): 483–489, 1992.

Grugni G, Moreni G, Guzzaloni G, Ardizzi A, De Medici C, Sartorio A, and Morabito F. No correlation between insulinemic levels and arterial hypertension in obese females. Minerva Endocrinol, 15 (2): 141–143, 1990.

Gwinup G and Elias AN. Hypothesis: Insulin is responsible for the vascular complications of diabetes. Med-Hypotheses, 34 (1): 1–6, 1991.

Haenel H. Phylogenesis and nutrition. Nahrung, 33 (9): 867–887, 1989.

Haffner SM, Stern MP, Hazuda HP, Mitchel BD, and Patterson JK. Incidence of type II diabetes in Mexican Americans predicted by fasting insulin and glucose levels, obesity, and body-fat distribution. Diabetes, 39; 283–288, 1990.

Haffner SM, Stern MP, Hazuda HP, Mitchel BD, and Patterson JK. Cardiovascular risk factors in confirmed prediabetic individuals. Does the clock for coronary heart disease start ticking before the onset of clinical diabetes? JAMA, 263 (21): 2893–2898, 1990.

Haffner SM, Ferrannini E, Hazuda HP, and Stern MP. Clustering of cardiovascular risk factors in confirmed prehypertensive individuals. Hypertension, 20 (1): 38–45, 1992.

Hallfrisch J. Metabolic effects of dietary fructose. FASEB J, 4 (9): 2652–2660, 1990.

Heaton KW, Marcus SN, Emmett PM, and Bolton CH. Particle size of wheat, maize, and oat test meals: effects on plasma glucose and insulin responses and on the rate of starch digestion in the liver. Am J Clin Nutr, 47 (4): 675–682, 1988.

Heber GL. The endocrinology of obesity. IN: Treatment of Obesity: A Multidisciplinary Approach, presented through the Department of Education at Harvard Medical School, Nov 7–9. Ed. by GL Blackburn, PN Benotti, and EA Mascioli, 1991.

Heller RF and Heller RF. Profactor-H (Elevated circulating insulin): The link to health risk factors and diseases of civilization. Medical Hypothesis 45: 325–330, 1995.

Heller RF and Heller RF. Hypertriglyceridemia in the normal-weight and overweight: Correcting a physical cause. Annual meeting of the American Institute of Nutrition, April 13, 1995.

Heller RF and Heller RF. Hyperinsulinemic obesity and carbohydrate addiction: The missing link is the carbohydrate frequency. Medical Hypotheses, 42: 307–312, 1994.

Heller RF and Heller RF. Hunger and cravings in the overweight: Correcting a physical cause. Annual meeting of the American Institute of Nutrition, April 27, 1994.

Heller RF and Heller RF. Dietary carbohydrates: The frequency factor. Annual meeting of the American Institute of Nutrition, April 30, 1993.

Himsworth HP. Diabetes mellitus: its differentiation into insulin-sensitive and insulin-insensitive types. Lancet: 127–130, 1936.

Himsworth HP and Kerr RB. Insulin-sensitive and insulin-insensitive types of diabetes mellitus. IN: Clinical Science Incorporating Heart, Vol 4, Ed. Lewis, Shaw and Sons Ltd, London: 119–152, 1939.

Hollenbeck C and Reaven GM. Variations in insulin-stimulated glucose uptake in healthy individuals with normal glucose tolerance. J Clin Endocrinol Metab, 64: 1169–1173, 1987.

Hollenbeck C, Coulston AM, and Reaven GM. Effects of sucrose on carbohydrate and lipid metabolism in NIDDM patients. Diabetes Care, 12 (1): 62–66, 1989.

Hrnciar J, Jakubikova K, and Okapcova J. How should we implement the basic principles of treatment of type 2 diabetes mellitus from the aspect of the hormone-metabolic syndrome X. Vnitr Lek, 38 (8): 729–737, 1992.

Hubner G, von Dorsche HH and Zuhlke H. Morphological studies of the effect of chromium-III-chloride on the islet cell organ in rats under the conditions of high and low fat diets. Anat Anz, 167 (5): 389–391, 1988.

Hud JA Jr, Cohen JB, Wagner JM, and Cruz PD Jr. Prevalence and significance of acanthosis nigricans in an adult obese population. Arch Dermatol, 128 (7): 941–944, 1992.

Ishiguro T, Sato Y, Oshida Y, Yamanouchi K, Okuyama M, and Sakamoto N. The relationship between insulin sensitivity and weight reduction in simple obese and obese diabetic patients. Nagoya J Med Sci, 49: 61–69, 1987.

Janka HU, Ziegler AG, Standl E, and Mehnert H. Daily insulin dose as a predictor of macrovascular disease in insulin treated non-insulin-dependent diabetics. Diabetes Metab, 13 (3 Pt 2): 359–364, 1987.

Jeejeebhoy KN, Chu RC, Marliss EB, Greenburg GR, and Bruce-Robertson A. Chromium deficiency, glucose intolerance and neuropathy reversed by chromium supplementation in a patient receiving long term total parenteral nutrition. Am J Clin Nutr, 30: 531–538, 1977.

Jenkins DJA. Nutrition and diet in management of diseases of the gastrointestinal tract: (D) colon. IN: Modern Nutrition in Health and Disease, 7th ed., ed. by ME Shils and VR Young, Lea & Febiger, Philadelphia: 1023–1066, 1988.

Jenkins DJA, Shapira N, Greenberg G, Jenkins AL, Collier GR, Poduch C, Wolever TM, Anderson RA, and Blendis LM. Low glycemic index foods and reduced glucose, amino acid, and endocrine responses in cirrhosis. Am J Gastroenterol, 84 (7): 732–739, 1989.

Jern S. Effects of acute carbohydrate administration on central and peripheral hemodynamic responses to mental stress. Hypertension: 18 (6): 790-797, 1991.

Johansson G. Four years experience with magnesium hydroxide in renal stone disease. Magnesium Bulletin, February, 1981.

Kakar F, Hursting SD, Henderson MM, and Thronquist MD. Dietary sugar and breast cancer: Epidemiologic evidence. Clin Nutr, 9: 68–71, 1990.

Kakar F, Thornquist MD, Henderson MM, Klein RD, Kozawa SM, Santisteben GA, Hursting SD, and Urban ND. The effect of dietary sugar and dietary antioxidants on mammary tumor growth and lethality in BALB/c mice. Clin Nutr, 9: 62–67, 1990.

Kannel WB, Wilson PW, and Zhang TJ. The epidemiology of impaired glucose tolerance and hypertension. Am Heart J, 121 (4 Pt 2): 1268–1273, 1991.

Kaplan, NM. The deadly quartet: Upper-body obesity, glucose intolerance, hypertriglyceridemia, and hypertension. Arch Intern Med, 149; 1514–20, 1989.

Kazumi T, Yoshino G, Matsuba K, Iwai M, Iwatani I, Matsushita M, Kasama T, Hosokawa T, Numano F, and Baba S. Effects of dietary glucose or fructose on the secretion rate and particle size of triglyceride-rich lipoproteins in Zucker fatty rats. Metab, 40 (9): 962–966, 1991.

Kemp K. Carbohydrate addiction. Practitioner, 190: 358–364, 1963.

Klurfeld DM, Lloyd LM, Welch CB, Davis MJ, Tulp OL, and Kritchevsky D. Reduction of enhanced mammary carcinogenesis in LA/N-cp (corpulent) rats by energy restriction. Proc Soc Exp Biol Med, 196 (4): 381–384, 1991.

Koop CE. The Surgeon General's Report on Nutrition and Health. U.S. Department Health and Human Services, Publication No. 88–50210: p: 111, 1988.

Koppel JD. Nutrition, diet, and the kidney. IN: Modern Nutrition in Health and Disease, 7th ed., ed. by ME Shils and VR Young, Lea & Febiger, Philadelphia: Ch 58: 1230-1268, 1988.

Kornhuber HH, Kornhuber J, Wanner W, Kornhuber A, and Kaiser-auer CH. Alcohol, smoking and body build: obesity as a result of the toxic effect of 'social' alcohol consumption. Clin Physiol Biochem, 7 (3–4): 203–216, 1989.

Kozlovsky AS, Moser PB, Reisner S, and Anderson RA. Effects of diets high in simple sugars on urinary chromium losses. Metab, 35 (6): 515–518, 1986.

Kumpulainen JT, Wolf WR, Veillon C, and Mertz W. Determination of chromium in selected United States diets. J Agric Food Chem, 27 (3): 490-494, 1979.

Lääkso M, Sarlund H, Salonen R, Suhonen M, Pyörälä K, Salonen JT, and Karhapää P. Asymptomatic atherosclerosis and insulin resistance. Atheroscler and Thromb, 11: 1068–1076, 1991.

Landin K. Treating insulin resistance in hypertension with metformin reduces both blood pressure and metabolic risk factors. J Intern Med, Feb; 229 (2): 181–7, 1991.

Landsberg L. Obesity, metabolism, and hypertension. Yale J Biol Med, 62 (5): 511–519, 1989.

Landsberg L. Insulin resistance, energy balance and sympathetic nervous system activity. Clin Exp Hypertens, 12 (5): 817–830, 1990.

Lange J, Arends S, and Willms B. Alcohol-induced hypoglycemia in type 1 diabetes. Medizinische Klinik, 86 (11): 551–554, 1991.

Lefebvre PJ and Scheen AJ. Hypoglycemia. In Diabetes Mellitus, Theory and Practice, ed. by H Rifkin and D Porte, Jr. Appleton & Lange, Stamford, CT: p. 896–910, 1990.

Leibel R.; Obesity and nutrient metabolism. Presented at the American Association for the Advancement of Science, May 26, 1984.

Leiter EH. Control of spontaneous glucose intolerance, hyperinsulinemia, and islet hyperplasia in nonobese C3H.SW male mice by Y-linked locus and adrenal gland. Metab, 37 (7): 689–696, 1988.

Leutenegger M. Theoretical aspects of the relationship between diabetic macroangiopathy and hyperinsulinism. Presse Med, 21 (28): 1324–1329, 1992.

Lillioja S, Mott DM, Howard BV, Bennett PH, Yki-Jarvinen H, Freymond D, Nyomba BL, Zurlo F, Swinburn B, and Bogardus C. Impaired glucose tolerance as a disorder of insulin action: Longitudinal and cross-sectional studies in Pima Indians. N Eng J Med, 318: 1217–1225, 1988.

Linder MC (ed.) Nutitional Biochemistry and Metabolism with Clinical Applications. Elsevier: New York, 1985.

Lindin K, Tengborn L, and Smith U. Treating insulin resistance in hypertension with metformin reduces both blood pressure and metabolic risk factors. J Intern Med, 229 (2): 181–187, 1991.

Linscheer WG and Vergroesen AJ. Lipids. IN: Modern Nutrition in Health and Disease, 7th ed., ed. by ME Shils and VR Young, Lea & Febiger, Philadelphia: 72–107, 1988.

Lithell H. Insulin resistance and cardiovascular drugs. Clin Exp Hypertens, 14 (1–2): 151–162, 1992.

Liu G, Coulson A, Hollenbeck C, and Reaven GM. The effect of sucrose content in high and low carbohydrate diets on plasma glucose, insulin, and lipid responses in hypertriglyceridemic humans. J Clin Endocrinol Metab, 59 (4): 636–642, 1984.

Lutz W. Life expectancy—the Japanese experience. Wein Med Wochenschr, 141 (7): 148–150, 1991.

Mahler RJ. Diabetes and hypertension. Horm Metab Res, 22 (12): 599–607, 1990.

Marshall S, Garvey WT, and Traxinger RR. New insights into the metabolic regulation of insulin action and insulin resistance: role of glucose and amino acids. FASEB J, 5: 3031–3036, 1991.

Marston RW and Peterkin BB. Nutrient content of the national food supply. Natl Food Rev, 9: 21–25, 1980.

MacDonald I. Carbohydrates. IN: Modern Nutrition in Health and Disease, 7th ed., ed. by ME Shils and VR Young, Lea & Febiger, Philadelphia: 38–51, 1988.

Melchoir JC, Rigaud D, Colas-Linhart N, Petiet A, Girard A, and Apfelbaum M. Immunoreactive beta-endorphin increases after an aspartame chocolate drink in healthy human subjects. Physiol Behav, 50 (5): 941–944, 1991.

Modan M, Halkin H, Almog S, Lusky A, Eshkol A, Sheft M, Shitrit A, and Fuchs Z. Hyperinsulinemia. A link between hypertension, obesity and glucose intolerance. J Clin Invest, 75: 809–817, 1985.

Modan M, Halkin H, Lusky A, Segal P, Fuchs Z, and Chetrit A. Hyper-insulinemia is characterized by jointly distributed plasma VLDL, LDL, and HDL levels. A population study. Atheroscler, 8 (3): 227–236, 1988.

Modan M and Halkin H. Hyperinsulinemia or increased sympathetic drive as links for obesity and hypertension. Diabetes Care, 14 (6): 470-487, 1991.

Molnar D. Insulin secretion and carbohydrate tolerance in childhood obesity. Klin Padiatr, 202 (3): 131–135, 1990.

Morgan JB, York DA, Wasilewska A, and Portman J. A study of the thermic responses to a meal and to a sympathomimetic drug (ephedrine) in relation to energy balance in man. Brit J Nutr 47: 21–32.

Mountjoy KG and Holdaway IM. Effect of insulin receptor down regulation on insulin-stimulated thymidine incorporation in cultured human fibroblasts and tumor cell lines. Cancer Biochem Biophys, 12 (2): 117–126, 1991.

Nader S. Polycystic ovary syndrome and the androgen-insulin connection. Am J Obstet Gynecol, 165 (2): 346–348, 1991.

National Research Council. Recommended Dietary Allowances, 10th ed., 1989. Food and Nutrition Board, Commission on Life Sciences, Washington, DC, National Academy Press: 241–243, 1989.

Niijima A, Togiyama T, and Adachi A. Cephalic-phase insulin release induced by taste stimulus of monosodium glutamate (umami taste). Physiol Behav, 48 (6): 905–908, 1990.

Nobels F and Dewailly D. Puberty and polycystic ovarian syndrome: the insulin/insulin-like growth factor I hypothesis. Fertil Steril, 58 (4): 655–666, 1992.

Noberasco G, Odetti P, Boeri D, Maiello M, and Adezati L. Malondi-aldehyde (MDA) level in diabetic subjects. Relationship with blood glucose and glycosylated hemoglobin. Biomed Pharma-cother, 45 (4–5): 193–196, 1991.

O'Dea K. Westernization and non-insulin-dependent diabetes in Australian aborigines. Ethn Dis, 1 (2): 171–187, 1991.

O'Dea K. Westernization, insulin resistance and diabetes in Aus-tralian aborigines. Med J Aust, 155 (4): 258–264, 1991.

O'Donnell MJ and Dodson PM. The non-drug treatment of hyperten-sion in the diabetic patient. J Hum Hypertens, 5 (4): 287–294, 1991.

Oh W, Gelardi NL, and Cha CJ. Maternal hyperglycemia in pregnant rats: its effect on growth and carbohydrate metabolism in the offspring. Metab, 37 (12): 1146–1151, 1988.

Ohlson LO, Larsson B, Bjorntorp P, Eriksson H, Szardsudd K, Welin L, Tibblin G, and Wilhelmsen L. Risk factors for type 2 (non-insulin-dependent) diabetes mellitus. Thirteen and one-half years of follow-up of the participants in a study of Swedish men born in 1913. Diabetologia, 31 (11): 798–805, 1988.

Olefsky JM. Obesity. IN: Harrison's Principles of Internal Medicine, 12th ed., ed. by Wilson JD, Braunwald D, Isselbacher KJ, Peters-dorf RG, Martin JB, Fauci AS and Root RK. McGraw Hill, Inc., Health Professions Division, New York, 1: 411–417, 1991.

Oral Contraceptives, Mead Johnson Laboratories. OVCON®50 OVCON®35 (Norethindrone and ethinyl estradiol tablets, UPS). A Bristol-Meyers Squibb Co. Evansville ID, 47721, 1990.

Passwater, RA. Supernutrition for healthy hearts, Dial Press, New York: 37–38, 1978.

Pedersen, O. Insulin resistance—a pathophysiological condition with numerous sequelae: non-insulin-dependent diabetes mellitus (NIDDM), android obesity, essential hypertension, dyspipi-demia and atherosclerosis. Ugeskr Laeger, 154 (20): 1411–1418, 1992.

Peterson CM and Jovanovic-Peterson L. Randomized crossover study of 40% vs. 55% carbohydrate weight loss strat with previous gestational diabetes mellitus and non-diabetic women of 130%-200% ideal body weight. J Amer Coll Nutr, 14 (4): 369–375, 1995.

Petrides AS and DeFronzo RA. Glucose metabolism in cirrhosis. H Hepatol, 8 (1): 107–114, 1989.

Pi-Sunyer FX. Obesity IN: Modern Nutrition in Health and Disease, 7th ed., ed. by ME Shils and VR Young, Lea and Febiger, Philadelphia: 795–816, 1988.

Pollare T, Vessby B, and Lithell H. Lipoprotein lipase activity in skeletal muscle is related to insulin sensitivity. Arterioscler Thromb, 11 (5): 1192–1203, 1991.

Pontremoli R, Zavaroni I, Mazza S, Battezzati M, Massarino F, Tixi-anello A, and Reaven GM. Changes in blood pressure, plasma triglyceride and aldosterone concentration, and red cell cation concentration in patients with hyperinsulinemia. Am J Hypertens, 4 (2 Pt 1): 159–163, 1991.

Poulter NR. Treatment of hypertension: a clinical epidemiologist's view. J Cardiovasc Pharmacol, 18 Suppl 2: S35–S38, 1991.

Prelevic GM, Wurzburger MI, Balint-Peric L, and Ginsberg J. Twenty-four-hour serum growth hormone, insulin, c-peptide and blood glucose profiles and serum insulin-like growth factor-I concentrations in women with polycystic ovaries. Horm Res, 37 (4–5): 125–131, 1992.

Prevention Total Health System®: Understanding vitamins and minerals, ed. by Editors of Prevention® Magazine, Rodale Press, Emmaus, Pennsylvania, 1984.

Proctor CA, Proctor TB, and Proctor B. Etiology and treatment of fluid retention (hydrops) in Menière's syndrome. Ear Nose Throat J, 71 (12): 631–635, 1992.

Proudler AJ, Felton CV, and Stevenson JC. Ageing and the response of plasma insulin, glucose and C-peptide concentrations to intravenous glucose in postmenopausal women. Clinical Science, 83: 489–494.

Randolph JF, Kipersztok S, Ayers JW, Ansbacher R, Peegel H, and Menon KM. The effect of insulin on aromatase activity in isolated human endometrial glands and stroma. Am J Obstet Gynecol, 157 (6): 1534–1539, 1990.

Randolph TG. Masked food allergy as a factor in the development and persistence of obesity. J Lab Clin Med, 32: 1547–1549, 1947.

Randolph TG. The descriptive features of food addiction. Quart J Studies Alcohol 17: 198–224, 1956.

Randolph TG and Moss RW. An Alternative Approach to Allergies, Lippincott and Crowell, New York, 1980.

Ravussin E and Bogardus C. Energy expenditure in the obese: Is there a Thrifty Gene? Infusionstherapie, 17: 108–112, 1990.

Ravussin E. Energy metabolism in obesity. Studies in the Pima Indians. Diabetes Care, 16 (1): 232–238, 1993.

Reaven GM. Role of insulin resistance in human disease. Diabetes, 37: 1595–1607, 1988.

Reaven GM and Hoffman BB. Hypertension as a disease of carbohydrate and lipoprotein metabolism. Am J Med, 87 (6A): 2S-6S, 1989.

Reaven GM. Insulin resistance and compensatory hyperinsulinemia: role in hypertension, dyslipidemia, and coronary heart disease. Am Heart J, 121 (4 Pt 2): 1282–1288, 1991.

Reaven, GM. Insulin resistance, hyperinsulinemia, and hypertriglyceridemia in the etiology and clinical course of hypertension. Am J Med, 90 (2A): 7S-11S, 1991.

Reaven GM. Role of insulin resistance in human disease. Diabetes, 37: 1595–1607, 1991.

Reaven GM. Relationship between insulin resistance and hypertension. Diabetes Care, 14 Suppl 4: 33–38, 1991.

Reiser S, Bickard MC, Hallfrisch J. Michaelis IV OE, and Prather ES. Blood lipids and their distribution in lipoproteins in hyperinsulinemic subjects fed three different levels of sucrose. J Nutr, 111: 1045–1057, 1981.

Reiser S, Powell AS, Scholfield DJ, Panda P, Ellwood KC, and Canary JJ. Blood lipids, lipoproteins, apoproteins, and uric acid in men fed diets containing fructose or high-amylose cornstarch. Am J Clin Nutr, 49 (5): 832–839, 1989.

Ri K. Study on insulin resistance in rats treated with estrogen and progesterone—assessment with euglycemic clamp technique. Nippon Naibunpi Gakkai Zasshi, 63 (6): 798–808, 1987.

Riales R. Effect of chromium chloride supplementation on glucose tolerance and serum lipids including high-density lipoprotein of adult men. Amer J of Clin Nutrition, 34 (12) 2670-8, 1981.

Rimm IJ and Rimm AA. Association between juvenile onset obesity and severe obesity in 73,532 women. Am J Public Health, 66: 479–481, 1976.

Robertson D, Frolich JC, Carr RK, Watson JT, Hollifield JW, Shand DG, and Oates JA. Effects of caffeine on plasma renin activity, catecholamines and blood pressure. N Eng J Med, 298 (4): 181–186; 1978.

Roden J. Insulin levels, hunger, and food intake: An example of feedback loops in body weight regulation. Health Psychol, 4: 1–18, 1985.

Rombauer IS and Rombauer Becker M. Joy of Cooking, New American Library, New York, 1964.

Rönnemaa T, Laakso M, Pyöräälä K, Kallio V, and Puukka P. High fasting plasma insulin is an indicator of coronary heart disease in non-insulin-dependent diabetic patients and nondiabetic subjects. Arterioscler-Thromb, 11 (1): 80-90, 1991.

Rossi-Fanelli F, Cascino A, and Muscaritoli M. Abnormal substrate metabolism and nutritional strategies in cancer management. JPEN J Parenter Enteral Nutr, 15 (6): 680-683, 1991.

Ruderman N. Exercise in therapy and prevention of type II diabetes. Implications for blacks. Diabetes Care, 13 (11): 1163–1168, 1990.

Rupp H. Insulin resistance, hyperinsulinemia, and cardiovascular disease. The need for novel dietary prevention strategies [editorial]. Basic Res Cardiol, 87 (2): 99–105, 1992.

Saad MF, Knowler WC, Pettitt DJ, Nelson RG, Mott DM, and Bennett PH. The natural history of impaired glucose tolerance in the Pima Indians. N Eng J Med, 319: 1500-1506, 1988.

Salomaa VV, Tuomilehto J, Jaucianien M, Korhonsen HJ, Stengard J, Uusitupa M, Pitkanen M, and Penttilla I. Hypertriglyceridemia in different degrees of glucose intolerance in a Finnish population-based study. Diabetes Care, 15 (5): 657–665, 1992.

Sato Y, Shiraishi S, Oshida Y, Ishiguro T, and Sakamoto N. Experimental atherosclerosis-like lesions induced by hyperinsulinism in Wistar rats. Diabetes 38: 91–96, 1989.

Scallet AC, Faris PL, Beinfeld MC, and Olney JW. Hypothalamic neurotoxins alter the contents of immunoreactive cholecystokinin in pituitary. Brain Res, 407 (2): 390-393, 1987.

Schneider DJ and Sobel BE. Augmentation of synthesis of plasminogen activator inhibitor type 1 by insulin and insulin-like growth factor type I: implications for vascular disease in hyperinsulinemic states. Proc Natl Acad Sci USA, 88 (22): 9959–9963, 1991.

Schroeder HA. The role of chromium in mammalian nutrition. Am J Clin Nutr, 21 (6): 230-244, 1968.

Schumann D. Post-operative hyperglycemia: clinical benefits of insulin therapy. Heart-Lung, 19 (2): 165–173, 1990.

Schwarz K and Mertz W. A glucose tolerance factor and its differentiation from factor 3. Arch Biochem Biophys, 72: 515–518, 1957.

Sechi LA, Melis A, Pala A, Marigliano A, Sechi G, and Tedde R. Serum insulin, insulin sensitivity, and erythrocyte sodium metabolism in normotensive and essential hypertensive subjects with and without overweight. Clin Exp Hypertens [A], 13 (2): 261–272, 1991.

Sharma AM, Ruland K, Spies KP, and Distler A. Salt sensitivity in young normotensive subjects is associated with a hyperinsulinemic response to oral glucose. J Hypertens, 9 (4): 329–335, 1991.

Shelepov VP, Chekulaev VA, and Pasha-Zade GR. Effect of putrescine on carbohydrate and lipid metabolism in rats. Biomed Sci, 1 (6): 591–596, 1990.

Shelmet JJ, Reichard GA, Skutches CL, Hoeldtke RD, Owen OE, and Boden G. Ethanol causes acute inhibition of carbohydrate, fat, and protein oxidation and insulin resistance. J Clin Invest, 81 (4): 1137–1145, 1988.

Shils ME. Enteral (tube) and parenteral nutrition support IN: Modern Nutrition in Health and Disease, 7th ed., ed. by ME Shils and VR Young, Lea & Febiger, Philadelphia: 1023–1066, 1988.

Sicree RA, Zimmet PZ, King HOM, and Coventry JS. Plasma insulin response among Nauruans: Prediction of deterioration in glucose tolerance over 6 yr. Diabetes, 36: 179–186, 1987.

Sidey FM. Role of the adrenal medulla in stress-induced hyperinsulinemia in normal mice and in mice infected with Bordetella pertussis or treated with pertussis toxin. J Endocrinol, 118 (1): 135–140, 1988.

Simonson DC. Hyperinsulinemia and its sequelae. Horm Metab Res Suppl, 22: 17–25, 1990.

Singer P and Baumann R. Glucose-induced or postprandial hyperinsulinemia in mild essential hypertension—an underestimated biochemical risk factor. Med Hypotheses, 34 (2): 257–164, 1991.

Skouby SO, Andersen O, Saurbrey N, and Kuhl C. Oral contraception and insulin sensitivity: in vivo assessment in normal women and in women with previous gestational diabetes. J Clin Endocrinol Metab, 64: 519–526, 1987.

Skouby SO, Andersen O, Petersen KR, Molsted-Pedersen L, and Kuhl C. Mechanism of action of oral contraceptives on carbohydrate metabolism at the cellular level. Am J Obstet Gynecol, 163 (1 Pt 2): 343–348, 1990.

Smith U, Gudbjornsdottir S and Landin K. Hypertension as a metabolic disorder—an overview. J Intern Med Suppl, 735: 1–7, 1991.

Somogyi JC and Nageli U. Antithiamine effect of coffee. Int J Vit Nutr Res, 46 (2): 149–153; 1976.

Sowers JR. Is hypertension an insulin-resistant state? Metabolic changes associated with hypertension and antihypertensive therapy. Am Heart J, 122 (3 Pt 2): 932–935, 1991.

Sowers JR, Standley PR, Ram JL, Zemel MB, and Resnick LM. Insulin resistance, carbohydrate metabolism, and hypertension. Am J Hypertens, 4 (7 Pt 2): 46S–472S, 1991.

Spring B, Chiodo J, Harden M, Bourgeois MJ, Mason JD, and Lutherer L. Psychobiological effects of carbohydrates. J Clin Psychiatry, 50 (5, Suppl): 27–33, 1989.

Spustova V. Insulin resistance as a risk factor in atherosclerosis. Vnitr Lek, 38 (11): 1105–1110, 1992.

Statistical Bulletin. Hypertension in the United States: 1960 to 1980 and 1987 estimates. Statistical Bulletin: 13–17, 1989.

Statistical Bulletin. Life expectancy remains at record level. Statistical Bulletin: 26–30, 1989.

Statistical Bulletin, 1989. Diabetes mortality update. Statistical Bulletin: 24–35 (Oct-Dec).

Staub HW, Reussner G, and Thiessen Jr R. Serum cholesterol. reduction by chromium in hypercholesterolemic rats. Sci, 165: 746–747, 1969.

Stern MP and Haffner SM. Body fat distribution and hyperinsulinemia as risk factors for diabetes and cardiovascular disease. Atheroscler, 6: 123–130, 1986.

Stern MP, Knapp JAA, Hazuda HP, Haffner SM, Patterson JK, and

Mitchell BD. Genetic and environmental determinants of type II diabetes in Mexican Americans. Is there a "descending limb" to the modernization/diabetes relationship? Diabetes Care, 14 (7): 649–654, 1991.

Stock S, Granstrom L, Backman L, Matthiesen AS, and Uvnas-Moberg K. Elevated plasma levels of oxytocin in obese subjects before and after gastric banding. Int J Obes, 13 (2): 213–222, 1989.

Stolar MW. Atherosclerosis in diabetes: the role of hyperinsulinemia. Metab, 37 (2 Suppl 1): 1–9, 1988.

Stoll BA and Secreto G. New hormone-related markers of high risk to breast cancer. Ann Oncol, 3 (6): 435–438, 1992.

Storlien LH, Kraegen EW, Jenkins AB, and Chisholm DJ. Effects of sucrose vs starch diets on in vivo insulin action, thermogenesis, and obesity in rats. Am J Clin Nutr, 47 (3): 420-427, 1988.

Storlien LH, Oakes ND, Pan DA, Kusunoki M, and Jenkins AB. Syndromes of insulin resistance in the rat. Inducement by diet and amelioration with benfluorex. Diabetes, 42 (3): 457–462, 1993.

Stout RW. Overview of the association between insulin and atherosclerosis. Metabolism, 34 (12): 7–12, 1985.

Stout RW. Insulin and atheroma. 20-year perspective. Diabetes Care, 13 (6): 631–654, 1990.

Stout RW. Insulin and atherogenesis. Eur J Epidemiol, 8 Suppl 1: 134–135, 1992.

Striffler JS, Polansky MM, and Anderson RA. Dietary Chromium improves IVGTT insulin and glucose responses in sucrose-fed Cr-deficient rats. (Abs 6285 in FASEB J 4/5–4/9): A2022, 1992.

Sugiyama Y. The role of insulin in reproductive endocrinology and perinatal medicine. Nippon Sanka Fujinka Gakkai Zasshi, 42 (8): 791–799, 1990.

Telander RL, Wolf SA, Simmons PS, Zimmerman D, and Haymond MW. Endocrine disorders of the pancreas and adrenal cortex in pediatric patients. Mayo Clin Proc, 61 (6): 459–466, 1986.

The Bantam Medical Dictionary, Bantam Books, New York, London, 1982.

Tepperman J and Tepperman H. Metabolic and Endocrine Physiology, fifth ed. p. 259, Year Book Medical Publishers, Inc., Chicago, 1987.

Thomas DE, Brotherhood JR, and Brand JC. Carbohydrate feeding before exercise: effect of glycemic index. Int J Sports Med, 12 (2): 180-186, 1991.

Thomassen A, Neilsen TT, Bagger JP, and Henningsen P. Effects of intravenous glutamate on substrate availability and utilization across the human heart and leg. Metab, 40 (4): 378–384, 1991.

Toepfer EW, Mertz W, Roginski EE, and Polansky MM. Chromium in foods in relation to biological activity. J Agr Food Chem, 21 (1): 69–73, 1973.

Troisi RJ, Weiss ST, Parker DR, Sparrow D, Young JB, and Landsberg L. Relation of obesity and diet to sympathetic nervous system activity. Hypertens, 17 (5): 669–677, 1991.

Tseng CH and Tai TV. Risk factors for hyperinsulinemia in chlorpropamide-treated diabetic patients: a three-year follow-up. J Formos Med Assoc, 91 (8): 770-774, 1992.

Tufts University Diet and Nutrition, Vol. 11, No. 5, July 1993.

Tweng CH and Tai TY. Risk factors for hyperinsulinemia in chloropropamide-treated diabetic patients: a three-year follow-up. J Formos Med Assoc, 91 (8): 770-774, 1992.

Uhde TW, Boulenger JP, Jimerson DC, and Post RM. Caffeine: Relationship to human anxiety, plasma MHPG and cortisol. Psychopharmacol-Bull., 20 (3): 426–430; 1984.

Urdl W, Desoye G, Schmon B, Hofmann HM, and Ralph G. Interaction between insulin and insulin-like growth factor I in the pathogenesis of polycystic ovarian disease. Ann NY Acad Sci, 626: 177–183, 1991.

Unterberger P, Sinop A, Noder W, Berger MR, Fink M, Edler L, Schmahl D, and Ehrhart H. Diabetes mellitus and breast cancer. A retrospective follow-up study. Onkologie, 13 (1): 17–20, 1990.

Vaaler S. Carbohydrate metabolism, insulin resistance, and metabolic cardiovascular syndrome. J Cardiovasc Pharmacol, 20 Suppl 8: S11–S14, 1992.

Vaisman N, Sklan D, and Dayan Y. Effect of semi-starvation on plasma lipids. Int J Obes, 14 (12): 989–996, 1990.

Valensi, P. Pathogenic role of hyperinsulinism in macroangiopathy. Epidemiological data. Presse Med, 21 (28): 1307–1311, 1992,

Van der Walt JG and Lingington MJ. A review of energy metabolism in producing ruminants. 2. Control of nutrient partitioning. J S Afr Vet Assoc, 61 (2): 78–80, 1990.

Van Itallie TB. Health implications of overweight and obesity in the United States. Ann Intern Med, 103 (6 Pt 2): 983–988, 1985.

Velek J. Karasova L, Pelikanova T, Sosna T, and Skibova J. Blood pressure and insulin resistance in type 2 diabetics. Vnitr Lek, 37 (9–10): 752–760, 1991.

Weaver JU, Kopelman PG, and Hitman GA. Central obesity and hyperinsulinemia in women are associated with polymorphism in the 5' flanking region of the human insulin gene. Eur J Clin Invest, 22 (4): 265–270, 1992.

Webster's New Twentieth Century Dictionary (unabridged), 2nd ed., World Publishing Co., New York, 1975.

Wendorf M. Diabetes, the ice free corridor, and the Paleoindian settlement on North America. Am J Phys Anthropol, 79 (4): 503–520, 1989.

Wendorf M and Goldfine ID. Archeology of NIDDM. Excavation of the "thrifty" genotype. Diabetes, 40 (2): 161–165, 1991.

Wendorf M. Archeology and the "thrifty" non insulin dependent diabetes mellitus (NIDDM) genotype. Adv Perit Dial, 8: 201–207, 1992.

White PJ, Cybulski KA, Primus R. Johnson DF, Collier GH, and Wagner GC. Changes in macronutrient selection as a function of dietary tryptophan. Physiol and Behav, 43: 73–77, 1988.

Wicklmayr M, Rett K, Baldermann H, and Dietze G. The kallikrein/kinin system in the pathogenesis of hypertension in diabetes mellitus. Diabetes Metab, 15 (5 Pt 2): 306–310, 1989.

Woods SC, Porte, Jr D, Bobbioni E, Ionescu E, Sauter JF, Rohner-Jeanrenaud F, and Jeanrenaud B. Insulin: its relationship to the central nervous system and to the control of food intake and body weight. Am J Clin Nutr, 42: 1063–1071, 1985.

Woteki CE, Walsh SO, Raper N, et al. recent trends and levels of dietary sugars and other caloric sweeteners, IN: Metabolic Effects of Utilizable Dietary Carbohydrates, ed. by S Reiser, Marcel Dekker, New York 1–27, 1982.

Yale, J. Taming the hunger hormone: is insulin the key to weight control? American Health, Jan-Feb, 1984.

Yam D, Fink A, Nir I, and Budowski P. Insulin-tumor interrelationships in thymoma bearing mice. Effects of dietary glucose and fructose. Br J Cancer, 64 (6): 1043–1046, 1991.

Young IS, Torney JJ, and Trimble ER. The effect of ascorbate supplementation on oxidative stress in streptozotocin diabetic rats. Free Radic Biol Med, 13 (1): 41–46, 1992.

Zavaroni I, Bonara E, Pagliara M, Dall'Aglio E, Luchetti L, Buonanno G, Bonati PA, Bergonzani M, Gnudi L, Passeri M, and Reaven GM. Risk factors for coronary artery disease in healthy persons with hyperinsulinemia and normal glucose tolerance. N Eng J Med, 320 (11): 702–706, 1989.

INDEX